Common Problems in the Newborn Nursery

Gilbert I. Martin • Warren Rosenfeld
Editors

Common Problems in the Newborn Nursery

An Evidence and Case-based Guide

Springer

Editors
Gilbert I. Martin
Citrus Valley Medical Center
West Covina, CA
USA

Warren Rosenfeld
Stony Brook University SUNY
Mount Sinai - South Nassau Medical Center
Oceanside, NY
USA

ISBN 978-3-319-95671-8 ISBN 978-3-319-95672-5 (eBook)
https://doi.org/10.1007/978-3-319-95672-5

Library of Congress Control Number: 2018957469

This Springer imprint is published by the registered company Springer Nature Switzerland AG
The registered company address is: Gewerbestrasse 11, 6330 Cham, Switzerland

Preface

The newborn baby is the most frequently hospitalized patient and represents 10% of all hospital admissions in the United States. Every day there are approximately 25,000 examinations, evaluations, and medical decisions made on patients with the diagnosis of "newborn." While, in general, the transition from intrauterine to extrauterine life is a normal physiologic event, newborns may present with a number of clinical challenges for the healthcare providers who are responsible for their care.

Speaking before national audiences on the subject *Common Problems in the Newborn Nursery* for over 20 years, we have discussed a wide variety of issues that arise for all of us who care for babies. We have chosen 21 of these topics for discussion in this book to help the reader discern the normal from the abnormal and the emergent from the non-emergent and to help the providers to make decisions concerning dilemmas that are encounter on a daily basis. The chapters are designed in an evidence and case-based format with questions that need to be answered by the reader. A dénouement and discussion follows each question and answer.

We have assembled a number of contributors with expertise in the care of newborns in the nursery. We hope the scenarios that are presented reflect the issues our readers are presented with in their daily nursery rounds. While the contributors' answers reflect a prudent and accepted approach, readers should also realize that there is often more than one right answer or approach to many of these clinical challenges.

We thank all of the contributors to this monograph and Portia Wong from Springer-Verlag for all of their expertise and assistance. In addition, our editorial assistant, Sandy Skelley provided much of the organizational and administrative support.

West Covina, CA, USA — Gilbert I. Martin
Oceanside, NY, USA — Warren Rosenfeld

Contents

Contributors

David H. Adamkin, MD Division of Neonatal Medicine, Department of Pediatrics, University of Louisville, Louisville, KY, USA

Joseph Ahdoot, MD Pacific Pediatric Cardiology Medical Group, Keck School of Medicine, Children's Hospital of Los Angeles, Los Angeles, CA, USA

David Geffen School of Medicine at UCLA, Mattel Children's Hospital, Los Angeles, CA, USA

Moris Angulo, MD SUNY/Stony Brook School of Medicine, Stony Brook, NY, USA

Division of Genetics, NYU Winthrop Hospital, Mineola, NY, USA

Henry H. Bernstein, DO, MHCM, FAAP General Pediatrics, Cohen Children's Medical Center and Zucker School of Medicine at Hofstra/Northwell, New Hyde Park, NY, USA

David A. Clark, MD Department of Pediatrics, Albany Medical Center, Albany, NY, USA

Avroy A. Fanaroff, MD, FRCP, FRCPCH Pediatrics, Division of Neonatology, Case Western Reserve School of Medicine and Eliza Henry Barnes Chair in Neonatology, Rainbow Babies and Children's Hospital, University Hospitals Cleveland Medical Center, Cleveland, OH, USA

Jonathan M. Fanaroff, MD, JD Pediatrics, Division of Neonatology, Case Western Reserve University School of Medicine, Rainbow Center of Pediatric Ethics, Neonatal Intensive Care Unit, Rainbow Babies and Children's Hospital, University Hospitals Cleveland Medical Center, Cleveland, OH, USA

Lincoln Ferguson, MD, MPH Department of Pediatrics, Mount Sinai South Nassau Medical Center, Oceanside, NY, USA

NYIT College of Osteopathic Medicine, Glen Head, NY, USA

Walter M. Fierson, MD, FAAO, FAAP Arcadia, CA, USA

Theresa M. Fiorito, MD Department of Pediatrics, Children's Medical Center at NYU Winthrop Hospital, Mineola, NY, USA

Jay P. Goldsmith, MD Division of Newborn Medicine, Department of Pediatrics, Tulane University School of Medicine, Tulane Lakeside Hospital for Women and Children, New Orleans, LA, USA

Mercedes E. Gonzalez, MD, FAAD Pediatric Dermatology of Miami, Department of Dermatology, University of Miami Miller School of Medicine, Miami, FL, USA

Herbert Wertheim College of Medicine, Florida International University, Miami, FL, USA

Stephany M. Guiles, MD Division of Newborn Medicine, Department of Pediatrics, Tulane University School of Medicine, Tulane Lakeside Hospital for Women and Children, New Orleans, LA, USA

Thomas A. Hooven, MD Department of Pediatrics, Vagelos College of Physicians and Surgeons, Columbia University, New York, NY, USA

Ranjith Kamity, MD, FAAP Department of Pediatrics, NYU Winthrop Hospital, Mineola, NY, USA

SUNY Stony Brook School of Medicine, Stony Brook, NY, USA

Kaitlin Kenaley, MD Division of Neonatology, Christiana Care Health System, Newark, DE, USA

Leonard R. Krilov, MD Department of Pediatrics, Children's Medical Center at NYU Winthrop Hospital, Mineola, NY, USA

Department of Pediatrics, State University of New York at Stony Brook School of Medicine, Stony Brook, NY, USA

Robert Loitz, MD Pacific Pediatric Cardiology Medical Group, Pasadena, CA, USA

Keck School of Medicine, University of Southern California, Los Angeles, CA, USA

Gilbert I. Martin, MD Neonatal Intensive Care Unit, Citrus Valley Medical Center–Queen of the Valley Hospital, West Covina, CA, USA

Loma Linda University Medical Center, Loma Linda, CA, USA

Gregory C. Martin, MD Banner University Medical Center Phoenix, Phoenix, AZ, USA

Department of Child Health, University of Arizona College of Medicine Phoenix, Phoenix, AZ, USA

Andrea C. Morris, DNP, RNC-NIC, CCRN, CNS Kaiser Permanente-Fontana, Fontana, CA, USA

Emily A. Morris, MD Neonatal-Perinatal Medicine, Vanderbilt University School of Medicine, Mildred Stahlman Division of Neonatology, Monroe Carell Jr. Children's Hospital, Nashville, TN, USA

Asif Noor, MD Department of Pediatrics, Children's Medical Center at NYU Winthrop Hospital, Mineola, NY, USA

Arielle L. Olicker, MD Pediatrics, Division of Neonatology, Case Western Reserve University School of Medicine, Rainbow Babies and Children's Hospital, University Hospitals Cleveland Medical Center, Cleveland, OH, USA

Lu-Ann Papile, MD Division of Neonatology, Department of Pediatrics, University of New Mexico Health Sciences Center, University of New Mexico, Albuquerque, NM, USA

Stephen A. Pearlman, MD, MSHQS Division of Neonatology, Christiana Care Health System, Newark, DE, USA

Sidney Kimmel College of Medicine of Thomas Jefferson University, Philadelphia, PA, USA

Richard A. Polin Department of Pediatrics, Vagelos College of Physicians and Surgeons, Columbia University, New York, NY, USA

Warren Rosenfeld, MD Department of Pediatrics, SUNY/Stony Brook School of Medicine, Stony Brook, NY, USA

Department of Pediatrics, Mount Sinai - South Nassau Medical Center, Oceanside, NY, USA

Smeeta Sardesai, MD, MS Ed, FAAP Keck School of Medicine, University of Southern California, Los Angeles, CA, USA

Bruce D. Sindel, MD Neonatal Intensive Care Unit, Pediatrix Medical Group, a MEDNAX Company, Citrus Valley Medical Center—Queen of the Valley Campus, West Covina, CA, USA

Western University of Health Sciences, Pomona, CA, USA

Ann R. Stark, MD Neonatal-Perinatal Medicine, Vanderbilt University School of Medicine, Mildred Stahlman Division of Neonatology, Monroe Carell Jr. Children's Hospital, Nashville, TN, USA

Stephanie Tong, MD General Pediatrics, Cohen Children's Medical Center and Zucker School of Medicine at Hofstra/Northwell, New Hyde Park, NY, USA

James S. Yeh, MD, FACS Department of Surgery, Citrus Valley Medical Center–Queen of the Valley Hospital, West Covina, CA, USA

Post-resuscitation Care of the Depressed Newborn

1

Stephany M. Guiles and Jay P. Goldsmith

Introduction

Newborns who are depressed at birth present a challenge to the practicing physician. A neonate may respond to resuscitation and seem to be improving at 5 or 10 min of age. However, it is often difficult to determine if there has been intrapartum asphyxia or other causes such as sepsis to account for the neonatal depression. Therefore, triage of the newborn to the appropriate nursery may be problematic. If the newborn is admitted to a NICU, multiple tests will be done, and maternal newborn bonding and perhaps breastfeeding will be affected. However, delay in diagnosis of a truly ill newborn may have significant consequences since potential therapies may be delayed. This is especially true for therapeutic hypothermia (TH), which has been shown to be most effective if initiated within the first 6 h of life [1, 2]. If this window of opportunity is missed, the newborn with intrapartum asphyxia may not benefit from the potential positive effects of this treatment.

This chapter will review the approach to the depressed newborn who is successfully resuscitated. It will guide the practicing physician in determining which newborns need more testing and treatment. The reader will be presented three cases, led through the appropriate physical evaluation and queried regarding which tests to order, how to evaluate those tests, and why they may be misleading. The determination of need for further evaluation, treatment, and possibly even transfer to a higher level of care will be discussed.

Case Presentation

A 40 and 5/7 weeks gestation male is born by emergency cesarean section for non-reassuring fetal status to a 22-year-old primigravida female. Upon rupture of membranes 4 h prior to delivery, meconium-stained amniotic fluid was noted. Fetal heart monitoring revealed multiple variable and late decelerations which led to the operative delivery under general anesthesia. The baby is born limp with a heart rate of 60 beats per minute (bpm). He is suctioned and intubated in the delivery room. No meconium is retrieved from below the vocal cords. Chest compressions are given for only 30 seconds, and his heart rate quickly increases to over 100 bpm. Over the next several minutes, he begins to have gasping respirations which become regular at 6 min of age and he is extubated. Pulse oximetry increases to 90% by 10 min of age, and oxygen is gradually weaned off to room air. Apgar scores of 1, 5, and 7 are assigned at 1, 5, and 10 min of age.

S. M. Guiles, MD · J. P. Goldsmith, MD (✉)
Division of Newborn Medicine, Department of Pediatrics, Tulane University School of Medicine, Tulane Lakeside Hospital for Women and Children, New Orleans, LA, USA

G. I. Martin, W. Rosenfeld (eds.), *Common Problems in the Newborn Nursery*,
https://doi.org/10.1007/978-3-319-95672-5_1

At this time you:

1. Allow baby to remain skin-to-skin with the mother.
2. Request umbilical cord gases from the obstetrical team.
3. Obtain arterial blood gas on baby.

The American Congress of Obstetricians and Gynecologists (ACOG) currently recommends umbilical cord blood analysis for high-risk deliveries (i.e., low 5-min Apgar score, severe intrauterine growth restriction, maternal thyroid disease, fetal heart rate tracing abnormalities, intrapartum fever, multiple gestation pregnancies, and cesarean deliveries for fetal distress) [3, 4]. As a physician involved in newborn care, it is important to be able to interpret umbilical cord gases correctly. The arterial cord gas can be a valuable representation of the fetal state prior to delivery [5–7]. A low arterial cord pH has been associated with adverse neurologic sequelae [8]. Using both the arterial and venous cord values, the clinician may be able to determine the intrapartum events leading to neonatal depression [4, 5, 9] (Table 1.1).

Answer: 2

Table 1.1 Normal arterial and venous cord blood gas values

	Venous cord blood normal range (Mean ± 2SD)	Arterial cord blood normal range (Mean ± 2SD)
pH	7.25–7.45	7.18–7.38
pCO2 (mmHg)	26.8–49.2	32.2–65.8
pO2 (mmHg)	17.2–40.8	5.6–30.8
$HCO3^-$	15.8–24.2	17–27
Base excess (BE)	0 to −8	0 to −8

From Pomerance [10]
Data are mean values ± 2 standard deviations (SD)
Note: "Normal" is arbitrarily defined as the mean ± two times the standard deviation (approximately 95.4% of a normally distributed population)
[a]Base excess, estimated from data
[b]1 kPa = 7.50 mmHg; 1 mmHg = 0.133 kPa

In order to be able to correctly interpret umbilical cord blood gases, one must understand the physiology of fetal-placental gas exchange. Oxygenated blood leaves the placenta and courses through the *umbilical vein* to deliver oxygen to the fetal tissues. Deoxygenated blood containing higher carbon dioxide and increased acids leaves the fetus through the two *umbilical arteries*. Carbon dioxide easily diffuses across the placenta, but acids (such as lactic acid) leave more slowly [4, 7].

Since it carries the oxygenated blood resulting from gas exchange with the maternal circulation, the umbilical venous gas represents both fetal and maternal acid/base status. Conversely, the umbilical artery transports deoxygenated blood from the fetal tissues back to the placenta and therefore is reflective of both the uteroplacental status and the fetal acid/base state [10]. Based on this physiology, the venous umbilical cord gas should have a higher pH and a lower pCO2 than the umbilical arterial cord gas [4–6, 10]. This is the opposite of what one would expect of venous and arterial gases in a newborn who has transitioned to the postpartum circulation (an obvious exception being transposition of the great arteries). Cord gases are an important window into the fetal state while in utero [4, 5, 7]. However, results can be misleading if only a venous sample is obtained, the blood samples are mishandled, or there has been obstruction to cord blood flow in the last several minutes prior to birth [5, 10].

The lab reports the cord blood gas revealing a pH of 7.14, pCO2 of 54, pO2 of 36, and base excess of −11.

At this time you:

1. Are reassured by the cord gas and allow the baby to breastfeed.
2. Request the obstetrical team or respiratory therapist to repeat sampling, obtaining both arterial and venous cord blood gases.
3. Obtain an arterial blood gas on the baby.

In the ideal situation, both arterial and venous umbilical cord blood will be sampled for blood gas analysis [4]. The umbilical artery pH should be at least 0.02 units lower than the vein [6, 11].

The normal umbilical arterial pCO2 is usually more than 4 mmHg greater than the vein [6, 11]. Therefore, if two cord gases are reported and the A-V difference is 0.02 units or less in the pH and <4 mmHg in the pCO2, then the two results are likely from the same vessel [6, 11]. Even if an arterial cord gas is not reported, one can usually estimate the extent of acidemia based on the venous pH. The venous pH is usually >0.02 to <0.10 higher than the arterial pH. For a venous pH of 7.06 or less, there is a greater than 50% probability of significant arterial acidemia (defined as a pH less than 7.0). For a venous pH of ≥7.14 to <7.17 there is an estimated 10% probability of significant arterial acidemia. Finally, for a venous pH of ≥7.17 to <7.23, there is an estimated 5% probability of significant arterial cord acidemia [12].

If only one cord blood gas is reported, it may be from the umbilical vein, as this vessel is larger and more easily sampled [4, 6, 10]. One clue that a single gas sample is of venous origin is the PaO2 value. If the reported PaO2 is >31 mmHg, it is highly likely to be a venous sample [10].

Umbilical cord gases can be drawn from a doubly clamped cord kept at room temperature up to 60 min after delivery with little change in pH or pCO2 [3–5]. However, cord gases are unreliable for lactate beyond 20 min after birth [5, 13]. If too much heparin is added to the specimen to prevent clotting, the acid/base results can be affected due to the acidotic properties of the compound [5]. Therefore, most cord blood-gas samples are collected in pre-heparinized syringes. Air bubbles in the specimen may also affect the results by erroneously increasing the pH and the pO2 and by decreasing the pCO2; however, with most modern blood-gas analyzers, results will not be reported when an air bubble is detected [10].

Delayed cord clamping is currently recommended for *vigorous* newborns [14, 15]. If blood gas analysis is performed in the setting of delayed cord clamping, it is important to consider its potential effect on acid-base status. Continued placental gas exchange and/or neonatal breathing can affect the cord blood gas results by decreasing the pH, base excess, and bicarbonate and by increasing the lactate and pCO2 [6, 16, 17]. Currently, it is recommended that immediate cord clamping takes place for the depressed newborn in order not to delay resuscitation [3, 14, 15, 18].

Answer: 2

You correctly interpret the first cord gas results as venous (high pO2) and ask the respiratory therapist to collect an arterial sample from the cord. She gives you the following results: pH 7.07, pCO2 62, pO2 9, and BE -15.

At this time you:

1. Are reassured by the cord gases (since the pH from both the artery and vein is >7.0) and continue standard newborn care.
2. You are concerned by the significant arterial cord acidosis and plan further evaluation.

Once the umbilical cord gas is proven valid (i.e., from the correct vessel, without air bubbles, and not affected by heparin), it may be used to evaluate intrapartum events [4, 5, 9].

Fetal acidosis may be the result of a sudden decrease in placental or umbilical blood flow from conditions such as cord compression or placental abruption [3]. Other potential causes for fetal acidosis include fetal anemia, placental insufficiency, maternal hypoxemia and hypoventilation, and chronic maternal conditions such as preeclampsia [3, 6, 19].

Cord compression, e.g., cord prolapse, decreases blood flow from the placenta to the fetus [4]. When the cord is subjected to compression, the thin-walled umbilical vein is more likely to collapse compared to the thick-walled umbilical arteries [10]. This may lead to a reassuring venous cord gas and acidotic arterial cord gas, underscoring the importance of obtaining both samples [4, 5, 7, 20].

In placental abruption there is decreased perfusion of the placenta. In contrast to umbilical cord compression, the arterial and venous cord blood pCO2 values will be similar although both can potentially be significantly acidotic [4, 9].

Uncommonly there may be a complete occlusion of all three vessels in the umbilical cord with resulting cessation of blood flow to and from the fetus. In this situation, both cord blood gases could appear to be normal, as they reflect the acid-base state immediately prior to the complete occlusion, although the newborn may be significantly acidotic [4, 10, 21].

Answer: 2

Despite the reassuring venous cord gas, you are concerned by the significant arterial cord acidosis and plan further evaluation. What other evaluations might you consider?

1. Neonatal arterial blood gas.
2. Obtain a cord or neonatal lactate level.
3. Perform a neurologic exam.

A systemic arterial blood gas should be obtained within the first hour of life in all depressed newborns. This will help to determine potential intrauterine events and may also reflect the adequacy of resuscitation. An arterial blood gas obtained within the first hour of life that demonstrates significant acidosis coupled with an abnormal neurologic exam can be used to guide time-sensitive treatments such as therapeutic hypothermia. A capillary blood gas (CBG) may be misleading in the first hours after birth since poor perfusion may depress the pH and make the base deficit appear higher. However, a normal CBG at this time is reassuring.

It is possible to obtain an arterial lactate from the umbilical cord. Elevated cord lactate levels may be used to predict the presence of hypoxic-ischemic encephalopathy (HIE) [22]. In the setting of fetal hypoxia, anaerobic metabolism results in the accumulation of lactic acid, resulting in a metabolic acidosis. Unlike volatile acids, such as carbon dioxide, lactic acid is removed at a slower rate by the placenta from the fetal circulation [4, 7, 10]. For this reason, cord lactate levels are thought to reflect fetal acidosis and may be used to help predict neurologic outcomes [22]. However, at this time there is no consensus on the cord lactate level that might predict adverse outcomes [6]. A neonatal arterial lactate might also be helpful in the absence of a reliable cord gas. Shah reported that a plasma lactate level >7.5 mmol/l within the first hour of life was associated with moderate or severe HIE with a sensitivity of 94% and specificity of 67% [23].

An umbilical cord metabolic acidosis in a healthy appearing, vigorous newborn does not predict poor neurologic outcomes [24, 25]. A newborn must also have an exam consistent with moderate to severe encephalopathy in order to consider the possibility of a neurologic insult and to meet criteria for TH [25]. Therefore a thorough evaluation, including a neurological examination, is essential to predict long-term outcomes.

Answer: 1, 3

The newborn's arterial blood gas at 55 min of life is pH = 7.22, pCO2 of 49, pO2 of 74, and BE −10. At this time you proceed with a neurologic exam. You observe the newborn has a weak cry and slowly withdraws his legs with stimulation. His arms and legs are extended and his hands are clenched bilaterally. He has a weak suck and an incomplete Moro reflex by spreading his arms and barely pulling them inward.

At this point you should:

1. Refer patient for therapeutic hypothermia.
2. Observe and re-examine baby in 2–4 h with repeat ABG.
3. Start passive cooling.
4. Order ultrasound of the brain.

The Sarnat staging system provides a methodical approach to the neurologic evaluation of a depressed newborn. It employs the following elements: level of consciousness, neuromuscular control including posture and muscle tone, reflexes, autonomic system responses, and the presence or absence of seizures [26] (Table 1.2).

The level of consciousness of the newborn is evaluated as hyperalert, lethargic, stuporous, or comatose. The hyperalert newborn often appears to be staring and irritable and may not sleep for up to 24 h. Per Sarnat, the lethargic newborn would be irritated when disturbed and would have a delayed but completed response to a stimulus. In the more severe cases, the level of

Table 1.2 Modified Sarnat staging system here

Stage	Stage 1	Stage 2	Stage 3
Level of consciousness	Hyperalert	Lethargic	Stuporous or comatose
Tone	Normal	Decreased	Flaccid
Posture	Mild distal flexion	Strong distal flexion, complete extension	Decerebrate posturing
Spontaneous activity	Normal or decreased	Decreased	No activity
Reflexes			
Suck	Weak	Weak	Absent
Moro	Strong, easily elicited	Incomplete	Absent
Autonomic system			
Pupils	Dilated	Constricted	Variable, nonreactive to light, unequal
Heart rate	Tachycardia	Bradycardia	Variable
Respiration		Periodic breathing	Apnea
Seizures	None	Common	Uncommon

Derived from [1, 26]

consciousness is described as stuporous. The stuporous newborn would only respond to painful stimuli by withdrawing or demonstrating decerebrate posturing [26]. Rarely, the newborn could be considered comatose with no arousal nor motor response [27]. When evaluating posture, distal flexion and full extension means that the extremities are extended and the wrists and digits, including the thumb, are flexed (i.e., cortical thumb), where the thumb is flexed and held across the palm. Hypotonia occurs when decreased resistance is met with passive movement of the extremities. Flaccid is described when no resistance is met. The Sarnat system (Table 1.2) has been modified to be used in evaluation of term and near-term newborns for therapeutic hypothermia [1].

Following birth asphyxia, a sequence of events may occur in the brain leading to cerebral injury and long-term neurodevelopmental impairment. Birth asphyxia occurs before, during, or after birth due to many causes including lack of placental blood flow and subsequent poor gas exchange leading to hypoxia and hypercapnia [28, 29]. There are three phases of cerebral injury: (1) primary phase, (2) latent phase, and (3) delayed phase [30, 31]. The primary phase occurs during the asphyxial event and results in hypoxia and decreased cerebral circulation with eventual neuronal cell swelling which, if the event was severe, may lead to necrosis and cell death [29, 31–33]. The latent phase begins with the return of cerebral circulation and occurs over hours 1–6, with partial recovery [32, 33]. The delayed phase occurs at 6–15 h following the hypoxic event, with secondary deterioration leading to neuronal death and clinical deterioration [30–32]. It is the latent phase, which occurs between hours one and six, which is considered the therapeutic window to prevent secondary deterioration and delayed neuronal death [2, 33].

Knowledge that interventions during the therapeutic window might halt neuronal death and positively affect long-term neurodevelopmental outcomes has been an impetus for research into potential treatments for HIE [34]. TH has been established as the standard of care for this condition [2]. With multiple trials, TH has been demonstrated to decrease both mortality and neurodevelopmental impairment among newborns with HIE [33, 35].

The neuroprotective effect of TH is achieved by lowering the core body temperature and subsequently reducing the metabolic rate of the brain in attempt to prevent neuronal cell death [33]. There are two different types of cooling systems for TH that have been studied with large randomized controlled trials: whole body (systemic) hypothermia and selective head hypothermia [1, 36–38]. Both systems are effective in reducing mortality and neurodevelopmental impairment in moderate to severe encephalopathic newborns [32, 33, 35].

In 2014, the American Academy of Pediatrics' Committee on Fetus and Newborn recommended that the decision to use TH should be guided by two validated protocols [39]. Two protocols that are currently used by a majority of institutions in the United States: the NICHD Protocol for Systemic Hypothermia [1] and the "CoolCap" Study for selective head hypothermia [36]. These protocols use slightly different criteria, which means it is very important for the generalist to be familiar with the specific protocol that is commonly used by their referral institution.

The following inclusion criteria are consistent across most protocols [1, 36–38]:

1. Gestational age greater than or equal to 36 weeks
2. Less than or equal to 6 h of life
3. One or more of the following:
   (a) A pH ≤ 7 or base deficit ≥ 16 on a cord gas or any blood gas within the first hour of life
   (b) A 10 min Apgar score of ≤ 5
   (c) Positive pressure ventilation for at least the first 10 min of life
4. An exam indicative of moderate or severe encephalopathy

Each protocol has different requirements to distinguish between moderate or severe encephalopathy by using Sarnat staging (see Table 1.2 above). Whole body hypothermia requires presence of seizures or one or more signs in three of six Sarnat categories [1]. In selective head hypothermia, a newborn is said to have moderate or severe encephalopathy if the level of consciousness is lethargic, stuporous, or comatose and the neurologic exam reveals one or more of the following: abnormal reflexes (including pupillary abnormalities or abnormal oculomotor reflexes), hypotonia, a weak or absent suck, or seizures [36].

Many referral centers that use the selective head cooling protocol require an amplitude electroencephalograph (aEEG) prior to initiation of cooling [36]. An aEEG is a bedside monitor that screens for abnormal brain activity as well as seizures [40].

Exclusion criteria generally include one or more of the following [1, 36–38]:

- Gestational age less than 36 weeks
- Greater than 6 h since birth
- Birthweight less than 1800 g
- Presence of a major congenital abnormality
- A moribund newborn

Some protocols also exclude newborns with gross hemorrhage [37] or intracranial hemorrhage [36].

TH should only be provided in an institution with a neonatal intensive care unit with the following capabilities: an approved and implemented standardized cooling protocol, the necessary equipment (including active controlled hypothermia equipment, core temperature monitoring, mechanical ventilation, EEG or aEEG, and MRI), the necessary subspecialty services (i.e., pediatric neurology), and the availability of long-term neurodevelopmental follow-up [39, 41].

The short therapeutic window (e.g., 6 h) creates a conundrum for outlying hospitals that often lack the capacity to do TH [42–44]. One solution has been to attempt to treat these newborns through passive and uncontrolled active cooling at these outlying hospitals until transport can be arranged [42–45]. Passive cooling involves discontinuing active warming activities by turning off the radiant warmer and removing blankets [45]. Uncontrolled active cooling involves briefly placing ice packs or cool gel packs on the newborn's chest and/or forehead [42, 45]. Both passive cooling and uncontrolled active cooling are risky endeavors, as they place newborns at high risk for severe hypothermia [42]. This is especially true for severely encephalopathic newborns due to their propensity for temperature dysregulation [43, 45]. Overcooling may result in bleeding, thrombosis, sepsis, and arrhythmias [46]. Many transport teams now have controlled active cooling devices that can be initiated on arrival to the outlying hospital [47]. Some centers will treat patients up to 24 h after injury, although a recent study showed no statistical improvement from newborns cooled beyond 6 h of life [48].

It is also important to avoid *hyperthermia* and hypoglycemia in asphyxiated newborns as they have been associated with increased brain injury and poorer outcomes [2, 41, 49–51].

The most common side effects of active controlled cooling are sinus bradycardia and thrombocytopenia [33].

Answer: 1

Denouement: This baby should be referred for TH if not available at your hospital. If you are uncertain that the patient meets criteria, repeat the exam and studies in 1 h and/or consult your neonatologist. Cranial ultrasound will not give any useful information at this early stage in the evolution of a possible HIE, but may demonstrate unexpected findings such as hemorrhage or hydrocephalus. Continued metabolic acidosis or an elevated arterial lactate (> 7.5 mmol/l) and continued hypotonia would tend to favor treatment with TH before 6 h of age.

Case Presentation

A 38 and 4/7 weeks gestation male is born by cesarean section for failure to progress to a 26-year-old primigravida female. Pregnancy was complicated by poor prenatal care. Membranes ruptured 14 h prior to delivery with clear amniotic fluid. At birth, the baby is limp with a heart rate of 80 bpm. He is noted to have poor respiratory effort and receives 2 min of positive pressure ventilation (PPV). After PPV, he begins to spontaneously breathe and his heart rate improves to 130; however, he continues to have poor tone. Apgar scores of 2, 5, and 7 are assigned at 1, 5, and 10 min of age. An unspecified cord blood gas shows a pH of 7.22, pCO_2 of 52, pO_2 of 18, and a base excess of −7. You are called to assess whether or not this patient qualifies for cooling.

You perform a history and physical exam and you realize that the history is not consistent with the criteria for TH although the newborn is encephalopathic on exam. Your staff have yet to perform the newborn's measurements including weight, length, and head circumference.

At this time you:

1. Turn off the radiant warmer and call the referral center.
2. Obtain head ultrasound since your referral center prefers one before cooling.
3. Ask staff to perform newborn measurements.

You obtain a head ultrasound preemptively since your referral institution prefers one before cooling. It reveals massive hydrocephalus. While writing your note, you realize the patient's head circumference is 39 cm > 99% while weight and length are 50%, 3290 g and 50 cm respectively.

This case emphasizes the importance of obtaining a full history, performing a complete physical exam, and adhering to the protocol's inclusion criteria for TH. Encephalopathy is a broad entity encompassing multiple etiologies all leading to a depressed mental state [52, 53]. As such, there is a broad differential for neonatal encephalopathy beyond hypoxic-ischemic events including sepsis, meningitis, congenital infection, inborn errors of metabolism, genetic disorders, intracranial abnormalities including perinatal stroke both ischemic and hemorrhagic, hydrocephalus, and neonatal epilepsy syndromes [54]. Therefore, only those newborns that meet the criteria for TH should be cooled. Performing TH on newborns that do not meet criteria could result in delayed or missed diagnoses, resulting in increased morbidity and mortality. Until HIE is confirmed, it has been advised to describe the newborn as having neonatal encephalopathy [53].

Some protocols recommend obtaining a head ultrasound prior to cooling which would have detected the abnormality in this case. The 39 cm head circumference (>99% for gestational age) is disproportionate to the newborn's weight and length, which were in the 50% for gestational age. The head ultrasound revealed undiagnosed hydrocephalus which explained the depressed Apgar scores, hypotonia, and decreased activity noted on the exam.

Answer: 2, 3

Newborns that possess an inborn error of metabolism can also demonstrate signs and symptoms of encephalopathy. They may be initially asymptomatic, as the placenta acts as a filter removing the byproducts of their deranged metabolism. Following birth, these patients may go on to develop lethargy and seizures. It is therefore reasonable to include serum ammonia and lactate levels in evaluating neonatal encephalopathy.

Newborns with sepsis can also be lethargic and may readily become acidotic. The early institution of antibiotics in these cases is critical. By evaluating the perinatal events, physical examination, the results of cord blood and post-birth blood gas analysis, and other laboratory evaluations, one can usually differentiate the various causes of neonatal encephalopathy.

Case Presentation

A 40 and 6/7 weeks gestation female is born by vaginal birth after cesarean (VBAC) delivery to a 32-year-old G2P1. Pregnancy was uncomplicated. Rupture of membranes occurred 28 h prior to delivery revealing clear amniotic fluid. The baby is limp with a heart rate of 70 bpm at birth. She remains apneic and receives PPV via self-inflating bag. Heart rate declines to 60 bpm despite ventilation corrective steps, and she is successfully intubated on the second attempt at 4 min of life. Her heart rate has declined to 40 bpm despite adequate ventilation. She receives 5 min of chest compressions. One dose of endotracheal tube epinephrine and one dose of intravenous epinephrine via an emergent umbilical line results in improvement of heart rate. Due to poor perfusion, she receives a 10 ml/kg normal saline bolus. Apgar scores are 1 at 1 min, 1 at 5 min, 3 at 10 min, 3 at 15 min, and 3 at 20 min. An arterial cord gas shows pH of 6.95/pCO2 83/pO2 19/HCO3 17.8/base excess −15.7. She is transferred to the newborn nursery for stabilization. Her temperature on admission is 37.4 °C, and she is placed under a radiant warmer on manual control. After continuous manual ventilation, an ABG is obtained at 50 min of life revealing pH 6.95, pCO2 66, pO2 26, HCO3 14, and base excess −19, and bedside glucose is 39 mg/dl. On exam, you note with arterial puncture she slowly responds by flexing her arms and demonstrates a facial grimace. Without stimulation she has decreased activity, poor tone, a weak suck, and equal but delayed Moro reflex, pupils appear constricted, heart rate is 120 bpm, and she is now spontaneously breathing above the ventilated breaths.

You call the referral center for transport. How would you proceed to stabilize the newborn while waiting for the transport team?

1. Make patient NPO, start D10W at 60 ml/kg/day, obtain blood culture, and start ampicillin and gentamicin.
2. Make patient NPO, start D10W at 100 ml/kg/day, obtain blood culture, and start ampicillin and gentamicin.
3. Make patient NPO and turn off radiant warmer. Do not start antibiotics.
4. Make patient NPO, turn off radiant warmer, give a 2 ml/kg bolus of D10 W and start D10W at 60 ml/kg/day, obtain blood culture, and start ampicillin and ceftazidime.

Birth asphyxia is the result of poor perfusion to the fetus from either decreased placental or umbilical blood flow [28]. In response, the fetal heart preferentially shunts blood to the vital organs, including the brain, the heart, and the adrenal glands, and, if prolonged, these organs can be adversely affected [24, 55]. Asphyxia can ultimately lead to HIE but can also cause electrolyte and endocrine disturbances, as well as dysfunction of the heart, kidneys, and/or liver [50, 56].

During the stabilization of the depressed newborn, the potential for multi-organ dysfunction should be considered. The depressed newborn should be made NPO, given a bolus of glucose, and started on dextrose containing intravenous fluids. Fluid restriction of 40–70 ml/kg/day is recommended to avoid fluid overload and to theoretically prevent worsening of cerebral edema [51, 56]. Careful fluid balance must be maintained, as too strict a fluid restriction can lead to hypovolemia with the worsening of acute kidney injury (AKI). Fluid restriction may also increase the risk of hypoglycemia which is associated with poorer neurodevelopmental outcomes [51].

Newborns with HIE should be screened for sepsis with a blood culture and receive empiric antibiotics. If nephrotoxic medications are used, such as gentamicin, it is important to monitor drug levels prior to the subsequent dose to ensure they are within the therapeutic range [51, 57]. If the patient is anuric or oliguric or has an elevated creatinine, nephrotoxic medications should, if possible, be avoided [51, 57]. Antibiotic regimens might include piperacillin-tazobactam or ampicillin and a third-generation cephalosporin such as ceftazidime.

Answer: 4

You obtain a point of care blood glucose which is 54 mg/dl. You make the newborn NPO and start D10W at 60 ml/kg/day. A blood culture is obtained and you have ordered ampicillin and ceftazidime. 15 min later, the nurse calls you to the bedside to evaluate jerking movement of the upper and lower extremities associated with increased blood pressure and oxygen desaturation.

At this time you:

1. Continue waiting for the transfer team.
2. Order 20 mg/kg Phenobarbital IV once stat.
3. Obtain BMP, Mg, and ionized Ca.

Neonatal seizures are defined as sudden, abnormal activity causing motor, behavioral, and/or autonomic dysfunction [27, 58]. They may present with tonic, clonic, or myoclonic movements or have a subtler presentation such as apnea, vital sign instability, or horizontal eye deviation with or without nystagmus [27]. With the advent of video EEG, it is now known that seizure-like activity can be easily misinterpreted [58]. Some activities that are characterized as clinical seizures do not show simultaneous EEG changes, and documented electrographic seizures do not always have stereotypical clinical activity [27]. This emphasizes the need for prolonged EEG monitoring [27]. If the newborn has seizure-like activity, the provider should screen for and correct electrolyte and metabolic derangements by obtaining a serum glucose, sodium, ionized calcium, and magnesium level [59]. If the clinician suspects seizures in a patient with HIE, it would be advisable to load with phenobarbital 20 mg/kg [27]. Phenobarbital is effective at suppressing clinical seizures, but electrographic seizures may be ongoing [27]. Therefore, it is important to transfer to a center with full neurologic monitoring capabilities through EEG or aEEG and the availability of neurologic consultation.

Answer: 2

The transport team arrives and successfully transfers the newborn to a higher level of care. The mother remains as an inpatient following her C-section. The following day, she asks how the referral center will evaluate her newborn for brain damage.

Your response to her:

1. That is a good question for the referral center.
2. Oftentimes an MRI will be performed within the first week.
3. A brain MRI will be performed and there will be developmental follow-up.

Following therapeutic hypothermia, an MRI is performed between 1 and 2 weeks of age to evaluate the extent of the injury and gather prognostic information for the family [2]. Injuries to the basal ganglia and thalamus are more likely to be associated with a poor prognosis than watershed injuries, and injury to posterior limb of the internal capsule is highly associated with a poor neurodevelopmental outcome [27, 60]. Although TH is associated with an improved MRI, a normal MRI does not preclude neurodevelopmental impairment [61]. Both normal MRIs and those with only mild injuries can be associated with neurodevelopmental impairment; therefore, it is important to be cautious when counseling families on prognosis [61].

Answer: 3

Clinical Pearls

- After successful resuscitation of a term or near-term neonate, the clinician should determine the cause of the neonatal depression.
- Evaluation of the resuscitated neonate should occur quickly since therapies (i.e., therapeutic hypothermia, antibiotics) are time sensitive.
- An umbilical cord blood gas with a PO2 of >31 mmHg has likely been obtained from the umbilical vein.
- Most (but not all) of the time an umbilical venous blood gas pH will be predictive of the umbilical artery pH.
- In the absence of a cord blood gas, an early arterial blood gas or arterial lactate level may assist in determining if the patient is a candidate for therapeutic hypothermia.
- Neurological evaluation of the neonate using a modified Sarnat scoring system will assist in determining if the baby is a candidate for therapeutic hypothermia.
- *H*yperthermia and hypoglycemia should be avoided in post-resuscitated neonates as they are synergistic with asphyxia injury.
- Apnea in a term neonate has a central nervous system etiology until proven otherwise.

Conflict of Interest Both authors declare they have no conflicts of interest with regard to the content of this manuscript.

References

1. Shankaran S, Laptook AR, Ehrenkranz RA, Tyson JE, McDonald SA, Donovan EF, et al. Whole-body hypothermia for neonates with hypoxic-ischemic encephalopathy. N Engl J Med. 2005;353(15):1574–84.
2. Shankaran S. Therapeutic hypothermia for neonatal encephalopathy. Curr Treat Options Neurol. 2012;14(6):608–19.
3. Nageotte MP. Intrapartum fetal surveillance. In: Creasy RK, Resnik R, editors. Creasy & Resnik's maternal-fetal medicine principles and practice. 7th ed. Philadelphia: Saunders; 2014. p. 488–506.
4. Armstrong L, Stenson BJ. Use of umbilical cord blood gas analysis in the assessment of the newborn. Arch Dis Child Fetal Neonatal Ed. 2007;92(6):F430–4.
5. Blickstein I, Green T. Umbilical cord blood gases. Clin Perinatol. 2007;34(3):451–9.
6. Higgins C. Umbilical-cord blood gas analysis Bronshoj. Denmark: Radiometer Medical ApS; 2014.
7. Thorp JA, Rushing RS. Umbilical cord blood gas analysis. Obstet Gynecol Clin N Am. 1999;26(4):695–709.
8. Malin GL, Morris RK, Khan KS. Strength of association between umbilical cord pH and perinatal and long term outcomes: systematic review and meta-analysis. BMJ. 2010;340:c1471.
9. Johnson JW, Richards DS. The etiology of fetal acidosis as determined by umbilical cord acid-base studies. Am J Obstet Gynecol. 1997;177(2):274–80. discussion 80-2
10. Pomerance J. Interpreting umbilical cord gases. 2nd ed. California: BNMG; 2012; (cordgases.com).
11. Westgate J, Garibaldi JM, Greene KR. Umbilical cord blood gas analysis at delivery: a time for quality data. Br J Obstet Gynaecol. 1994;101(12):1054–63.
12. Cantu J, Szychowski JM, Li X, Biggio J, Edwards RK, Andrews W, et al. Predicting fetal acidemia using umbilical venous cord gas parameters. Obstet Gynecol. 2014;124(5):926–32.
13. Armstrong L, Stenson B. Effect of delayed sampling on umbilical cord arterial and venous lactate and blood gases in clamped and unclamped vessels. Arch Dis Child Fetal Neonatal Ed. 2006;91(5):F342–5.
14. Practice CoO. Committee opinion no. 684: delayed umbilical cord clamping after birth. Obstet Gynecol. 2017;129(1):e5–e10.
15. Weiner GM, Zaichkin J, Kattwinkel J. Textbook of neonatal resuscitation. 7th ed. Elk Grove Village: American Academy of Pediatrics, American Heart Association; 2016. Xii
16. Valero J, Desantes D, Perales-Puchalt A, Rubio J, Diago Almela VJ, Perales A. Effect of delayed umbilical cord clamping on blood gas analysis. Eur J Obstet Gynecol Reprod Biol. 2012;162(1):21–3.
17. Wiberg N, Källén K, Olofsson P. Delayed umbilical cord clamping at birth has effects on arterial and venous blood gases and lactate concentrations. BJOG. 2008;115(6):697–703.
18. WHO. Guideline: delayed umbilical cord clamping for improved maternal and infant health and nutrition outcomes. Geneva: World Health Organization; 2014.
19. Liston R, Sawchuck D, Young D, Canada SoOaGo, Program BCPH. Fetal health surveillance: antepartum and intrapartum consensus guideline. J Obstet Gynaecol Can. 2007;29(9 Suppl 4):S3–56.
20. Pomerance J. Umbilical cord blood gases casebook. Interpreting umbilical cord blood gases, V. J Perinatol. 1999;19(6 Pt 1):466–7.
21. Pomerance J. Umbilical cord blood gases casebook. Interpreting umbilical cord blood gases, VII. J Perinatol. 2000;20(5):338–9.

22. Allanson ER, Waqar T, White C, Tunçalp Ö, Dickinson JE. Umbilical lactate as a measure of acidosis and predictor of neonatal risk: a systematic review. BJOG. 2017;124(4):584–94.
23. Shah S, Tracy M, Smyth J. Postnatal lactate as an early predictor of short-term outcome after intrapartum asphyxia. J Perinatol. 2004;24(1):16–20.
24. King TA, Jackson GL, Josey AS, Vedro DA, Hawkins H, Burton KM, et al. The effect of profound umbilical artery acidemia in term neonates admitted to a newborn nursery. J Pediatr. 1998;132(4):624–9.
25. Hafström M, Ehnberg S, Blad S, Norén H, Renman C, Rosén KG, et al. Developmental outcome at 6.5 years after acidosis in term newborns: a population-based study. Pediatrics. 2012;129(6):e1501–7.
26. Sarnat HB, Sarnat MS. Neonatal encephalopathy following fetal distress. A clinical and electroencephalographic study. Arch Neurol. 1976;33(10):696–705.
27. Volpe JJ. Neurology of the newborn. 5th ed. Philadelphia: Saunders/Elsevier; 2008. xiv
28. Levene MI, de Vries LS. Hypoxic-ischemic encephalopathy. In: Martin RJ, Fanaroff AA, editors. Fanaroff and Martin's neonatal-perinatal medicine: diseases of the fetus and infant. 9th ed. St. Louis: Elsevier/Saunders; 2011. p. 952–71.
29. Rainaldi MA, Perlman JM. Pathophysiology of birth asphyxia. Clin Perinatol. 2016;43(3):409–22.
30. Gunn AJ. Cerebral hypothermia for prevention of brain injury following perinatal asphyxia. Curr Opin Pediatr. 2000;12(2):111–5.
31. Gunn AJ, Thoresen M. Hypothermic neuroprotection. NeuroRx. 2006;3(2):154–69.
32. Douglas-Escobar M, Weiss MD. Hypoxic-ischemic encephalopathy: a review for the clinician. JAMA Pediatr. 2015;169(4):397–403.
33. Jacobs SE, Berg M, Hunt R, Tarnow-Mordi WO, Inder TE, Davis PG. Cooling for newborns with hypoxic ischaemic encephalopathy. Cochrane Database Syst Rev. 2013;31(1):CD003311.
34. Gunn AJ, Laptook AR, Robertson NJ, Barks JD, Thoresen M, Wassink G, et al. Therapeutic hypothermia translates from ancient history in to practice. Pediatr Res. 2017;81(1–2):202–9.
35. Tagin MA, Woolcott CG, Vincer MJ, Whyte RK, Stinson DA. Hypothermia for neonatal hypoxic ischemic encephalopathy: an updated systematic review and meta-analysis. Arch Pediatr Adolesc Med. 2012;166(6):558–66.
36. Gluckman PD, Wyatt JS, Azzopardi D, Ballard R, Edwards AD, Ferriero DM, et al. Selective head cooling with mild systemic hypothermia after neonatal encephalopathy: multicentre randomised trial. Lancet. 2005;365(9460):663–70.
37. Simbruner G, Mittal RA, Rohlmann F, Muche R, nnnT P. Systemic hypothermia after neonatal encephalopathy: outcomes of neo.nEURO.network RCT. Pediatrics. 2010;126(4):e771–8.
38. Azzopardi DV, Strohm B, Edwards AD, Dyet L, Halliday HL, Juszczak E, et al. Moderate hypothermia to treat perinatal asphyxial encephalopathy. N Engl J Med. 2009;361(14):1349–58.
39. Papile LA, Baley JE, Benitz W, Cummings J, Carlo WA, Eichenwald E, et al. Hypothermia and neonatal encephalopathy. Pediatrics. 2014;133(6):1146–50.
40. Glass HC, Wusthoff CJ, Shellhaas RA. Amplitude-integrated electro-encephalography: the child neurologist's perspective. J Child Neurol. 2013;28(10):1342–50.
41. Manley BJ, Owen LS, Hooper SB, Jacobs SE, Cheong JLY, Doyle LW, et al. Towards evidence-based resuscitation of the newborn infant. Lancet. 2017;389(10079):1639–48.
42. O'Reilly KM, Tooley J, Winterbottom S. Therapeutic hypothermia during neonatal transport. Acta Paediatr. 2011;100(8):1084–6. discussion e49
43. Hallberg B, Olson L, Bartocci M, Edqvist I, Blennow M. Passive induction of hypothermia during transport of asphyxiated infants: a risk of excessive cooling. Acta Paediatr. 2009;98(6):942–6.
44. Kendall GS, Kapetanakis A, Ratnavel N, Azzopardi D, Robertson NJ, Group CoRS. Passive cooling for initiation of therapeutic hypothermia in neonatal encephalopathy. Arch Dis Child Fetal Neonatal Ed. 2010;95(6):F408–12.
45. Fairchild K, Sokora D, Scott J, Zanelli S. Therapeutic hypothermia on neonatal transport: 4-year experience in a single NICU. J Perinatol. 2010;30(5):324–9.
46. Hoehn T, Hansmann G, Bührer C, Simbruner G, Gunn AJ, Yager J, et al. Therapeutic hypothermia in neonates. Review of current clinical data, ILCOR recommendations and suggestions for implementation in neonatal intensive care units. Resuscitation. 2008;78(1):7–12.
47. Chaudhary R, Farrer K, Broster S, McRitchie L, Austin T. Active versus passive cooling during neonatal transport. Pediatrics. 2013;132(5):841–6.
48. Laptook AR, Shankaran S, Tyson JE, Munoz B, Bell EF, Goldberg RN, et al. Effect of therapeutic hypothermia initiated after 6 hours of age on death or disability among newborns with hypoxic-ischemic encephalopathy: a randomized clinical trial. JAMA. 2017;318(16):1550–60.
49. Thoresen M. Supportive care during neuroprotective hypothermia in the term newborn: adverse effects and their prevention. Clin Perinatol. 2008;35(4):749–63. vii
50. Shankaran S. The postnatal management of the asphyxiated term infant. Clin Perinatol. 2002;29(4):675–92.
51. Sweetman DU, Riordan M, Molloy EJ. Management of renal dysfunction following term perinatal hypoxia-ischaemia. Acta Paediatr. 2013;102(3):233–41.
52. Kurinczuk JJ, White-Koning M, Badawi N. Epidemiology of neonatal encephalopathy and hypoxic-ischaemic encephalopathy. Early Hum Dev. 2010;86(6):329–38.
53. Executive summary: neonatal encephalopathy and neurologic outcome, second edition. Report of the American college of obstetricians and gynecologists' Task force on neonatal encephalopathy. Obstet Gynecol. 2014;123(4):896–901.
54. Martinello K, Hart AR, Yap S, Mitra S, Robertson NJ. Management and investigation of neonatal

encephalopathy: 2017 update. Arch Dis Child Fetal Neonatal Ed. 2017;102(4):F346–F58.

55. Leone TA, Finer NN. Shock: a common consequence of neonatal asphyxia. J Pediatr. 2011;158(2 Suppl):e9–12.
56. Kecskes Z, Healy G, Jensen A. Fluid restriction for term infants with hypoxic-ischaemic encephalopathy following perinatal asphyxia. Cochrane Database Syst Rev. 2005;20(3):CD004337.
57. Durkan AM, Alexander RT. Acute kidney injury post neonatal asphyxia. J Pediatr. 2011;158(2 Suppl):e29–33.
58. Shetty J. Neonatal seizures in hypoxic-ischaemic encephalopathy – risks and benefits of anticonvulsant therapy. Dev Med Child Neurol. 2015;57(Suppl 3):40–3.
59. Gomella TL, Cunningham MD, Eyal FG. Neonatology: management, procedures, on-call problems, diseases, and drugs. 6th ed. New York: McGraw-Hill Medical; 2009. xviii, 894 p.
60. Merhar SL, Chau V. Neuroimaging and other Neurodiagnostic tests in neonatal encephalopathy. Clin Perinatol. 2016;43(3):511–27.
61. Rollins N, Booth T, Morriss MC, Sanchez P, Heyne R, Chalak L. Predictive value of neonatal MRI showing no or minor degrees of brain injury after hypothermia. Pediatr Neurol. 2014;50(5):447–51.

Newborn Birth Injuries

2

Smeeta Sardesai

Introduction

Birth injuries, although declining due to improvements in obstetric care and prenatal diagnosis, remain a significant cause of neonatal morbidity and mortality and are a source of great concern for the parents, obstetricians, pediatricians, and other healthcare providers.

There is a wide spectrum of birth injuries that range from minor and self-limited to severe. Often injuries occur due to risk factors such as macrosomia, prematurity, forceps delivery, vacuum extraction, abnormal fetal presentation, prolonged labor, and precipitous delivery [1, 2], but damage can also occur in utero before initiation of birth process and in the absence of any identifiable risk factors.

At times, signs and symptoms may not be apparent immediately after birth due to the presence of other associated clinical problems. Some injuries may become more evident at the time of or after discharge. In order to initiate appropriate treatment, it is important for clinicians to remain alert to the possibility that birth injuries may become apparent even after newborns are discharged from the hospital.

S. Sardesai, MD, MS Ed, FAAP
Keck School of Medicine, University of Southern California, Los Angeles, CA, USA
e-mail: sardesai@usc.edu

In most cases, management of soft tissue injuries requires only careful observation and follow-up. However, in other instances such as subgaleal hemorrhage, early recognition and immediate intervention is required for survival.

It is important that clinicians are able to recognize and manage birth injuries and provide appropriate counseling to parents regarding prognosis. Misdiagnosis and/or mistreatment can have significant impact on both short-term and long-term well-being of a child. Counseling of parents regarding the severity of birth injuries and associated prognosis helps in establishing expectations regarding the outcome and avoiding misunderstandings.

Case Presentation

You are evaluating a 12-h-old male neonate with estimated gestational age of 38 weeks, birth weight 3.8 kg with a scalp swelling, weakness, and pallor of the body. The mother G1P0 received antenatal care in a private hospital, kept all appointments, and used only the prescribed medications. She delivered vaginally by vacuum extraction; Apgar score was 7/8. Physical examination revealed a hypotonic, pale infant with diminished peripheral pulses and a weak cry. The anterior fontanelle was full, and a fluctuant mass with bruised skin on the posterior aspect of the head was noted.

G. I. Martin, W. Rosenfeld (eds.), *Common Problems in the Newborn Nursery*,
https://doi.org/10.1007/978-3-319-95672-5_2

At this time, you think the swelling on the scalp is:

1. Caput succedaneum
2. Cephalohematoma
3. Subgaleal hemorrhage
4. Subarachnoid hemorrhage

Extracranial injuries (Fig. 2.1) occur above the parietal layer of the skull. They include caput succedaneum, cephalohematoma, subgaleal hemorrhage, and skull fractures.

Caput Succedaneum

Caput succedaneum (Fig. 2.2) is characterized by a vaguely demarcated area of edema over the scalp that was the presenting part during a vertex delivery. The edema is due to a serosanguinous fluid collection a few millimeters thick above the periosteum that presents as a soft tissue swelling of the scalp. Because of the location external to the periosteum, it may extend across the suture lines and can be confused with subgaleal hemorrhage, the more serious form of extracranial injury. Careful assessment is necessary to avoid misdiagnosis, which can have potentially catastrophic results. Firm, constant pressure in one spot is the easiest way to elicit the characteristic pitting edema of caput succedaneum.

Caput succedaneum is easily differentiated from a cephalohematoma as the swelling is above the periosteum and crosses the suture lines although occasionally a bilateral cephalohematoma can be difficult to distinguish from a caput succedaneum.

Cephalohematoma

A cephalohematoma is subperiosteal collection of blood caused by rupture of diploic blood vessels that traverse from skull to periosteum. Repeated buffeting of the fetal skull against the maternal pelvis during a prolonged or difficult labor and mechanical trauma from forceps or vacuum devices during delivery have been implicated [1]. Cephalohematomas may not be apparent at birth and may develop incrementally during

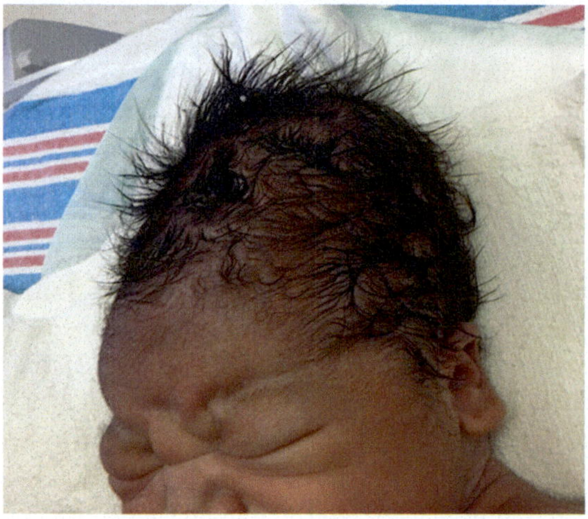

Fig. 2.2 Newborn at 10 min of life with caput succedaneum

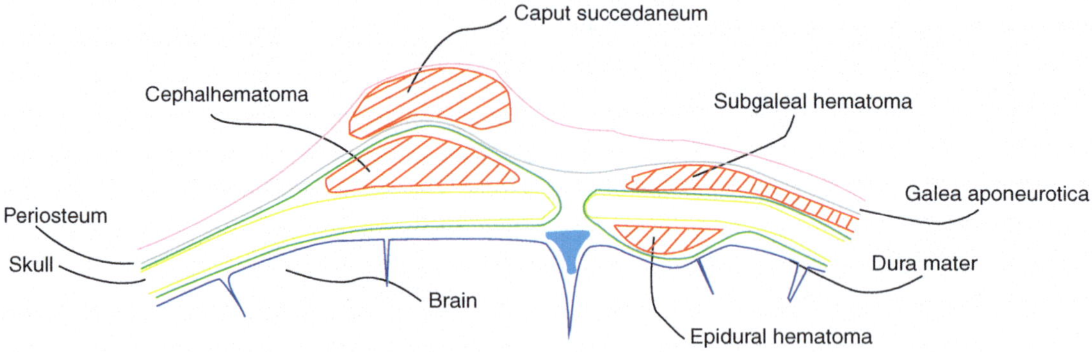

Fig. 2.1 Extracranial injuries in the planes of the scalp

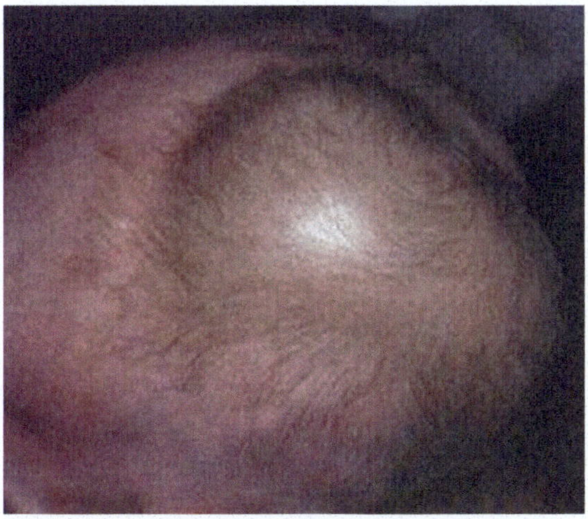

Fig. 2.3 Unilateral left parietal cephalohematoma

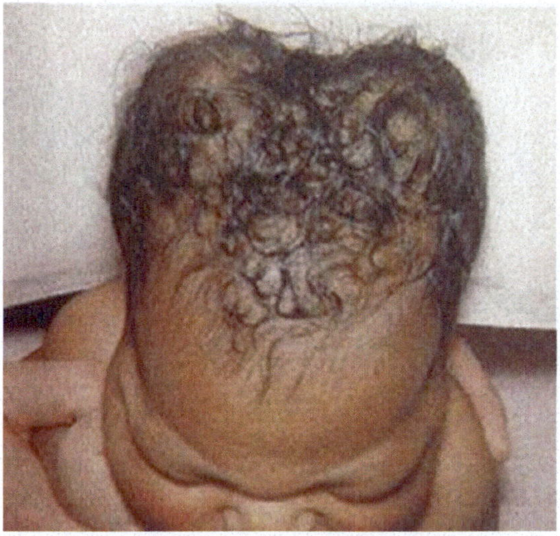

Fig. 2.4 Bilateral parietal cephalohematomas

the first 24 h of life and present as either a unilateral (Fig. 2.3) or bilateral (Fig. 2.4) palpable mass, often over a parietal or occipital bone.

Because the blood is subperiosteal, the swelling does not extend across the suture lines and is the distinguishing feature of cephalohematoma.

Subgaleal Hemorrhage

A subgaleal hemorrhage (SGH) is a potentially fatal lesion that results from bleeding under the epicranial aponeurosis. The epicranial aponeurosis is a sheet of fibrous tissue that extends from the orbital ridges anteriorly to the nape of the neck posteriorly and to the level of the ears laterally, creating a subgaleal or subaponeurotic space. Thus, SGH can spread across the entire calvarium. SGH is most often associated with vacuum-assisted deliveries which may produce a shearing force to the scalp, thereby tearing large emissary veins. This risk increases further in deliveries in which both forceps and vacuum extraction are used [1]. Infants with SGH present initially with pallor, poor tone, and fluctuant swelling on the scalp that can rapidly result in shock [3]. As the hemorrhage progresses, it may displace the ears anteriorly, and periorbital edema may develop (Fig. 2.5). Other symptoms may include signs of pain, particularly when the head or scalp is manipulated.

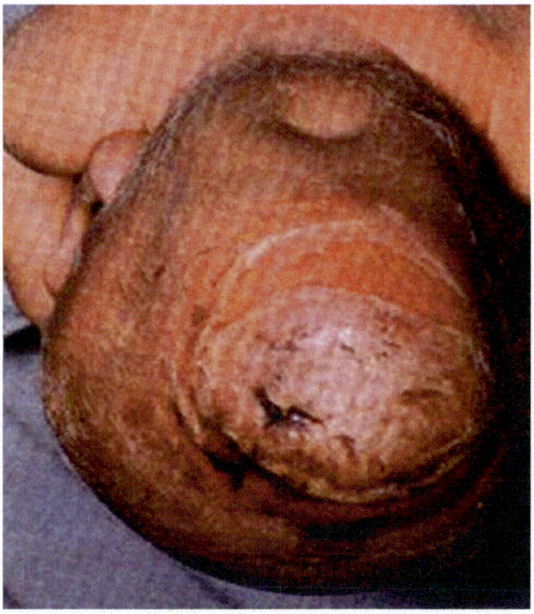

Fig. 2.5 Severe scalp edema and abrasion of the scalp in an infant with subgaleal hemorrhage delivered by vacuum extraction

In any extensive SGH, an underlying bleeding disorder such as thrombocytopenia, vitamin K deficiency, hemophilia, and disseminated intravascular coagulation must be considered in the etiology. Clotting abnormalities not only predispose the infant to bleeding but also may contribute to the extension of a relatively insignificant

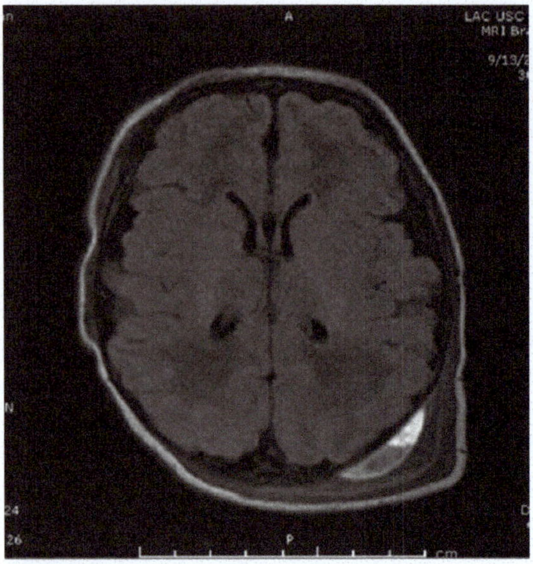

Fig. 2.6 MRI of the brain showing cephalohematoma beneath subgaleal hematoma

hemorrhage into a larger, more serious loss of blood. A coagulopathy may be related to consumption of clotting factors and platelets by the hematoma [4].

The infant in the vignette was found to have subgaleal hemorrhage and a cephalohematoma on MRI scan as seen in (Fig. 2.6).

Answer: 3

At this time you are concerned about:

1. Anemia
2. Jaundice
3. Infection
4. Shock from blood loss

It is rare to have significant blood loss or jaundice with caput. Blood loss in cephalohematoma is limited by periosteal attachment to the scalp bone.

Jaundice in infants with cephalohematoma and SGH is common but not in the first 24 h, usually occurs later than classic physiologic hyperbilirubinemia following the breakdown of the red blood cells (RBCs) in the cephalohematoma and in the SGH.

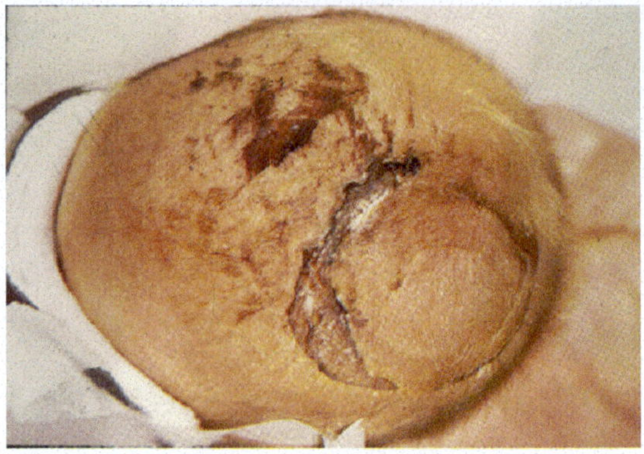

Fig. 2.7 Infant with scalp abrasion and infection following vacuum delivery

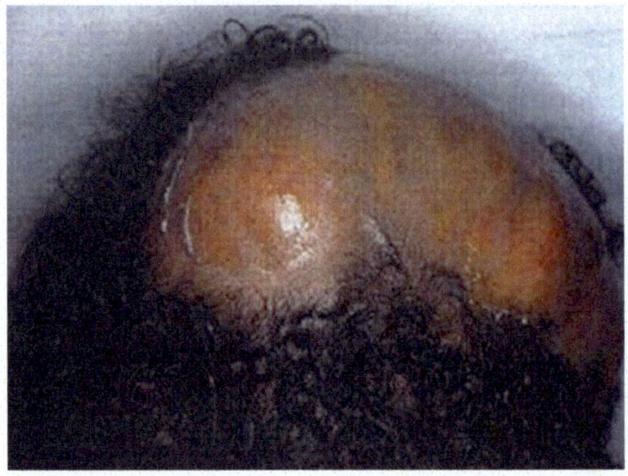

Fig. 2.8 Infant with infected cephalohematoma

Physicians should be aware that caput, cephalohematoma, and SGH are rare but potential sites for infection which may be caused either by direct traumatic scalp lesions (Fig. 2.7) or hematogenous extension [5]. Infected cephalohematoma presents as erythematous, fluctuant, painful mass that may have expanded from its baseline size (Fig. 2.8). Imaging with computed tomography (CT) or magnetic resonance imaging (MRI) may be helpful in making the diagnosis. Untreated infected cephalohematomas and SGH may lead to osteomyelitis, epidural abscess, or subdural empyema, and hence appropriate antibiotic treatment and surgical debridement are necessary when an infection occurs.

The subgaleal area is not limited by sutures, and therefore there are no barriers to prevent extension of bleeding, and hence a massive hemorrhage can quickly occur. The subaponeurotic space can hold up to 260 ml of blood (newborn's estimated blood volume is 80–100 ml/kg). Most subgaleal hemorrhages develop slowly over several hours to days. Mean age at onset of symptoms is 9 h but may occur sooner if hemorrhage is severe. Extracranial swelling with associated tachycardia and pallor should be a concern for blood loss and hypovolemic shock. Early recognition and management of this injury are crucial for good outcomes [6].

Answer: 4

How would you manage this patient?

1. Observation
2. Blood transfusion
3. Normal saline transfusion
4. Skull radiograph
5. Immediate CT/MRI scan

Management differs for each of the extracranial lesion. In cases of caput, the swelling subsides over the next few days, and observation is all that is necessary. In cases of uncomplicated cephalohematomas, no specific treatment is indicated, but anemia and hyperbilirubinemia may be treated as needed. The lesion gets absorbed within 2 weeks to 3 months. If neurologic symptoms develop or concerns regarding the possibility of a depressed skull fracture exist, a CT scan or MRI may be indicated to rule out intracranial pathology [7]. The skull radiographs below (Fig. 2.9a, b) show diffuse soft tissue swelling and do not offer lot of information unless there is underlying skull fracture.

Treatment of SGH includes carefully monitoring for the classic triad of clinical findings including tachycardia, a falling hematocrit, and increasing head circumference in the first 24–48 h after birth. These factors are particularly important in those infants who are considered stable enough to allow admission to the normal newborn nursery [6].

For infants presenting with shock, volume resuscitation is required. This may be achieved with normal saline, packed RBCs, fresh frozen plasma, and coagulation factors (if indicated). Treatment should not be delayed awaiting CT or

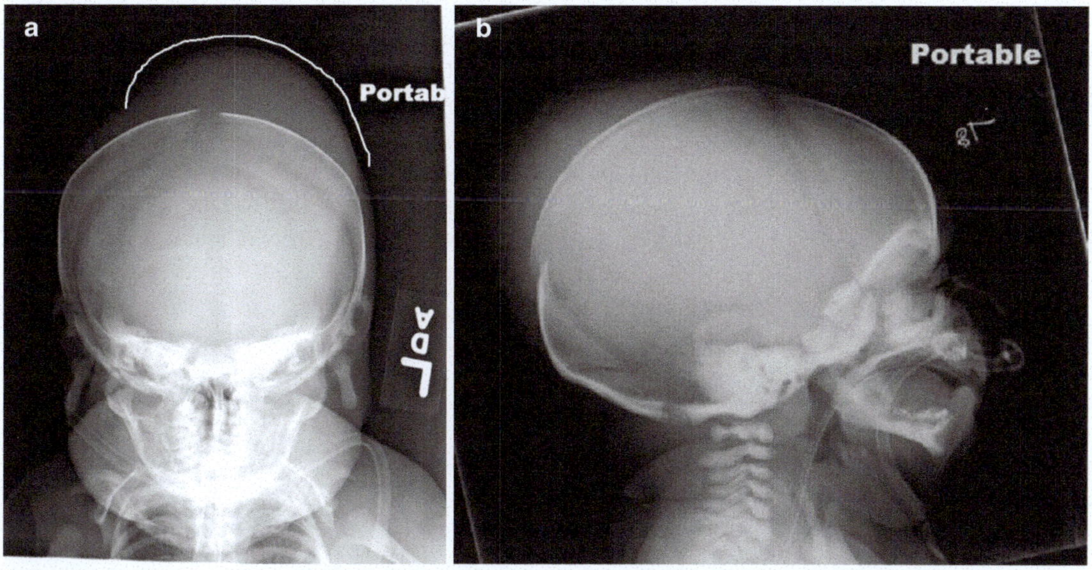

Fig. 2.9 (**a**) AP radiograph of the skull showing diffuse soft tissue swelling of the scalp that crosses sutures and that is especially prominent over the left frontoparietal region. The findings were felt to be most compatible with a subgaleal hematoma. (**b**) Lateral radiographs of the skull demonstrate diffuse soft tissue swelling of the scalp that crosses sutures and that is especially prominent over the left frontoparietal region. The findings were felt to be most compatible with a subgaleal hematoma

MRI confirmation. Stabilization of the infant is the immediate priority. Unrecognized hypovolemic shock can greatly diminish the chances of survival for infant with SGH [6]. This infant was effectively treated with two normal saline boluses and a blood transfusion for hypovolemic shock from blood loss. When discharged careful follow-up is necessary.

Answers: 2 and 3

What are some of the long-term complications you may observe during follow-up in this infant?

1. Alopecia
2. Calcification

Rarely in infants with caput succedaneum, a non-scarring distinct pattern of annular hair loss, commonly referred to as halo scalp ring, has been reported [8]. This is thought to be due to prolonged pressure on the scalp by the cervical os during or before the delivery.

Cephalohematoma may become calcified and cause bony deformities of the skull [9]. Persistent calcification that is not resolved by 6 months may need surgical excision.

Alopecia and calcification need to be evaluated during follow-up and may not be apparent during discharge from nursery.

Answers: 1 and 2

The above case presentations and questions provide information on various aspects of neonatal extracranial hemorrhage. Their distinguishing features are summarized in Table 2.1 below. (Table 2.1).

Case Presentation

A nurse from normal nursery calls you because she noted a large depression over the right parietal bone in a 4-h-old 3500 g infant born to a primiparous woman following a vertex vaginal delivery at 37 weeks of estimated GA. The obstetric history is significant for prolonged labor. The delivery was assisted with midforceps and vacuum extraction. Physical examination is remarkable for a 4 × 5 cm depression of the skull in the right temporoparietal region and a full anterior fontanelle. Neurological examination was normal.

At this time, you:

1. Order skull radiograph
2. Order ultrasound of the head
3. Order CT scan

Physical exam in this infant is consistent with depressed skull fracture. Depressed fractures are visible, palpable indentations in the smooth contour of the skull, like dents in a Ping-Pong ball. Depressed skull fractures are due to the inward buckling of the skull bones and are often associated with forceps-assisted deliveries. While the diagnosis is made by a plain radiograph of the head (Fig. 2.10), imaging with CT (Fig. 2.11) is required to determine the presence or absence of bone fragments in the cerebrum or associated intracranial injury [10, 11].

Linear skull fractures usually affect the parietal bones. They often are associated with cephalohematomas (Fig. 2.12). Linear skull fractures

Table 2.1 Distinguishing features of neonatal extracranial hemorrhage

Features	Caput succedaneum	Cephalohematoma	SGH
Location	At point of presentation, crosses suture lines	Over parietal bones Limited by sutures	Beneath epicranial aponeurosis Extends from orbit to nape of the neck
Findings	Vaguely demarcated Pitting edema	Distinct margins Initially firm Fluctuant after 48 h	Firm to fluctuant Crepitus, fluid waves
Timing	Max size at birth Resolves 48–72 h	Increases after birth for 12–24 h Resolves 2–3 weeks	Increases after birth, resolves 2–3 weeks
Blood loss	Minimal	Rarely severe	May be massive
Complications	Alopecia	Anemia, jaundice, infection, calcification	Hypovolemic shock, anemia, jaundice, infection

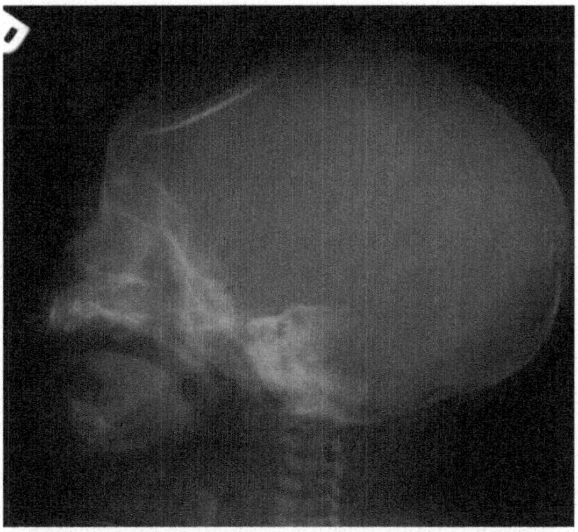

Fig. 2.10 Lateral skull radiograph showing the right parietal depressed skull fracture

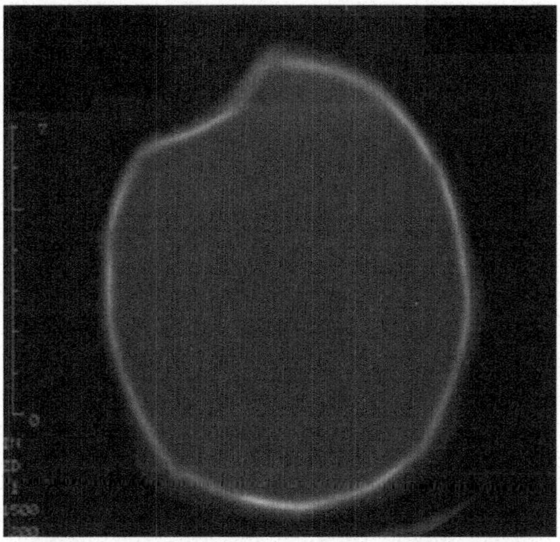

Fig. 2.11 CT of the infant with depressed skull fracture

are clinically not apparent and require no treatment [6, 10, 11].

Answers: 1 and 3

How would you manage the infant in this case?

1. Neurosurgical consultation
2. Observation only

Management depends on presence or absence of neurologic sequelae. Neurologic findings

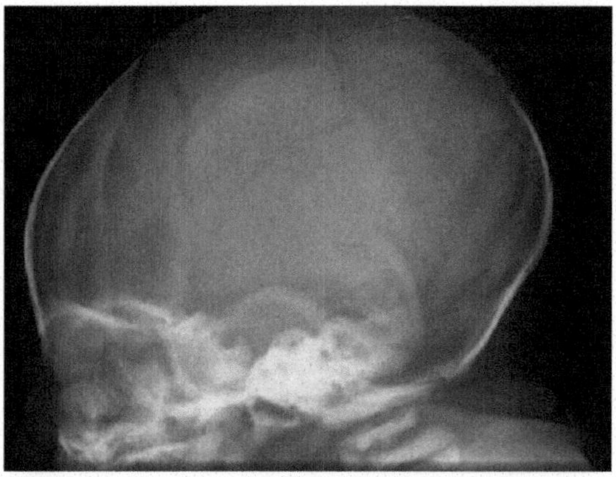

Fig. 2.12 Skull X-ray lateral view of infant with linear skull fracture (arrows)

due to skull fractures in infants born via normal spontaneous vaginal delivery are rare. These cases resolve spontaneously as in this case. Neurosurgical consultation was obtained, but no intervention was done as baby had no neurologic symptoms. Fracture reduction is done when the depth of buckling is more than 1 cm or baby has neurologic signs [6, 10, 11]. Parental reassurance and repeat skull radiographs for follow-up were done in this case.

Rarely, in an infant with linear skull fracture, a leptomeningeal cyst from a dural tear may occur [12]. Abnormally rapid head growth should raise suspicion for a leptomeningeal cyst in baby who had linear skull fracture. Infants with leptomeningeal cyst need to be referred to neurosurgery.

In this case neurosurgical consultation was obtained, and infant was observed closely for neurologic sequelae.

Answer: 1

Case Presentation

You are asked to evaluate a term male newborn with asymmetric facial movements when crying. The neonate was born to a 35-year-old, G1p0 mother with a birth weight of 3700 g and an Apgar score of 8/9 at 1 and 5 min. respectively. Baby was delivered vaginally after a prolonged

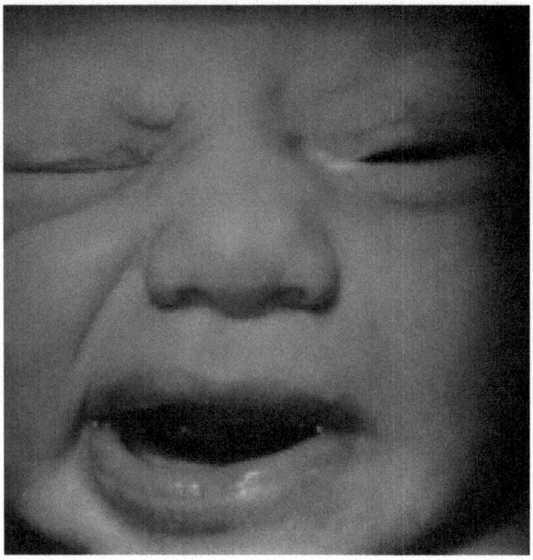

Fig. 2.13 Infant with left facial nerve palsy. (Adapted from Physical assessment of the newborn: a comprehensive approach to the art of physical examination, fifth edition, chapter 5. Springer Publishing Company)

labor. At birth, the infant was noted to have left palpebral fissure wider than the right and absence of nasolabial fold on the left side. You notice that when the infant cries there is deviation of angle of mouth to right and the left eye did not close completely. There is no forehead wrinkling and complete absence of facial movements on the left side (Fig. 2.13).

You examine the baby and conclude he has:

1. Right central facial palsy
2. Left central facial palsy
3. Right peripheral facial palsy
4. Left peripheral facial palsy

Peripheral facial nerve damage produces total facial paralysis on the involved side of the face. A central lesion will affect only the lower half of the face due to the fact that the corticobulbar fibers to the forehead and upper half of the face are distributed bilaterally. This patient has no movement of the forehead or periorbital eye muscles on the left. In addition there is flattening of the left palpebral fissure and movement of the mouth to the right (which may seem to be a drooping of the right side of the mouth). The entire left side of the face is involved, and so this baby has a left peripheral facial nerve palsy.

Answer: 4

At this time, you would:

1. Call a neurologist
2. Transfer the baby to neonatal intensive care unit

There is no emergency to call a neurologist. Congenital facial nerve paralysis should be differentiated from traumatic facial nerve paralysis as early as possible as this determines the course of the disease process and treatment plan, and therefore transfer of the baby to the NICU would be appropriate.

Answer: 2

How would you manage this patient?

1. Attention to eye care
2. Attention to feeding
3. Consult an ophthalmologist

Immediate medical treatment of facial paralysis requires attention to eye care. Infant should be managed with artificial tears to prevent dryness of the affected eye and eye padding to protect corneas [2].

This infant roomed in with the mother. Artificial tears and eye padding was provided to protect the eye from corneal abrasions. Baby was observed for feeding difficulties, as the ability to suck may be impaired due to inability to contract the lower facial muscles on the affected side. Infant was discharged on day 3 of life with significant improvement in facial nerve weakness. Parents were informed about this benign self-limiting condition and need for adequate eye care. Infant gradually improved in the follow-up clinic.

Answers: 1 and 2

Case Presentation

You are evaluating a 4200 g newborn infant with decreased movement of the right arm. The mother is 35 years old, G2P1, and her perinatal history includes difficult prolonged labor, shoulder dystocia, vertex presentation, vacuum extraction, and traction on the neck during delivery. Physical examination of the right arm revealed an adducted shoulder, internally rotated upper arm, extended elbow, pronated forearm, and flexed wrist. The infant had mild respiratory distress.

At this time, most likely cause for the decreased movement of the right arm is:

1. Erb's palsy
2. Klumpke's palsy
3. Pseudoparalysis from clavicle fractures
4. Pseudoparalysis from humerus fractures
5. Phrenic nerve palsy

When an infant is born with brachial plexus palsy (BPP), the condition generally is apparent from birth. Physical finding of the arm hanging limply from the shoulder is typical for BPP. In a common scenario as described in this case, the baby is large for gestational age and is the product of a difficult delivery to a multiparous woman, requiring the use of vacuum or forceps [13].

Clinical presentation of BPP can be classified according to the site of the nerve injury. Injury to the upper trunk involves nerve roots (C5–C6), middle trunk (C7), and lower trunk (C8–T1). Total BPP affects nerves at all levels (C5–T1).

Erb-Duchenne Palsy refers to an injury of the upper brachial plexus nerve roots (C5, C6, and C7) leading to loss of motion around the shoulder and ability to flex the elbow. Isolated lesion of upper trunk (C5–C6) is known as Erb's palsy. Infants with Erb's palsy classically have a "waiter's tip" limb posture characterized by adduction and internal rotation of the affected arm with extended elbow, pronated forearm and flexed wrist (Fig. 2.14).

Klumpke's palsy refers to an injury of the lower brachial plexus nerve roots (C8–T1). The infant with Klumpke's palsy holds the arm supinated, with the elbow bent and the wrist extended, often described as "beggar's hand" [14].

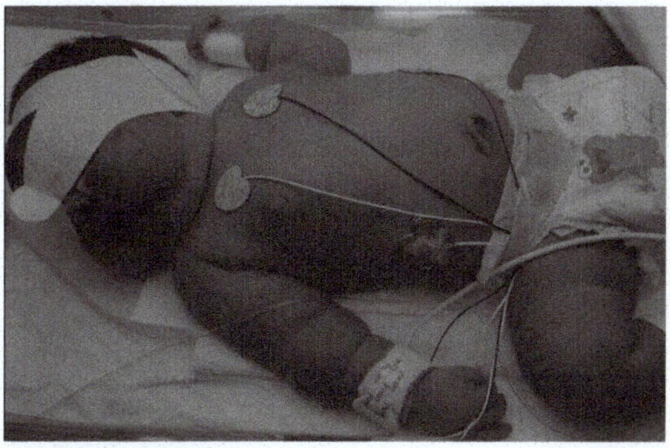

Fig. 2.14 Infant with right-sided upper plexus injury (Erb's palsy)

The infant with complete BPP (C5–T1) typically lies with the arm held limply at his/her side. In infants with Klumpke's palsy and total plexus lesions (C5–T1), careful examination of the child's eye should be performed for presence of Horner's syndrome (i.e., miosis, ptosis, anhidrosis), which suggests injury to the stellate ganglion.

The Moro, grasp, asymmetric tonic neck, and biceps reflexes should be evaluated, and any sensory loss in corresponding dermatomes should be noted. Deep tendon reflexes (DTRs) in the affected arm are absent, and the Moro response is asymmetrical, with no active abduction of the ipsilateral arm.

Injury to phrenic nerve with ipsilateral diaphragmatic paralysis should be considered in a newborn with BPP that has tachypnea and requires oxygen. Diagnosis of phrenic nerve injury is made by a chest radiograph (Fig. 2.15), which shows elevated diaphragm on the affected side. Real-time ultrasonography at the bedside can reveal abnormal motion of the affected hemidiaphragm and confirm the diagnosis [15]. Infant with phrenic nerve injury may require continuous positive airway pressure (CPAP) or mechanical ventilation and may even need surgical plication of diaphragm.

The most common symptom associated with a clavicle fracture in a newborn is fussiness or crying with movement of the affected arm due to pain in the clavicle. Decreased movements of the

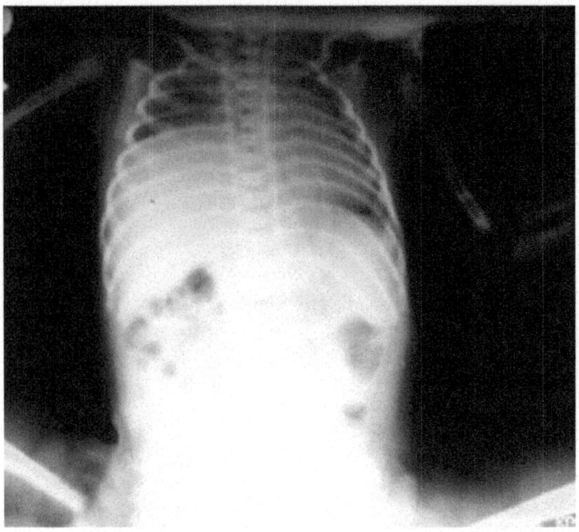

Fig. 2.15 CXR of infant with elevated right hemidiaphragm from phrenic nerve injury. (Reproduced with unrestricted permit from J Pediatr Neurosci. 2012 Sep–Dec; 7(3): 225–227)

affected upper limb due to pain (pseudoparalysis) and asymmetric Moro reflex is the most common indicator of the injury. This can be differentiated from BPP, because tendon reflexes remain intact following isolated clavicular fractures.

Infants with humeral fractures (Fig. 2.16) also present with decreased movement of the affected arm, decreased Moro reflex, localized swelling and crepitation, and an increased pain response with palpation and movement of the arm. Any infant with a humeral fracture should be evaluated for brachial plexus injury, as this is a common associated finding.

The infant in the vignette was diagnosed to have Erb's palsy. On physical examination, it was noted that baby was fussy and cried with movement of the affected limb. There was crepitus and swelling over the right clavicle as well.

Answers: 1 and 3

At this time, you look for:

1. Fracture or injury to the humerus
2. Fracture of the clavicle

The clavicle is the most commonly fractured bone in the neonate. Although, fractured clavicles are often associated with difficult vaginal delivery, they also occur in infants who are products of a normal spontaneous vaginal or cesarean delivery.

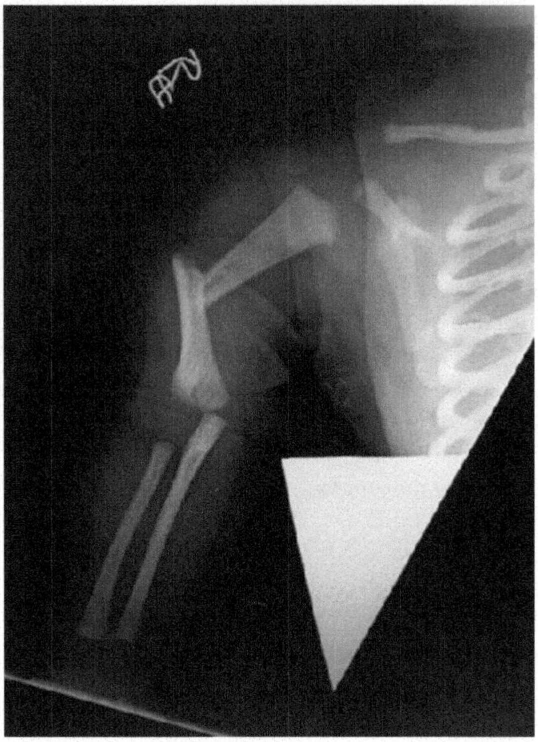

Fig. 2.16 Radiograph showing mid-shaft diaphyseal oblique fracture of right humerus

Clavicle fractures should be considered in any infant with BPP or infant presenting with decreased upper extremity movement. Infants with a clavicle fracture may be asymptomatic or be crying with passive movements of the affected extremity. Presence of crepitation, swelling, palpable bony irregularity, and/or bruising over the affected clavicle may be present in some infants.

Displaced fracture of the clavicle (Fig. 2.17) is accompanied by physical findings mentioned above in the immediate post-delivery period, whereas nondisplaced clavicle fracture (Fig. 2.18) may remain asymptomatic and diagnosis may be missed or delayed until there is a formation of a visible or palpable callous.

Diagnosis is confirmed with radiography (Fig. 2.17), where a clear fracture is usually readily identified.

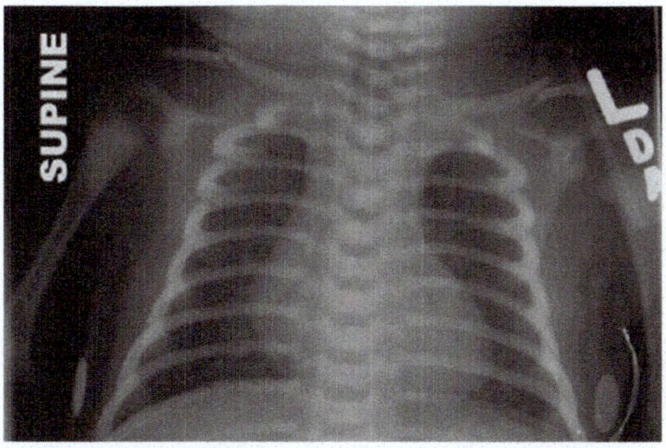

Fig. 2.17 CXR of infant with bilateral displaced clavicle fracture

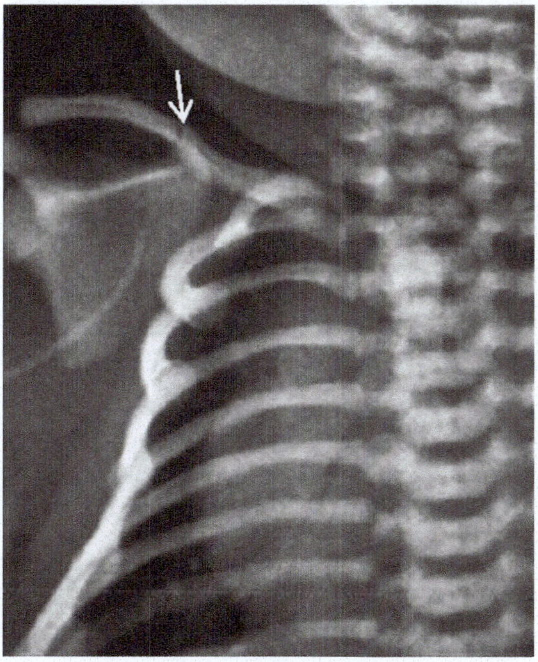

Fig. 2.18 CXR of infant with nondisplaced clavicle fracture (arrow)

Clavicle fractures in infants heal spontaneously with no long-term sequelae. In most cases, especially the asymptomatic ones, parental reassurance and gentle handling are all that are required [6, 10]. Analgesics may be given to decrease the pain. In infants with pseudoparalysis, the affected side can be placed in a long-sleeved garment and pinned to the chest with the elbow at 90 ° of flexion for 2 weeks. In infant with lack of tenderness and callus formation detected on physical examination, a repeat radiograph at 2 weeks of age is not necessary.

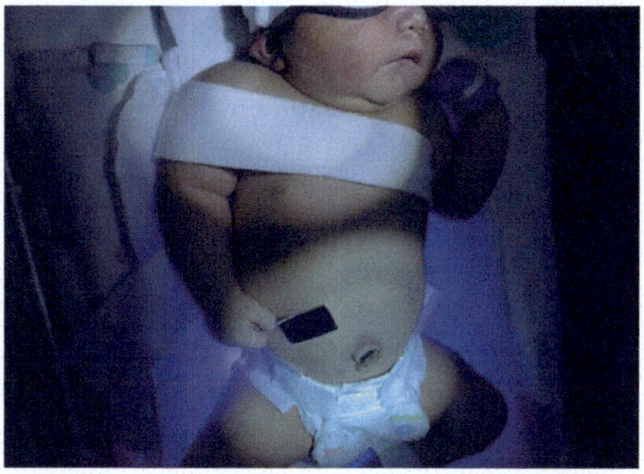

Fig. 2.19 Infant with a sling for right humeral fracture

Humeral fracture is also associated with pain response with palpation and movement of the arm, localized swelling, crepitation, and decreased Moro reflex. The diagnosis is generally made by a plain radiograph of the arm (Fig. 2.16). Because proximal epiphysis in the newborn is entirely cartilaginous, it is radiolucent; thus ultrasound evaluation may be more useful in proximal epiphyseal fracture of the humerus. Immobilization of the affected arm (Fig. 2.19) with the elbow in 90 ° flexion to prevent rotational deformities is the best treatment [6, 10]. Callus formation usually occurs in 7–10 days. A repeat radiograph can be performed at 3–4 weeks post-injury to confirm healing of humeral fracture. Reassurance to the parents that angulation will remodel as the infant grows should be provided.

Infants with decreased upper extremity movement should be evaluated for BPP, clavicle, and humeral fracture, as these lesions sometimes accompany each other.

Answer: 2

How would you manage the brachial plexus injury in this patient?

1. Discharge with follow-up in 1 week
2. MRI with follow-up with neurology
3. Follow-up with referral to physical therapy

Initial management of infant with BPP includes careful evaluation as the diagnosis of BPP is made from clinical findings. Observe the newborn for respiratory distress due to possible diaphragmatic de-innervation from phrenic nerve injury. Evaluate for signs of Horner's syndrome if the diagnosis is Klumpke's palsy. The neurologic examination should include observation of spontaneous movements, passive and active range of motion, stimulated motor and sensory responses, and assessment of Moro, grasp, and asymmetric tonic neck reflexes.

Since spontaneous recovery occurs in almost 90% of patients with Erb's palsy, outpatient follow-up within a week is appropriate. Physical therapy with passive range of motion exercises should be considered if no improvement is noted in 7–10 days.

Neuroimaging with high-resolution MRI can be considered in infants with no improvement. Follow-up with a neurologist is recommended to establish baseline loss of function and to monitor the improvement.

Full, spontaneous recovery is expected for infants showing some improvement within the first 2 weeks; partial recovery can be expected if initial improvement takes 4–6 weeks, and if no improvement is appreciated by 3 months of age, surgery may be attempted to improve the prognosis [16]. Surgical intervention may include nerve reconstruction or the transfer of other nerves to the affected area.

Answer: 1

Case Presentation

You are examining a 48-hour-old baby girl whose parents are anxious to go home. The baby is 8 lb., 6 oz., 38 weeks gestational age. The mother is 30 years old, G2P1. Her obstetric history and pregnancy are uneventful. Due to maternal preference for "natural" child birth, she delivered vaginally despite a breech presentation. On physical examination, you note that her feet are still bruised and she has new findings of erythematous, indurated plaques on her right posterior shoulder (Fig. 2.20) which were not there on her first physical exam soon after birth.

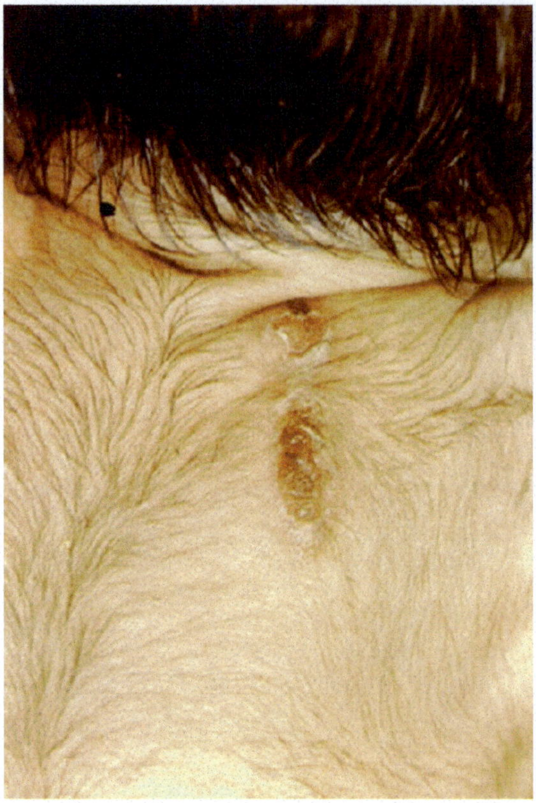

Fig. 2.20 Infant with fat necrosis

At this time you suspect:

1. Congenital melanocytic nevi
2. Superficial streptococcal infection
3. Fat necrosis
4. Café au lait spots

This infant has subcutaneous fat necrosis (SFN) which is a benign condition occurring in the neonatal period, characterized by inflammation and necrosis of subcutaneous fat tissue and typically presenting with subcutaneous purple-bluish hard nodules. Nodules may evolve with subcutaneous calcifications. SFN usually occurs in full-term infants over the trunk, arms, buttocks, thighs, and cheeks as firm, mobile, erythematous nodules and plaques following tissue trauma. The lesions are frequently tender with a taut and shiny skin.

Answer: 3

At this time, you:

1. Discharge the patient with follow-up within 24 h
2. Hold discharge and order selective blood tests

Full sepsis workup is not indicated in absence of risk factors for sepsis. At this time, holding the discharge would be most appropriate pending blood test result.

Answer: 2

How would you manage this case?

1. Draw serum calcium levels.
2. Skin biopsy of the lesion.
3. Start antibiotics pending blood test results.
4. You reassure the parents that it is just a bruise.

SFN is not just a bruise and these babies need blood test and close follow-up. In some infants, liquefied fat may present as fluctuant bullae or extensive calcification within the lesions. SFN may be complicated by hypercalcemia in some infants [17]. Uncomplicated SFN does not require treatment, but occurrence of hypercalcemia does require treatment. All neonates with subcutaneous fat necrosis should have their serum calcium level monitored regularly during the episode and during follow-up. Hypercalcemia usually develops when the subcutaneous fat necrosis begins to resolve, but the onset of hypercalcemia can be delayed several months after the development of skin manifestations which emphasizes the importance of prolonged follow-up.

Babies with hypercalcemia may present with irritability, constipation, poor weight gain, calcification of the kidneys, and, very rarely, heart rhythm disturbance, so treatment of SFN focuses on management of hypercalcemia.

Hypercalcemia may be treated by increased fluid intake, low-calcium milk feeds, furosemide, corticosteroids, and bisphosphonates [18].

In most cases, SFN is a self-limited process; the skin nodules and plaques spontaneously regress within weeks to a few months without cutaneous sequelae although cutaneous scarring and atrophy may occur at sites of involuted lesion. Serum calcium levels were done prior to discharge on this infant.

Answer: 1

How would you manage the bruising on the feet of this baby?

1. Observation only.
2. Do a CBC.
3. Do a coagulation panel.
4. Do bilirubin levels.

Bruising and petechiae may be noted on the presenting parts of the newborn. In this case there is bruising of the feet due to breech presentation. Bruising of the scrotum in frank breech presentation warrants testicular evaluation; similarly bruised eyelids warrant a full eye evaluation. Bruising is usually self-limiting and resolves spontaneously within 1 week, but significant bruising can be a major risk factor for severe hyperbilirubinemia. Observation with reevaluation within 2–3 days of hospital discharge to assess the infant for progressive jaundice is most appropriate in this case.

Answer: 1

Clinical Pearls

1. All newborns born after abnormal fetal presentations require a thorough pediatric examination.
2. Cesarean section does not eliminate the possibility of birth trauma, especially when prior attempts have been made at delivery with vacuum extraction or forceps.
3. The extracranial injuries of caput succedaneum and cephalohematoma usually

resolve spontaneously without any intervention.
4. Subgaleal hemorrhage can result in massive blood loss and, if not detected and managed appropriately, may lead to shock and death.
5. Clinical signs of an extremity fracture include crepitus, pain, swelling, and decreased limb movement.
6. Most clavicular and skull fractures resolve spontaneously and can be managed conservatively with observation alone.
7. CT of the head is indicated for a depressed skull fracture.
8. Upper arm palsy (Erb-Duchenne) caused by damage to the fifth and sixth cervical nerve roots is the most common peripheral nerve injury.
9. It is important to distinguish traumatic facial nerve palsy from congenital hypoplasia of the depressor anguli oris muscle.

References

1. Lyons J, Pressey T, Bartholomew S, Liu S, Liston RM, Joseph KS. Canadian perinatal surveillance system (Public Health Agency of Canada). Delivery of breech presentation at term gestation in Canada, 2003–2011. Obstet Gynecol. 2015;125(5):1153–61.
2. Demissie K, Rhoads GG, Smulian JC, et al. Operative vaginal delivery and neonatal and infant adverse outcomes: population based retrospective analysis. BMJ. 2004;329(7456):24–9.
3. Benaron DA. Subgaleal hematoma causing hypovolemic shock during delivery after failed vacuum extraction: a case report. J Perinatol. 1993;13:228.
4. Rosenberg AA. Traumatic birth injury. NeoReviews. 2003;4(10):e270–6.
5. Miedema CJ, et al. Primarily infected cephalhematoma and osteomyelitis in a newborn. Eur J Med Res. 1999;4:8.
6. Akangire G, Carter B. Birth Injuries in Neonates. Pediatr Rev 2016;37(11):451–462.
7. Mangurten HH, Puppala BL. Birth injuries. In: Fanaroff AA, Martin RJ, Walsh MC, editors. Fanaroff and Martin's neonatal-perinatal medicine, vol. 1. 10th ed. Philadelphia: Elsevier/Saunders; 2015. p. 407–35.
8. Tanzi EL, Hornung RL, Silverberg NB. Halo scalp ring. A case series and review of the literature. Arch Pediatr Adolesc Med. 2002;156(2):188–90. https://doi.org/10.1001/archpedi.156.2.188.
9. Wong CH, Foo CL, Seow WT. Calcified cephalohematoma: classification, indications for surgery and techniques. J Craniofac Surg. 2006;17(5):970–9.
10. Uhing MR. Management of birth injuries. Clin Perinatol. 2005;32(1):19–38.
11. Dupuis O, Silveira R, Dupont C, et al. Comparison of "instrument-associated" and "spontaneous" obstetric depressed skull fractures in a cohort of 68 neonates. Am J Obstet Gynecol. 2005;192(1):165–70.
12. Djientcheu VP, Njamnshi AK, Ongolo-Zolo P, Kobela M, Rilliet B, Essomba A, Sosso MA. Growing skull fractures. Childs Nerv Syst. 2006;22:721–5.
13. Volpe KA, Snowden JM, Cheng YW3, Caughey AB. Risk factors for brachial plexus injury in a large cohort with shoulder dystocia. Arch Gynecol Obstet. 2016;294(5):925–9. Epub 2016 Apr 4.
14. Otto Heise C, et al. Neonatal brachial plexus palsy. Arq Neuropsiquiatr. 2015;73(9):803–8.
15. Murty VSSY, Ram KD. Phrenic nerve palsy: a rare cause of respiratory distress in newborn. J Pediatr Neurosci. 2012;7(3):225–7. https://doi.org/10.4103/1817-1745.106487.
16. Yang LJ. Neonatal brachial plexus palsy – management and prognostic factors. Semin Perinatol. 2014;38(4):222–34.
17. Mahé E, Girszyn N, Hadj-Rabia S, Bodemer C, Hamel-Teillac D, De Prost Y. Subcutaneous fat necrosis of the newborn: a systematic evaluation of risk factors, clinical manifestations, complications and outcome of 16 children. Br J Dermatol. 2007;156(4):709–15.
18. Shumer DE, Thaker V, Taylor GA, Wassner AJ. Severe hypercalcaemia due to subcutaneous fat necrosis: presentation, management and complications. Arch Dis Child Fetal Neonatal Ed. 2014;99(5):F419–21.

3 Visual Diagnosis in the Newborn

David A. Clark

Introduction

Physical findings in the newborn are variable and often subjective. Some important disorders have subtle clinical signs, and some overt signs are inconsequential. This chapter will provide an overview of pertinent newborn physical findings which are apparent to the healthcare provider. The chapter is organized in the same fashion as a physical examination is often performed initially. Head shape and hair pattern and abnormalities of the mouth and neck are the first conditions discussed. Later in the chapter, anomalies of the umbilical cord, abdomen, back, and extremities are presented. As some of the potential material is addressed in other chapters, this chapter will not discuss newborn birth injuries (Chap. 2), dermatological conditions in the newborn (Chap. 4), the late preterm infant (Chap. 5), ambiguous genitalia and problems with sexual differentiation (Chap. 19), and common problems of the newborn eye (Chap. 20).

D. A. Clark, MD
Department of Pediatrics, Albany Medical Center, Albany, NY, USA
e-mail: ClarkD@mail.amc.edu

Case Presentation

You are asked to evaluate a "funny looking baby" born at term gestation last evening. On examination the baby has multiple findings.

Which of the following is associated with significant genetic disease?

1. Unilateral (right hand) simian crease
2. Small preauricular pit
3. Low-set ears without posterior rotation
4. Stalked (extra) digits on each fifth finger
5. None of the above

Although each of the features is determined by various sites of the human genome, none of them signal clinically significant disease. Commonly they are familial and anticipated by parents who often have the same traits. Your next step is to speak with the parents and examine them if necessary. They or their previous children may have the same physical finding, and if they have developed normally, the parents can be reassured that it is very unlikely that their baby has clinically significant disease [1].

Answer: 5

Several basic principles are important to remember in evaluating the baby. There is a broad range of "normal." Attractive parents do not always have attractive children and vice versa.

G. I. Martin, W. Rosenfeld (eds.), *Common Problems in the Newborn Nursery*,
https://doi.org/10.1007/978-3-319-95672-5_3

Abnormal symmetrical features are a hallmark of major syndromes. A child with trisomy 21 does not have unilateral abnormal eye findings. Asymmetric physical traits may be due to a local process (e.g., hemangioma) affecting limb development or due to intrauterine constriction.

There is great variability in size, shape, and position of the ears. The cartilage is soft and an edge of the ear may fold over. As the cartilage stiffens over the next few weeks, the ear will return to the expected shape. Approximately 1% of newborns have a small dimple (pit) in front of the ear. These pits rarely become infected. A low-set ear is defined as an entire ear that is below a straight line drawn from the inner canthus of the eye to the outer canthus and extended posteriorly. Alternatively, a low-set ear may be defined as one that the ear canal is below a line drawn from the outer canthus to the base of the occiput. Most clinicians prefer the former definition as it is easier to measure. Of much greater significance is the posterior rotation of the ear which is associated with many genetic syndromes including trisomies 18 and 13 [1]. Figure 3.1a, b illustrate a low-set ear with posterior rotation. This baby with Goldenhar syndrome also has a smaller anterior duplicate earlobe and an enlarged mouth. A unilateral simian crease is a common finding and of no clinical significance. Bilateral simian hand creases are less common, but in the absence of other physical findings in a baby who is not growth restricted, it is most likely benign.

Stalked (extra) digits on the fifth finger of each hand are a common familial trait. After consulting with the family, they may be removed. If there is a bony attachment, additional digits, or fused digits, the risk of significant genetic disease is increased [2].

Case Presentation

After a brief trial of labor, a primigravid mother is found to have her fetus in a transverse lie. A C-section is performed and she delivers a large for gestational age boy. She is concerned about the shape of his head which seems excessively elongated with a ridge on top (Fig. 3.2).

You tell her which of the following:

1. Large babies always have funny shaped heads.
2. Prolonged labor commonly causes excess molding of the skull.
3. Abnormal fusion of one or more sutures may cause the ridge.
4. Her pelvic structure forced the head into the abnormal shape.

In breech and elective cesarean deliveries where the head has not been engaged in the pel-

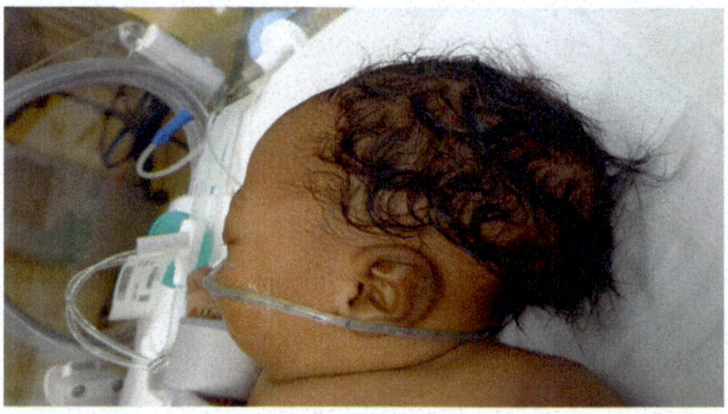

Fig. 3.2 Head elongation

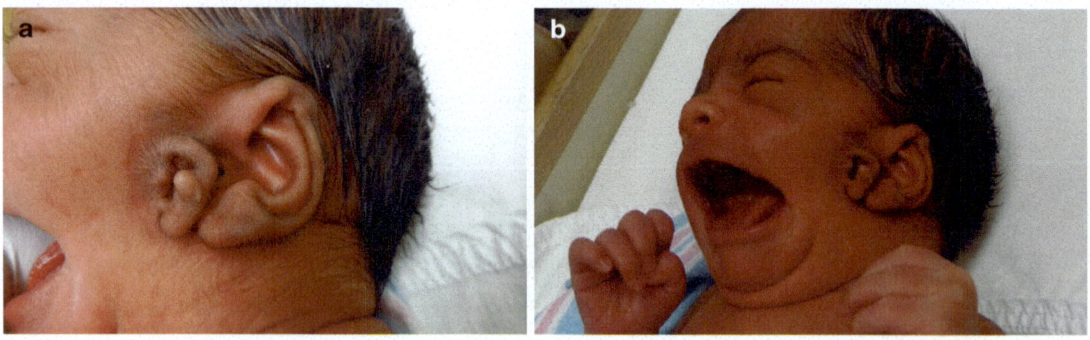

Fig. 3.1 (**a**) Ears. (**b**) Ears and mouth

vis, the newborn's head should be spherical. The shape of a newborn's head should be approximately spherical [3]. Scalp edema is common [4].

At birth and for the first week, the edges of the parietal bones commonly overlap the frontal and occipital bones resulting in small anterior and posterior fontanelles [5]. The bones gradually separate and suture lines and fontanelles should be palpable by the first office visit.

Molding of the head occurs in virtually all term newborns who are born after labor and from a vertex position. The change in shape is more profound in firstborn infants and in babies whose heads were engaged in the pelvis for a prolonged time. The pressure of the pelvic ischial spines on the head during a vertex vaginal delivery causes flattening of the forehead with tapering of the parietal bones to a depressed occiput. In a face or brow presentation, there is a prominent forehead.

The baby, in the case above, has a ridge due to craniosynostosis of the sagittal suture. The head growth will be asymmetric and will be further distorted unless the suture is surgically reopened [6].

Answer: 3

Craniosynostosis results from the premature fusion of one or more cranial sutures. It may be due to a primary defect of ossification [7]. More commonly there is failure of brain growth which allows secondary fusion. The misshapen head results from restricted skull growth based on which sutures have fused. Maternal smoking increases the incidence [8]. Primary craniosynostosis is associated with many syndromes [9].

Variations of fused sutures are:

1. Scaphocephaly (sagittal) – flattened side to side
2. Brachycephaly (bilateral coronal) – flattened front to back
3. Plagiocephaly (anterior-coronal, posterior-lambdoid) – flattened top of the skull
4. Trigonocephaly (metopic) – triangle-shaped skull

Case Presentation

A newborn has light-colored scalp hair over a depigmented area (Fig. 3.3a).

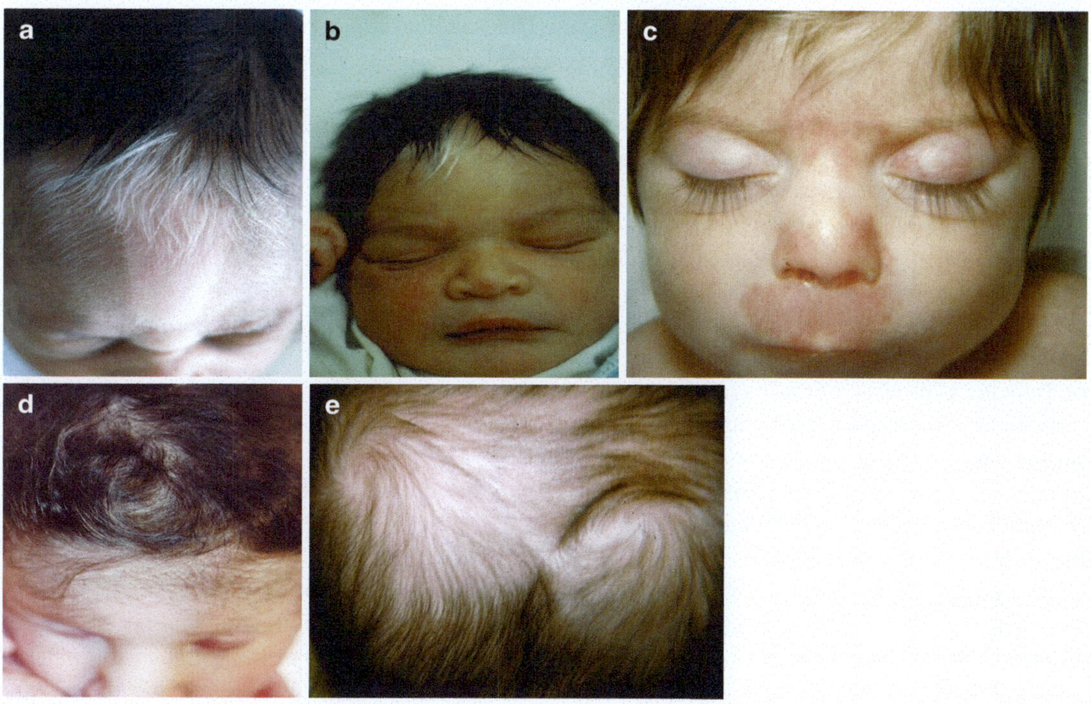

Fig. 3.3 (**a**) Piebaldism. (**b**) Waardenburg syndrome. (**c**) Hypertrichosis, long eyelashes. Cornelia de Lange syndrome. (**d**) Scalp hair anterior. (**e**) Scalp hair – double whorl

He is at greatest risk for:

1. Hearing loss
2. Melanoma
3. Discordant hair growth
4. Childhood alopecia
5. None of the above

Scalp hair is variable in volume, consistency, and pattern. Hair color expresses the pigmentation of the skin beneath it. Hair over a patch of light-pigmented skin will be light also but has no association with answers 1–4 above. Conversely, hair growing over a scalp melanoma will often be darker than surrounding scalp hair.

Answer: 5

A "white" forelock over a patch or normally pigmented skin is a classic sign of Waardenburg syndrome which often has associated progressive hearing loss (Fig. 3.3b). Decreased hair pigmentation is a prominent feature of albinism and untreated phenylketonuria [10].

The scalp hair should be distributed symmetrically with a visible neck, a break in hair between the hair of the scalp and the lateral eyebrow, a break between the eyebrows, and a single posterior hair whorl [11].

A low posterior hairline and short neck are associated with many syndromes including Turner syndrome (45X) fetal hydantoin syndrome, Cornelia de Lange syndrome, and Noonan syndromes. All of them are associated with developmental delay [1].

Hypertrichosis overlying the temple and melding into the eyebrow is a classic sign of both the Treacher Collins and Fraser syndromes.

Synophrys (unibrow) often with a low frontal hairline and luxuriant eyelashes is common in Cornelia de Lange syndrome, trisomy 18, fetal hydantoin syndrome, and Fanconi syndrome (Fig. 3.3c).

The majority of newborns have a single posterior scalp hair whorl. The expected location is posterior with 14% midline, 56% slightly to the left of midline, and 30% to the right of midline. Hair whorls in front of the ears, very lateral on the scalp, and just above the forehead are unusual variants seen in multiple syndromes with developmental delay [11] (Fig. 3.3d).

A double hair whorl is unusual and often familial. In the absence of any family member with a double hair whorl, the hair whorl which is derived from the ectoderm germ layer may be associated with an underlying brain underdevelopment (Fig. 3.3e).

Case Presentation

A mother complains that breastfeeding is painful. You examine the baby's mouth and find a tooth in the midline gum line of the mandible (Fig. 3.4a).

Your first step should be:

1. Consult a pediatric dentist.
2. Obtain an X-ray of the mandible.
3. Extract the tooth yourself.
4. Assure the mother that it will fall out by itself within the next week.

A natal tooth is a rare finding. Approximately 10% are a "false" tooth with no root structure. This calcified cap may be shed and possibly aspirated. The other 90% are normal primary teeth that have erupted early. An X-ray should be obtained to differentiate the two. A dentist should remove the tooth to allow comfortable breastfeeding. If the tooth has a root, it is a primary tooth, and the eruption and spacing of other primary teeth may be affected. It may be associated with various syndromes, including Ellis-van Creveld, Hallermann-Streiff, Pierre Robin, and Sotos [12].

Answer: 2

Other findings in the mouth include:

1. Bohn nodules – Remnants of salivary gland tissue as a result of cystic degeneration. They are found along the lingual and buccal ridges and at the junction of the hard and soft palate. These are <3 mm in size and are filled with keratin and resolve spontaneously (Fig. 3.4b).

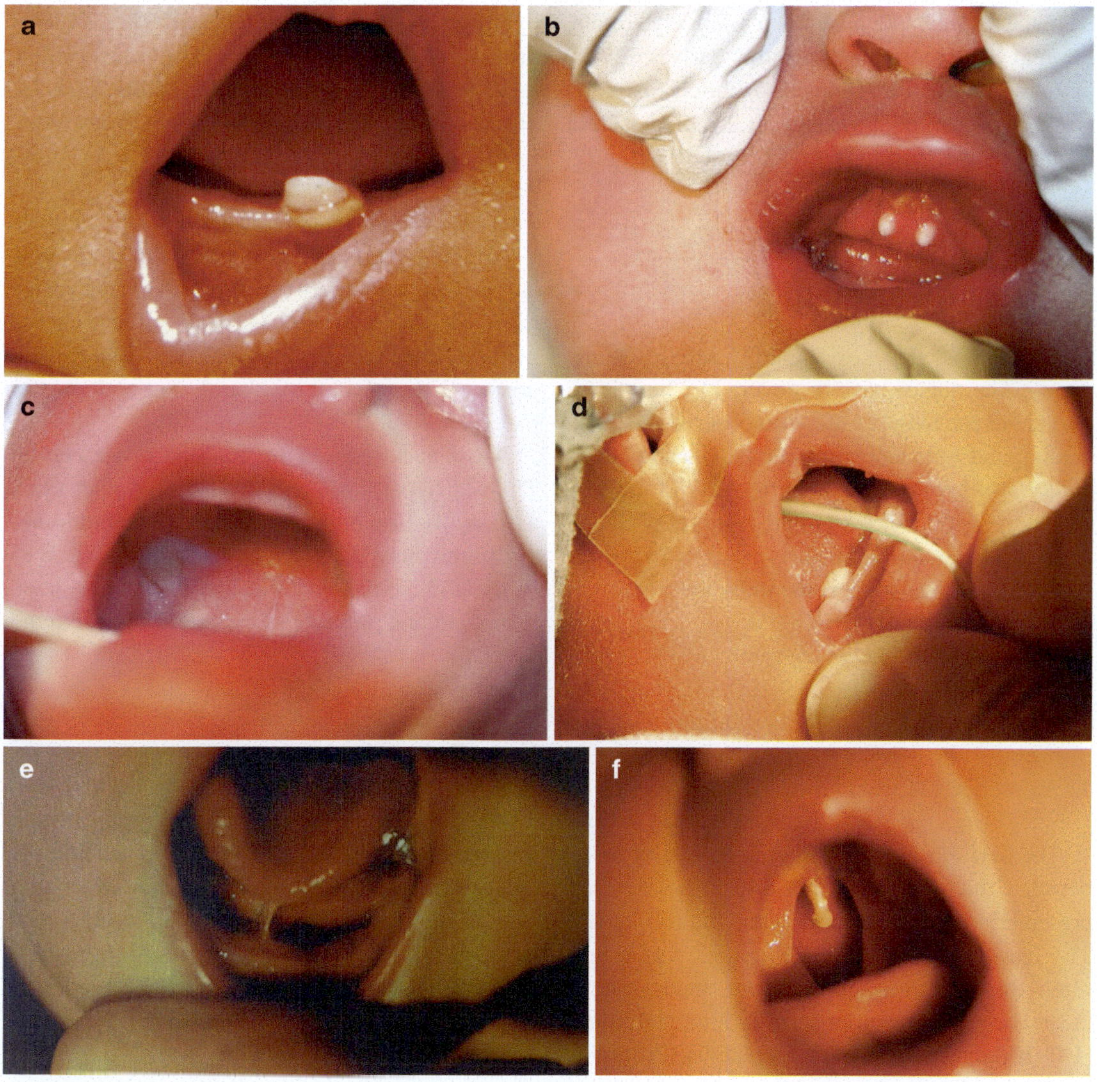

Fig. 3.4 (**a**) Neonatal tooth. (**b**) Bohn nodules. (**c**) Epstein pearls. (**d**) Ranula. (**e**) Ankyloglossia. (**f**) Absent uvula – submucous cleft palate

2. Epstein pearls – Also called gingival cysts, this is a white vesicle (<3 mm) lined with thin epithelium often on the center of the palate. They resolve spontaneously (Fig. 3.4c).
3. Ranula – Mucous retention cysts (mucoceles) on the floor of the mouth. They can be simple or more complex. These are usually disorders of the salivary glands. Surgical removal or marsupialization is sometimes required (Fig. 3.4d).
4. Tongue-tie (ankyloglossia) – Is a congenital oral anomaly where there is usually a short lingual frenulum connecting the underside of the tongue to the floor of the mouth. These almost always stretch soon after birth. Feeding difficulties are variable and there have been reports of elocution defects later on in childhood. Surgical intervention is may be warranted (Fig. 3.4e).
5. Uvula – A projection from the posterior end of the soft palate is composed of connective tissue, glandular tissue and some muscle fibers. It occasionally is bifurcated (bifid) especially if a cleft palate is present. A uvula may also be absent. Swallowing and feeding should be observed carefully (Fig. 3.4f).

In the vicinity, the nose has a relatively simple external structure which in the early embryo fuses in the midline. Delayed or failed fusion is rarely limited to the nose and often includes cleft lip and palate, common features of trisomy 13 Syndrome.

Case Presentation

A term newborn is reportedly breastfeeding poorly. The nurses have discovered a "lump" on the side of the baby's neck. You observe the baby feeding and note tachypnea as well as some difficulty swallowing. The neck mass is in the lateral neck, is soft and fluid filled, and is non-tender with a bluish hue (Fig. 3.5).

These findings suggest the mass is:

1. A thyroglossal duct cyst
2. A thyroid mass
3. A pneumomediastinum herniating into the neck
4. A cyst derived from lymphoid tissue

The first three clinical findings are midline or between the sternocleidomastoid muscles. This presentation is classic for a cystic malformation. The mass is derived from lymphoid tissue and often dissects into the posterior mediastinum [13]. The most common form is lymphangioma [14]. It may compress the esophagus (difficulty swallowing) and encompass the trachea resulting in a limited airway and tachypnea [15]. A cystic hygroma may be associated with Turner syndrome or Noonan syndrome. The more prominent masses are often discovered by prenatal ultrasonography.

Answer: 4

The treatment options currently include surgical resection, but there is a small chance of recurrence [16]. If the baby is stable, other options include sclerosing agents such as bleomycin, doxycycline, ethanol, picibanil, and sodium tetradecyl sulfate [17–19].

Most neck masses are midline or nearly so. Thyroid hyperplasia and thyroglossal duct cysts are usually firm and are very rare. A pneumomediastinum may dissect into the midline neck or further. These babies are usually very sick given the extent and pressure of the mediastinum in the chest.

Case Presentation

You attend the delivery of a poorly controlled diabetic who is delivered by C-section at 38 -week gestation due to fetal macrosomia and poor fetal heart rate reactivity. There was spontaneous rupture of the membranes 26 h prior to delivery. The baby boy weighs 4.4 kg, is covered with vernix (Fig. 3.6), and although initially depressed responds well to tactile stimulation and drying. Resuscitation is not necessary.

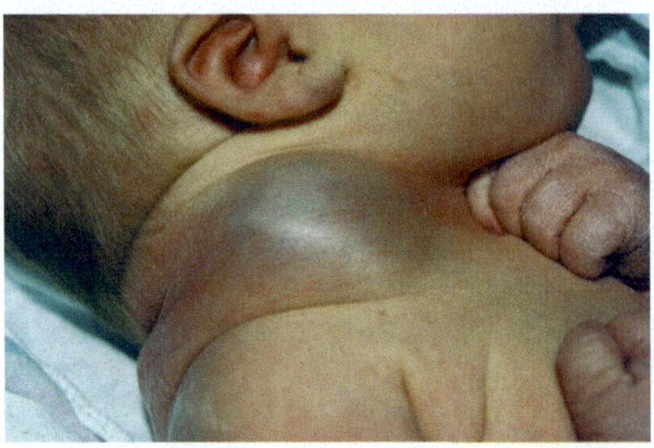

Fig. 3.5 Cystic hygroma

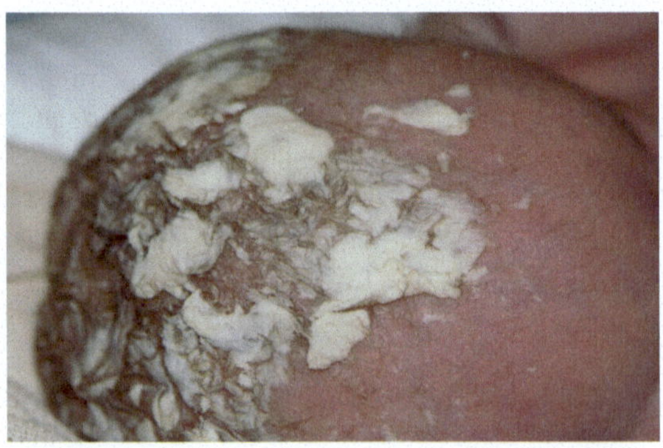

Fig. 3.6 Vernix

He is at greatest risk for which of the following?

1. Neonatal diabetes
2. Surfactant deficiency
3. Sepsis
4. Malrotation of the intestines
5. None of the above

Neonatal diabetes is a rare condition and the neonates are severely growth retarded. Some of the components of vernix are antibacterial, and there is no association with excess vernix and sepsis or intestinal malrotation.

This large for gestational age baby is at risk for numerous metabolic problems including hypoglycemia and hypocalcemia. The excess fetal growth is due to fetal hyperglycemia provoking an excess of fetal insulin, which stimulates somatic growth. At birth the baby's transplacental glucose source abruptly stops and the insulin provokes the hypoglycemia.

Answer: 2

The primary component of vernix is:

1. Water
2. Carbohydrates
3. Complex lipids
4. Proteins

The excess vernix is associated with surfactant deficiency. Vernix caseosa is a complex biofilm that protects the developing fetal skin from the changing composition of the amniotic fluid. It is a biofilm composed of water (81%), lipid (9%), and proteins (10%). It includes shed periderm and sebaceous secretions [20]. Lipids include cholesterol, ceramides, triglycerides, phospholipids, and sterol esters. There are 41 different proteins in vernix; 25 are unique and found nowhere else in the body. Some of these proteins are anti-infectious – defensins, lactoferrin, calprotectin, lysozyme, and neutrophil lipocalin to name a few. It begins to shed at ~34-week gestation in response to increasing surfactant shed from maturing fetal lung into the amniotic fluid [21]. Amniotic fluid aspirated at term produces more lung inflammation because of the lipids originating from the vernix.

Answer: 1

LGA babies born to diabetic mothers are at increased risk for malformations, primarily cardiac, central nervous system, limb anomalies, intestinal obstruction, and situs inversus, not malrotation of the intestines.

Case Presentation

A 1-week-old baby girl born at term returns to your office at 21 days with a persistent umbilical cord (Fig. 3.7).

The most appropriate treatment is:

1. Exploration and then excision with a sterile scalpel
2. Cautery with silver nitrate
3. Referral for evaluation by a surgeon
4. Oral antibiotics

A persistent cord commonly has a blood supply. A surgeon may need to explore it for an intra-abdominal component. The umbilical cord is composed of a glycoprotein matrix (Wharton's

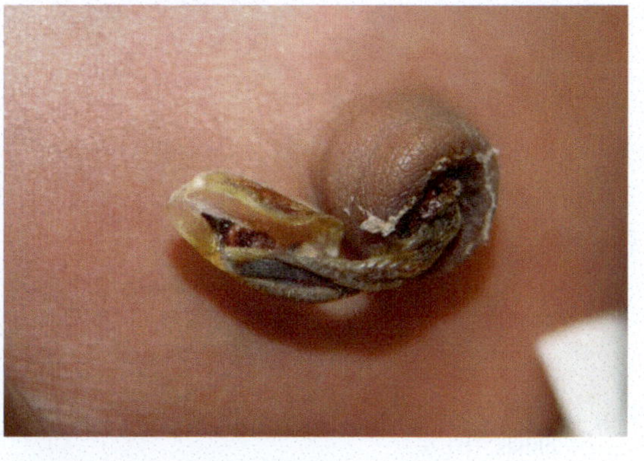

Fig. 3.7 Delayed cord shedding – 16 days

jelly) suspended in 90% water. There are three vessels, a vein and two arteries arising from each of the iliac arteries. The arteries coil around the vein in a counterclockwise rotation thought to be derived from the rotation of the bowel entering the abdomen from the coelomic cavity. Lack of rotation may be associated with malrotation of the intestines.

The cord dries rapidly in less than 4 days and is colonized with bacteria which attract neutrophils which in turn release chemokines (e.g. lysozyme) cleaving the dried cord by 8–10 days [22]. Neutropenia, leukocyte adhesion deficiency, and interleukin kinase deficiency are possibilities. Failure of neutrophils to respond and therefore a persistent cord is a prominent feature of a very rare x-linked syndrome exclusive to males and not pertinent to this female baby. Enthusiastic cleansing of the cord with alcohol delays colonization and thwarts ingress of neutrophils, delaying the shedding of the dried cord. Almost all other persistent cords are due to a continued blood supply. Surgical exploration has found peritoneum, omphalocele with or without intestine, a patent urachus, a urachal cyst, hemangiomas, AV malformation, and redundant skin [23].

Answer: 3

Case Presentation

A full-term infant is born to a mother with no prenatal care. Labor is protracted and a cesarean section is performed. At delivery, the healthcare providers note shiny intestines to the right of the umbilicus. There is no covering membrane over the intestines.

The above scenario is most compatible with:

1. Gastroschisis
2. Omphalocele

Major abdominal defects are often discovered prenatally. A gastroschisis is an abdominal wall defect almost always positioned to the right of but not involving the umbilical cord. The intestine is exposed to amniotic fluid which beyond 34-week gestation contains solubilized vernix and other compounds which induce intestinal adhesions and serosal inflammation. Although both defects are managed by similar surgical repairs, the inflamed intestine of a baby with a gastroschisis (Fig. 3.8a) is more likely to have motility problems.

An omphalocele results from a failure of the midgut to return from the yolk sac to the abdomen. It involves the umbilical cord and is usually enclosed in a sack protecting the bowel from

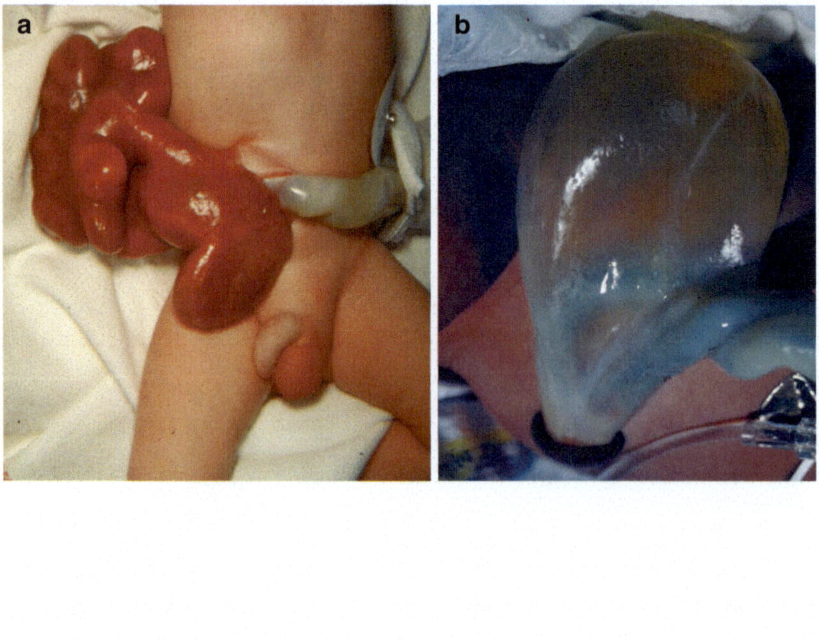

Fig. 3.8 (**a**) Gastroschisis. (**b**) Omphalocele

exposure to amniotic fluid (Fig. 3.8b). They are commonly associated with genetic defects especially the trisomy syndromes [1].

Case Presentation

Shortly after entering the room to examine a baby boy in the presence of his mother, she removes the baby's sock from the right foot. The mother asks "where is my baby's right great toe" (Fig. 3.9)?

Which is your most appropriate response?

1. It is a common variation of development of the foot.
2. It is an inherited congenital anomaly.
3. It was accidentally removed during delivery by C-section.
4. It was amputated by an amniotic band.

Most anomalies of limbs associated with syndromes are bilateral [24]. Numerous syndromes have focused on specific chromosomal or gene abnormalities that have associated limb defects. The anomalies include arachnodactyly, fractures, short limbs, limb reduction, brachydactyly, clinodactyly of the fifth finger, thumb hypoplasia or a triphalangeal thumb, radius aplasia, metacarpal and metatarsal hypoplasia, polydactyly, syndactyly, elbow dysplasia, and patella dysplasia. Newborns with any of these limb anomalies often have other physical findings that should trigger a genetic evaluation for the myriad of autosomal recessive disorders.

Small strips of amnion may project into the amniotic fluid especially with oligohydramnios. They wrap around rapidly growing small body parts, primarily limbs, and constrict blood flow. Deformities, unusual fusions, and less commonly amputations occur.

Answer: 4

Case Presentation

A newborn has multiple areas of darker pigmentation in a line below the normal nipple and extending into the axilla on both sides (Fig. 3.10).

You council the mother that:

1. They are normal variants.
2. They will fade over time.
3. All but the normally located nipple need to be surgically removed.
4. Only the axillary accessory nipples may need to be removed.

Supernumerary nipples may be found up to seven pairs. They result from the incomplete regression of the embryonic mammary ridge (milk line). The true nipples are usually normal. The distal nipples are progressively less pigmented and rarely have underlying tissue [25].

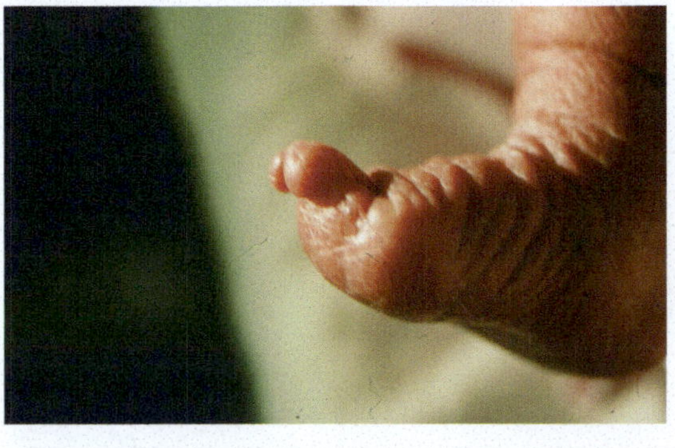

Fig. 3.9 Absent great toe, amniotic band

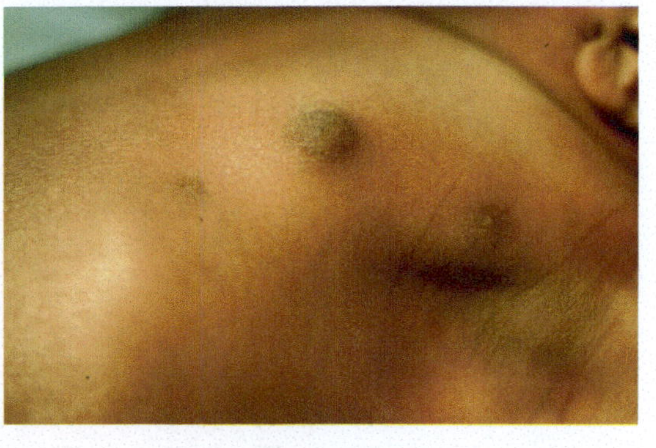

Fig. 3.10 Supernumerary nipples

There is a very rare association with various kidney and urinary tract malformations [26]. The axillary nipples tend to be more pigmented and often have breast tissue. This tissue may hypertrophy at puberty and may produce small amounts of milk postpartum. Given the sheltered location and excess heat, there is malignant potential. For these reasons, early surgical removal of axillary accessory nipples may be appropriate.

Case Presentation

A nurse in the regular nursery notes a "bump" on a baby's back when changing a diaper.

You examine the baby and find a midline closed skin-covered lesion in the lumbosacral region (Fig. 3.11a).

What is the most appropriate next step?

1. MRI/CT scan of the lower back
2. Neurosurgery consultation
3. Pediatric oncology consultation
4. Initiate antibiotics

Midline defects on the back, especially in the lumbar region, almost always involve a defect in the spine and often a significant defect of the spinal cord [27]. Neural tube defects are commonly affecting approximately 1500 babies each year in the United States. This incidence has decreased in the last 15 years due to supplemental folate administered to pregnant women especially prenatally and in the early first trimester [28, 29]. Although neural tube defects include anencephaly, encephalocele, and other anomalies of the head, this discussion will be limited to lesions of the lower back.

This case is a common presentation for a sacrococcygeal teratoma. It must be differentiated from a neural tube defect by proper imaging.

Answer: 1

Some defects are exposed to the level of nerve tissue. Others have minimal covering. Nearly all have a significant risk of infection. Careful sterile technique should allow protection of the defect and allow prompt imaging (MRI, CT) to determine the extent of the defect. A pediatric neurologist and pediatric neurosurgeon should be consulted promptly. All of the defects of the lower back have a high prevalence of lower extremity motor dysfunction, commonly with bladder and anal dysfunction in addition.

The variations include:

1. Spina bifida – spinal dysraphism, usually without neurologic sequelae
2. Meningoschisis – Exposed nerve tissue.
3. Meningocele – Spinal cord with a fluid-filled cover.
4. Meningomyelocele – The fluid filled sac contains nerve tissue.
5. Lipomeningomyelocele – Fat tissue is included in the defect.
6. Hemangio-meningocoele – Nerve tissue embedded in a midline hemangioma.

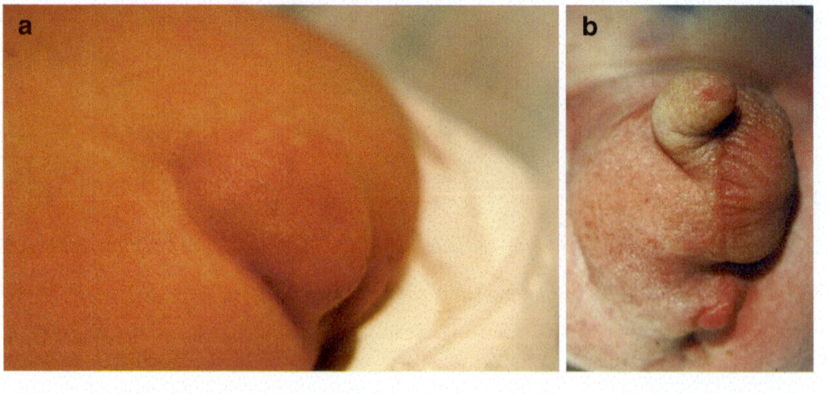

Fig. 3.11 (**a**) SC teratoma. (**b**) Anterior sacrococcygeal teratoma

A sacrococcygeal teratoma (Fig. 3.11b) is a unique tumor of the lower lumbar-sacral spine and coccyx which contains a mixture of tissue from all three embryonic germ lines. Rarely the tumor can be anterior filling the pelvis and extending into the gonads. This tumor may be massive and lethal and is often very difficult to resect.

Clinical Pearls

1. Any abnormal physical finding may be familial. Examine the parents.
2. Symmetrical abnormalities are more commonly associated with a significant genetic abnormality; e.g., a unilateral simian palm crease is common and not associated with serious genetic disease.
3. Although low-set ears may be clinically significant, if the ears are also posteriorly rotated, a syndrome is likely.
4. Vernix is a very complex lipid and protein biofilm that protects the fetal skin from the changing composition of amniotic fluid.
5. Increasing amniotic fluid surfactant in the last 6 weeks of gestation facilitates fetal shedding of vernix.
6. Abnormal hair on the head associated with syndromes includes synophrys and more than one scalp whorl.
7. If there is no root on a neonatal tooth, it should be extracted.
8. A dried umbilical cord that has not been shed by 2 weeks almost always has a persistent blood supply and may warrant evaluation by a pediatric surgeon.

References

1. Adams D, Clark DA. Common genetic and epigenetic syndromes. Pediatr Clin N Am. 2015;62(2):422–6.
2. O'Brien, J, Rinehart, T, et al. Glob libr women's med, (ISSN: 1756-2228) 2009; DOI https://doi.org/10.3843/GLOWM.10147.
3. Cunningham ML, Heike CL. Evaluation of the infant with an abnormal skull shape. Curr Opin Pediatr. 2007;19(6):645–51.
4. Furdon SA, Clark DA. Differentiating scalp swelling in the newborn. Adv Neonatal Care. 2001;1(1):22–7.
5. Slater BJ, Lenton KA, Kwan MD, Gupta DM, Wan DC, Longaker MT. Cranial sutures: a brief review. Plastic reconstructive. Surgery. 2008;121(4):170e–8e.
6. Panchal J, Uttchin V. Management of craniosynostosis. Plast Reconstr Surg. 2003;111(6):2032–48.
7. Cohen MM Jr, et al. Craniosynostosis: diagnosis, evaluation, and management. 2nd ed. Oxford: Oxford University Press; 2000. p. 316–53.
8. Honein MA, Rasmussen SA. Further evidence for an association between maternal smoking and craniosynostosis. Teratology. 2000;62(3):145–6.
9. Kimonis V, Gold JA, Hoffman TL, Panchal J, Boyadjiev SA. Genetics of craniosynostosis. Semin Pediatr Neurol. 2007;14(3):150–61.
10. Clark DA. Neonates and infants at risk for hearing and speech disorders. Top Lang Disord. 1989;10(1):1–12.
11. Furdon SA, Clark DA. Scalp hair characteristics in the newborn infant. Adv Neonatal Care. 2003;3(6):286–96.
12. Clark-Gambelunghe M, Clark D. Sensory development. Pediatr Clin N Am. 2015;62(2):367–84.
13. Perkins JA, Manning SC, Tempero RM, Cunningham MJ, Edmonds JL Jr, Hoffer FA, et al. Lymphatic malformations: current cellular and clinical investigations. Otolaryngol Head Neck Surg. 2010;142(6):789–94.
14. de Serres LM, Sie KC, Richardson MA. Lymphatic malformations of the head and neck. A proposal for staging. Arch Otolaryngol Head Neck Surg. 1995;121(5):577–82. http://reference.medscape.com/medline/abstract/7727093.
15. Bloom DC, Perkins JA, Manning SC. Management of lymphatic malformations. Curr Opin Otolaryngol Head Neck Surg. 2004;12(6):500–4.
16. Ozen IO, Moralioglu S, Karabulut R, et al. Surgical treatment of cervicofacial cystic hygromas in children. J Otorhinolaryngol Relat Spec. 2005;67(6):331–4.
17. Giguere CM, Bauman NM, Smith RJ. New treatment options for lymphangioma in infants and children. Ann Otol Rhinol Laryngol. 2002;111(12 Pt 1):1066–75.
18. Acevedo JL, Shah RK, Brietzke SE. Nonsurgical therapies for lymphangiomas: a systematic review. Otolaryngol Head Neck Surg. 2008;138(4):418–24.
19. Impellizzeri P, Romeo C, Borruto FA, Granata F, Scalfari G, De Ponte FS, et al. Sclerotherapy for cervical cystic lymphatic malformations in children. Our experience with computed tomography-guided 98% sterile ethanol insertion and a review of the literature. J Pediatr Surg. 2010;5(12):2473–8.
20. Singh G, Archana G. Unraveling the mystery of vernix caseosa. Indian J Dermatol. 2008;53(2):54–60.
21. Narendran V, Wickett RR, Pickens WL, Hoath SB. Interaction between pulmonary surfactant and vernix: a potential mechanism for induction of amniotic fluid turbidity. Pediatr Res. 2000;48(1):120–4.

22. Clark DA. Wither the umbilical cord. Pediatr Rev. 1995;9(12):1–2.
23. Donlon CR, Furdon SA, Clark DA. Look before you clamp: delivery room examination of the umbilical cord. Adv Neonatal Care. 2002;2(1):19–26.
24. Clark DA, Thompson JE. Atlas of Neonatology. Philadelphia/Pennsylvania: W.B. Saunders Co.; 1999.
25. Mimouni F, Merlob P, Reisner SH. Occurrence of supernumerary nipples in newborns. Am J Dis Child. 1983;137(10):952–3.
26. Grotto I, Browner-Elhanan K, Mimouni D, Varsano I, Cohen HA, Mimouni M. Occurrence of supernumerary nipples in children with kidney and urinary tract malformations. Pediatr Dermatol. 2001;18(4):291–4.
27. National Center on Birth Defects and Developmental Disabilities. Neural tube defects (annual report) (PDF). US Centers for Disease Control and Prevention. 2012.
28. Goh YI, Koren G. Folic acid in pregnancy and fetal outcomes. J Obstet Gynaecol. 2008;28(1):3–13.
29. Li F, Watkins D, Rosenblatt DS. Vitamin B-12 and birth defects. Mol Genet Metab. 2009;98(1–2):166–72.

Common Dermatological Conditions

4

Mercedes E. Gonzalez

Introduction

Newborn Skin

Shortly after birth (and removal of the vernix caseosa), the skin of a full-term neonate is typically soft and smooth. There are a variety of physiologic skin conditions that appear in the first few days to weeks of life that disappear in a short time. For example, desquamation of newborn skin, which appears as fine thin scaling, begins in the first 1–2 days of life and may not be complete until 3 weeks of age. Cutis marmorata, a bluish-purple lacy mottling of the skin, occurs in the first 1–2 days of life and is a reflection of immature temperature regulation in the skin that then normalizes in the first few months of life.

In addition to physiologic skin changes, there are a number of skin eruptions and skin lesions that can be present at birth and are often the source of anxiety and concern for parents. Birthmarks can present as a red, blue, brown-black, or white lesion; they can be flat or raised and hairy or warty and occur as single or multiple lesions or distributed over a segment of the body. Fortunately, regardless of color or shape, the vast majority of congenital skin lesions or "birthmarks" are a benign, isolated finding and parents can be reassured. Similarly, there are several skin eruptions that are common in the first few weeks of life that are benign and self-limited. It is critical to differentiate these benign and self- limited conditions, from those that require further work-up and systemic treatment. The following clinical cases describe several common skin conditions seen in newborns and discuss their appropriate work-up and management.

Case Presentation

The mother of an otherwise healthy 2-day-old boy born via natural spontaneous vaginal delivery, with Apgar scores of 9 and 9 calls for a pediatrician prior to discharge. She is concerned about several scattered pink blotchy macules, papules, and few pustules on his face and trunk as shown (Fig. 4.1). He is otherwise well.

What is the most likely diagnosis?

1. Transient neonatal pustular melanosis
2. Erythema toxicum neonatorum
3. Congenital cutaneous candidiasis
4. Bacterial folliculitis

This case demonstrates a typical presentation of erythema toxicum neonatorum (ETN). ETN is a common, benign, self-limiting skin eruption

M. E. Gonzalez, MD, FAAD
Pediatric Dermatology of Miami, Department of Dermatology, University of Miami Miller School of Medicine, Miami, FL, USA

Herbert Wertheim College of Medicine, Florida International University, Miami, FL, USA

G. I. Martin, W. Rosenfeld (eds.), *Common Problems in the Newborn Nursery*,
https://doi.org/10.1007/978-3-319-95672-5_4

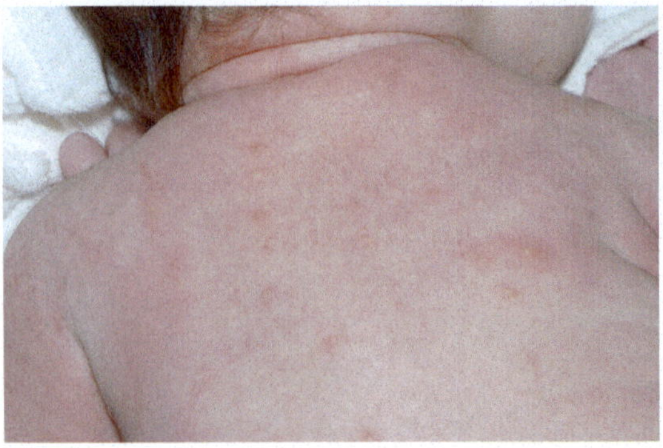

Fig. 4.1 Erythema toxicum neonatorum on the trunk of a newborn. Note the typical pink papules with surrounding erythema

seen in full-term newborns. It is more common in term neonates and is rare in premature babies. Skin lesions usually present at 3–4 days of age but can be seen as early as the first 24 h and up to 10 days of age. Lesions start as splotchy pink macules that evolve to having a central papule or pustule and self-resolve without sequelae. They are typically found on the face, trunk, and extremities with notable sparing of the palms and soles. The diagnosis is usually made clinically and a biopsy is rarely necessary. Table 4.1 [1] shows other diagnoses and helpful clinical and laboratory features for distinguishing between them.

Answer: 2

How would you counsel the parents?

1. Treatment with topical antifungals is required
2. Treatment with topical corticosteroids is required
3. Treatment with topical antibiotics is required
4. No treatment is required

You can reassure parents that although we do not know exactly what causes this eruption, it is a benign, self- limiting condition which heals without sequelae. New crops of lesions can appear for 5–7 days, but each individual lesion resolves in 1–2 days and does not recur. No treatment is required. The presence of this eruption is not linked to future skin disease.

Answer: 4

How can a definitive diagnosis be made?

1. A skin biopsy
2. A potassium hydroxide (KOH) prep
3. A bacterial culture
4. Clinical recognition

The diagnosis is usually made clinically. A Wright's stain [combination of acid dye (red "eosin") and a basic dye (blue "methylene blue")] on a skin scraping would highlight eosinophils, and occasionally there is associated peripheral eosinophilia. A skin biopsy is rarely necessary, however if performed would show a dense infiltrate (usually perifollicular) and subcorneal pustules composed of eosinophils.

Answer: 4

Case Presentation

You stop in to check on a 10-h-old baby whose delivery you attended that morning. On examination, the baby appears well. On the skin you notice scattered superficial pustules without surrounding redness. Some of these pustules have ruptured, leaving a circular rim of scale and/or a peeling edge (collarette). There are also scattered hyperpigmented macules on the face and a few pustules on his palms.

How do you explain this condition to the baby's family?

1. This is an infection that he acquired in utero.
2. This is a non-worrisome condition that will go away on its own.
3. This is an infection that he acquired during delivery.
4. This is the result of trauma during delivery.

Transient neonatal pustular melanosis (TNPM, *syn transient neonatal pustulosis, lentigines neonatorum*) is an idiopathic, benign, self-limiting skin eruption that occurs in 5% of darkly pigmented neonates. It is much less common in Caucasian newborns. Skin lesions are typically

Table 4.1 Differential diagnosis of neonatal vesiculopustular eruptions

Diagnosis	Typical age of onset	Clinical features	Diagnosis/laboratory
Erythema toxicum neonatorum (ETN)	DOL 1–2	Common, ~50% of full-term neonates	Clinical diagnosis; Wright stain (skin and peripheral blood smear): eosinophils; bacterial and viral cultures are negative
		Small papules and pustules surrounded by a flare of erythema	
		Spares palms and soles	
Transient pustular melanosis	Birth	Lesions progress through 3 phases: superficial pustules, collarettes of scale, hyperpigmented macules	Clinical diagnosis; gram stain shows neutrophils, bacterial culture is negative
		Widespread involvement including the palms and soles	
Congenital candidiasis	Birth–6 days	Monomorphic papulovesicles that evolve to pustules typically on face, palms, and soles; can be widespread or only involve the nail	Fungal stain shows pseudohyphae and budding yeast
		Majority present at birth	
Neonatal candidiasis	>1 week	Scaly red patches, papules, satellite pustules	Fungal stain shows pseudohyphae and budding yeast
		Affects diaper area and oral mucosa, intertriginous areas	
Miliaria rubra	1–12 weeks	Monomorphic small pink papules and pustules in areas that are wrapped or heated; or areas covered with thick emollients	Clinical based on appearance and location; when in doubt culture can rule out candida or other infection
Neonatal acne (a.k.a. neonatal cephalic pustulosis)	3–4 weeks	Pink papules and pustules, notably lack of comedones; typically on the face but can extend to scalp, shoulders, and upper back	Clinical diagnosis; potassium hydroxide (KOH) scraping may demonstrate yeast

present at birth and can be found anywhere on the skin but have a predilection for chin, neck, back, and legs. Lesions are often seen on palms and soles. These eruptions evolve through three characteristic phases. In the first phase, variably sized (2–10 mm) superficial pustules with minimal or no surrounding erythema are seen. In the second phase, there are faint hyperpigmented macules with fine collarettes of scale at sites of ruptured pustules. In the third phase, brown hyperpigmented macules, representing post-inflammatory hyperpigmentation, are seen at sites of previous pustules. These light brown macules may persist for months. The first two phases may occur in utero [2].

Answer: 2

How do you make the diagnosis?

1. A skin biopsy
2. A KOH preparation
3. A bacterial culture
4. Clinical recognition

The diagnosis of TPNM is usually made clinically; a gram stain and/or biopsy is rarely necessary. When in doubt or when the surrounding erythema is significant and an infection is considered, a swab of pustule contents for gram stain and culture can be helpful. A gram stain would show neutrophils and a bacterial culture is typically negative. A KOH preparation is not indicated. A skin biopsy would show spongiosis and intra- or subcorneal pustules containing neutrophils, fibrin, and rarely eosinophils. See Table 4.1 for the differential diagnosis of TPNM.

Answer: 4

What is the treatment?

1. Topical antifungal
2. Topical corticosteroid
3. Topical antibiotic
4. No treatment is required

Infants with TPNM are otherwise well and no treatment is necessary. Parents should be reassured that the eruption will self-resolve without sequelae. The residual hyperpigmented lesions will resolve but may take up to several months.

Answer: 4

Case Presentation

A one-week-old presents with yellow discoloration and thickening of the nail plates of several fingernails as shown in Fig. 4.2. Her mother states that these have been present since birth.

Analysis of the fingernail is most likely to show?

1. Gram-positive cocci
2. Pseudohyphae and budding yeast
3. Hyperkeratosis and parakeratosis
4. Neutrophils and fungal hyphae

Thickening and yellow discoloration of the nail plates may be the only manifestation of congenital cutaneous candidiasis (CCC). Histologic examination with a periodic acid-Schiff (PAS) stain of the nail plate is most likely to reveal pseudohyphae and budding yeast typical of *Candida albicans* infection. Gram-positive cocci would be seen in bacterial nail infections, and neutrophils and fungal hyphae are seen in dermatophyte infection of the nail. Hyperkeratosis and parakeratosis are seen in nail psoriasis.

Answer: 2

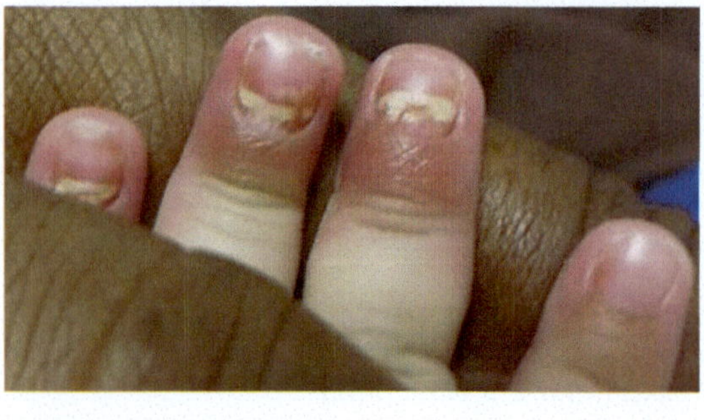

Fig. 4.2 Congenital cutaneous candidiasis present in several fingernails

How does congenital cutaneous candidiasis (CCC) present on the skin?

1. Vesicles on an erythematous base on mucous membranes
2. Superficial pustules some coalescing, extensor surfaces and palms and soles
3. Pink eczematous plaques with overlying yellow crusty scale
4. Papules, pustules, and desquamation in the diaper area

The typical rash of CCC consists of generalized 2–4 mm pink macules, papules, and/or pustules that evolve and sometimes coalesce into larger "lakes of pus." [3] Lesions are in different stages contributing to the appearance of diffuse erythema with overlying desquamation or a fine scale. The back, extensor surfaces, and skin folds are the typical areas affected, but the diaper area and oral mucosa are relatively spared. CCC often involves palms and soles (in contrast to ETN and TNPM) [3]. As in the case presented, some neonates have yellow discoloration and transverse ridging of the nail plates as the only manifestation of congenital cutaneous candidiasis. Congenital cutaneous candidiasis (as opposed to neonatal candidiasis) occurs earlier in life, presenting at birth or up to DOL 6. The diaper area and oral mucosa are spared. Table 4.2 highlights the key differences between congenital cutaneous candidiasis and neonatal candidiasis. Papules, pustules, and desquamation in the diaper area are typical of neonatal candidiasis. Vesicles on an erythematous base are seen in herpes simplex. Pink eczematous plaques with overlying yellow crusty scale are seen in infantile seborrheic dermatitis. Papules, pustules, and desquamation in the diaper area are typical of neonatal candidiasis.

Answer: 2

What is the treatment of CCC?

1. Intravenous antifungals and intravenous antibiotics until culture results are in
2. Intravenous antifungals for 10 days

Table 4.2 Key differences between congenital cutaneous candidiasis and neonatal/infantile candidiasis

	Congenital cutaneous candidiasis	Neonatal/infantile candidiasis
Onset of skin lesions	Birth up to DOL 6	2 weeks of life
Acquisition	Rare	Common
	Acquired in utero	Acquired through the birth canal or postnatally
Risk factors	Prematurity, foreign body in cervix, premature rupture of membranes, maternal history of vaginal candidiasis	Maternal history of vaginal candidiasis
Clinical features	Small pink macules and papules that evolve into pustules and desquamate	Scaly red macules, papules, and pustules usually localized to the intertriginous areas (body folds) with characteristic "satellite pustules" outside the folds
	Papules, pustules and desquamation often present at birth	
	Lesions are often at various stages	Affects diaper area (diaper dermatitis), oral mucosa (oral thrush), and intertriginous areas
	Widespread including palms and soles	
	Yellow discoloration and thickening of nail may be the only manifestation	
Diagnosis	Gram stain is negative KOH reveals budding yeast and pseudohyphae Fungal cultures from blood, urine, and CSF are usually negative	

Treatment	Depends on gestational age:
	  <1500 gm or <27 weeks: bacterial, fungal, viral cultures; and IV antifungal is required
	  Full term, healthy
	    Topical antifungal
	    Any systemic symptoms: IV antifungals
		Topical antifungals usually sufficient
		Watch premature and low birth weight infants closely
		Use systemic antifungals if any sign of systemic infection
		Cases with oral candidiasis, recurrent or recalcitrant cases may require systemic antifungal therapy, such as nystatin solution or oral fluconazole

3. Depends on age and hemodynamic status of neonate
4. Topical antifungals only

Treatment of CCC depends on the newborn's gestational age and hemodynamic status. Premature neonates less than 1500 g or less than 27 weeks' gestation will require bacterial, fungal, and viral cultures and should be treated with empiric IV antifungal therapy [4]. If the neonate is full term and hemodynamically stable, topical antifungals such as clotrimazole or ketoconazole cream to affected areas on skin twice daily should suffice. For affected nails, topical antifungals such as ketoconazole 2% cream twice daily should clear the infection in several months. In a cohort of mostly premature neonates, prompt systemic antifungal treatment at the time of presentation and treatment duration for $\geq$14 days prevented fungal dissemination and mortality. Delaying systemic treatment, use of oral or topical nystatin, and treating for <10 days was associated with dissemination of candida to the bloodstream [5]. Fortunately, systemic dissemination of cutaneous infection is rare occurring in ~5% of affected neonates; however, if there is any sign of systemic infection, there should be a low threshold for starting IV antifungals [4].

Answer: 3

Case Presentation

A 3-week-old baby boy is brought into your newborn follow-up clinic because his mother is concerned he has acne. He is otherwise well and thriving. On exam you note tiny superficial pustules and pinpoint pink papules on the posterior neck, scalp at the hairline, and her upper back (Fig. 4.3).

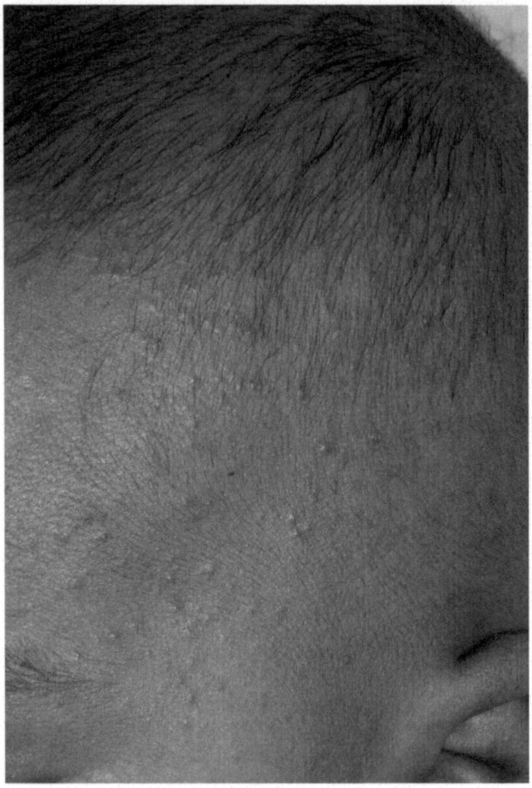

Fig. 4.3 Miliaria rubra on the scalp of a neonatal boy

What is the diagnosis?

1. Neonatal acne
2. Miliaria rubra
3. Seborrheic dermatitis
4. Transient neonatal pustular melanosis

Miliaria rubra is a common condition that is usually seen after the first week of life. Miliaria occurs more commonly in the neonatal period due to the immaturity of the sweat (eccrine) ducts which results in obstruction. Superficial obstruction results in miliaria crystallina, which is a clear superficial pinpoint vesicle with no surrounding pinkness. A slightly deeper obstruction of the eccrine duct results in miliaria rubra, a small papulovesicle with surrounding erythema, as demonstrated in this patient. Miliaria is more common in warmer climates. Typical lesions are located on the forehead, scalp, posterior neck, and upper back as opposed to neonatal acne where lesions are found on nose and cheeks. Pustules are usually sterile. Conditions that can look similar to miliaria are listed in Table 4.1. Neonatal acne presents with acneiform papules and pustules and occurs on the face, commonly on the cheeks. Seborrheic dermatitis is characterized by pink eczematous plaques with greasy yellow scaling.

Answer: 2

How do you treat and counsel the family?

1. This condition is lifelong and will come and go
2. Use topical antibiotic ointments twice daily until clears
3. This condition spontaneously improves without treatment
4. This condition will improve if dairy is eliminated from the diet

You can reassure parents that miliaria is a benign self-limited condition which can be caused by excessive swaddling, heat, fever, and occlusive dressings. These factors trigger obstruction of the premature eccrine sweat ducts and the resultant fluid accumulation in the dermis leads to an inflammatory response that is seen clinically as the surrounding redness on the skin. This condition spontaneous resolves with cooling and continued avoidance of triggers described above. It is important to counsel the family to use lightweight cotton clothing and to avoid overuse of occlusive emollients. Miliaria usually resolves later in infancy; topical antibiotics and removal of dairy do not treat miliaria.

Answer: 3

Case Presentation

A 2-week-old infant girl presents with a smooth, 1.5 cm circular patch of smooth alopecia on the scalp as shown (Fig. 4.4). Her parents report that it was a superficial erosion at birth and healed quickly. The surrounding hair appears normal.

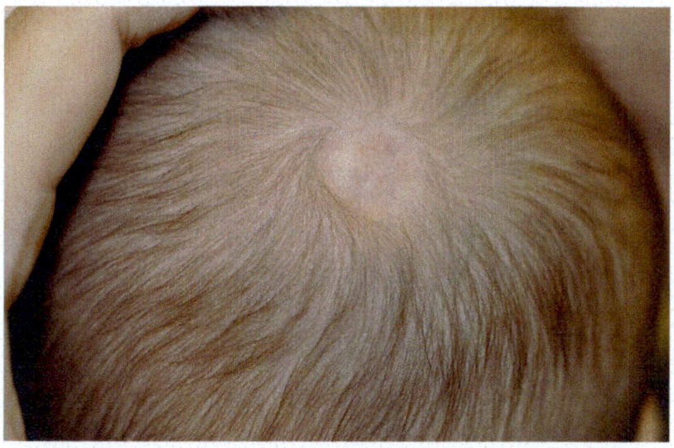

Fig. 4.4 Aplasia cutis congenita on the scalp

She was born via normal spontaneous vaginal delivery without the use of instrumentation.

What is the diagnosis and what is the cause?

1. Superficial abrasion from trauma during delivery
2. Nevus sebaceous
3. Ulcerated infantile hemangioma
4. Aplasia cutis congenita

Aplasia cutis congenita (ACC) is a congenital defect that results from a localized area of absent skin at birth. There is absence of the epidermis and dermis in the affected area, but occasionally underlying subcutaneous tissue, bone, and dura can also be missing. ACC is usually seen on the scalp as a single well-circumscribed area of alopecia. Less commonly, ACC presents as multiple areas of alopecia on the scalp or can be found on the face, trunk, or extremities. Most cases of ACC are sporadic and the exact etiology is unknown. A popular hypothesis suggests that ACC is the result of compromised vasculature of the placenta [6].

While the scenario above describes a typical patient with ACC, other common presentations at birth include a well-formed hairless scar and ulceration with a granulating base, a superficial erosion, or a translucent, glistening membrane ("membranous aplasia cutis" – uncommon variant). Lesions are usually sharply demarcated, oval, circular, or stellate and measure 1–3 cm in diameter [6].

Answer: 4

What is the management of ACC and is an additional work-up necessary?

1. A skin biopsy should be performed
2. Surgical correction is highly recommended
3. Depends on size, location, and presence of "hair collar."
4. MRI/MRA of head and neck

When a lesion of ACC is identified, a detailed and complete physical exam should be performed. ACC is an isolated defect in the majority of cases, but it can be associated with other developmental anomalies or be a feature of a variety of syndromes. In addition, a ring of long, dark hair around membranous aplasia cutis (the hair collar sign) is thought to herald an underlying neural tube defect. If the lesion appears large, deep, or stellate or if it is located in the midline, a radiologic evaluation to assess for an underlying defect is necessary [6]. In this case, a complete physical exam was normal and the lesion was small with no surrounding thick "hair collar" and not located in the midline. Therefore no additional work- up was needed.

When ACC presents with a superficial wound at birth, simple wound care with gentle cleansing, ointments, or antibiotic ointments and nonstick dressings will help heal most small defects quickly. The prognosis of ACC is excellent and most lesions heal completely in the first weeks to months of life. Lesions may heal with scarring. Alopecia may be of cosmetic concern when large or in a highly visible area. Most scars become inconspicuous as the hair and scalp grow. However large or very obvious scars may require plastic surgery correction in the future.

Answer: 3

Case Presentation

You are examining a 2-day-old baby girl at mother's bedside and notice a 3 cm oval, thin, yellow-tan hairless plaque as shown (Fig. 4.5). Her mother is now concerned and asks if it will need to be removed.

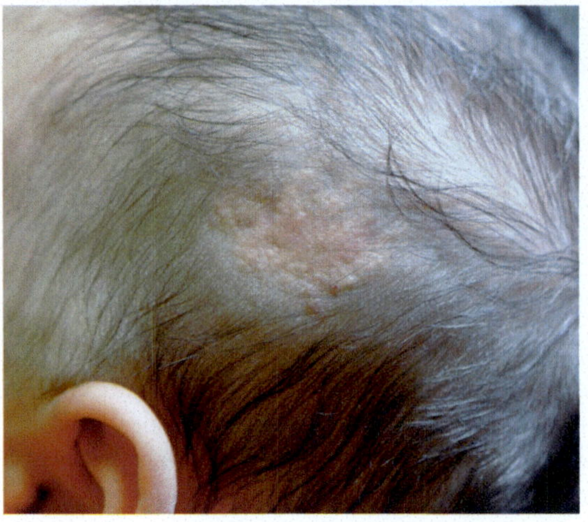

Fig. 4.5 Nevus sebaceous on the scalp

What is the diagnosis?

1. Nevus sebaceous
2. Aplasia cutis congenita
3. Congenital melanocytic nevus
4. Congenital alopecia

A nevus sebaceous (NS) is an easily recognizable yellow- to tan-colored, hairless, thin plaque that has a fine pebbly surface. An NS is a common congenital benign tumor predominantly composed of large and malformed sebaceous glands. NS can occur anywhere on the body but greater than 95% of lesions occur on the head and neck, most often on the scalp. Although usually localized, as in this patient, occasionally, a more extensive NS along the lines of Blaschko can be present. In such instances, NS can be associated with ocular or CNS abnormalities. NS occurs sporadically. If a dermatoscope is available, visualizing bright yellow dots and an absence of hair follicles can help make the definitive diagnosis, before the characteristic features become apparent.

Answer: 1

What is the natural history of a nevus sebaceous?

1. Rapid growth in the first year of life followed by involution
2. Spontaneous regression
3. Remains quiescent in childhood and thickens at puberty
4. Remains a flat hairless plaque throughout life

An NS is thought to result from a defect in cutaneous embryologic development; its exact etiology is unknown. Lesions are usually yellow to tan and mildly elevated with a pebbly surface at birth. Occasionally, NS can be thicker or have papillomatous projections, simulating a wart. It can also present as a large pedunculated lesion at birth. After infancy, lesions flatten, become more inconspicuous, and grow proportionately with the child. At puberty, under the influence of androgens, NS thicken, become darker yellow or brown, more papular or verrucous, and can be friable or itchy. Warty growths, representing secondary adnexal neoplasms, may develop within a NS during adolescence or later. The area will remain hairless.

Answer: 3

What is your recommendation for management?

1. Immediate complete excision
2. Clinical observation yearly
3. Complete surgical excision around puberty
4. Skin biopsy if growths appear within the lesion

When an NS is identified, the first step should be a complete physical examination to assess for other congenital defects and determine the extent of NS. Complete surgical removal remains the treatment of choice for NS given the concern for warty proliferation, permanent alopecia, and the development of secondary tumors after puberty. More recent investigations have shown that the risk of developing a malignant neoplasm within an NS is quite low [7]. Recommendations for timing of excision vary. Advantages of removing the lesions in infancy are greater laxity of tissues, smaller size of the lesion, and removal of any cosmetic impact on the developing child. The main disadvantage to early removal is the need for general anesthesia. Most often, smaller NS are removed in late childhood, prior to the onset of puberty, when the patient is able to cooperate with excision under local anesthesia. At this time the NS has not yet thickened under the influence of androgens. In cases of an extensive or widespread NS, a thorough medical history and physical examination should be performed with special attention to the ocular, neurologic, and musculoskeletal systems. Radiologic evaluation and further work-up should be symptom directed. Various ablative treatments including cryotherapy and electrodessication have been used to treat NS, but these do not remove the risk of neoplasia and can still leave areas of alopecia.

Answer: 3

Case Presentation

You are examining a 2-day-old newborn boy who was born with the lesion shown (Fig. 4.6). On examination, this area measures 3 × 2 cm and is a homogeneous brown color with smooth borders. He is otherwise well, and there is no family history of skin cancer or skin disease.

What is the diagnosis?

1. Epidermal nevus
2. Congenital melanocytic nevus
3. Café au lait patch
4. Mongolian spot

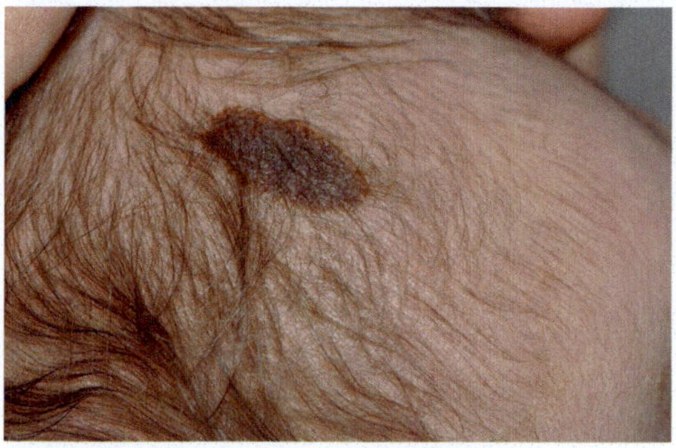

Fig. 4.6 Medium-sized congenital melanocytic nevus on the scalp

The lesion shown is a medium-sized congenital melanocytic nevus. Nevi present at birth or those that develop within the first 2 years of life are considered congenital melanocytic nevi (CMN). CMN have melanocytes that are located deeper down into the dermis surrounding hair follicles and nerves than those in acquired nevi and have characteristic dermoscopic features. CMN are classified according to their predicted final adult size as small, medium, or large. Small CMN have a final size of <1.5 cm in largest diameter. Medium CMN have a final size of 1.5–20 cm in greatest diameter. Large (or giant) CMN have a predicted adult size of >20 cm (equivalent to ≥9 cm on the head of an infant or ≥6 cm on the body of an infant). A newer classification scheme proposed in 2013 has further subdivided medium (M1: 1.5–10 cm; M2 > 10–20 cm) and large (L1″ > 20–30 cm; L2 > 30–40 cm) categories and added a "giant" category for lesions >40–60 cm (G1) and those >60 cm (G2). In addition, descriptive features such as heterogeneity, hypertrichosis, surface rugosity, and number of satellite lesions were added to the categorization schema to better describe CMN and provide more specific melanoma risk earlier in life [8]. Small or medium CMN are common and occur in 1–3% of neonates, whereas large CMN are estimated to occur in 1 in 20,000–50,000 neonates [9].

Answer: 2

What changes can occur in CMN over time?

1. Darkening
2. Hair growth
3. Thickening
4. All of the above

At birth, CMN present as tan to light or dark brown/black, flat or raised macules or papules of varying size that then enlarge in proportion to the child's growth. Over time CMN, can become darker or lighter in color, develop a mottled pigmentation, increase in thickness, and even spontaneously regress. Surface changes such as hypertrichosis, verrucous changes, and proliferative nodules can also occur.

Answer: 4

What is your recommendation for monitoring and treatment?

1. Complete excision as soon as possible
2. Regular clinical monitoring with discussion about risks and benefits of excision
3. Monitoring by parents at home
4. Excise completely around puberty

Information from larger cohort studies suggests that prophylactic removal of small and medium CMN is not recommended if there are no concerning features and no obstacles to monitoring, because the risk of melanoma is low [10]. Lifetime melanoma risk in small- and medium-sized CMN is 1% and typically presents after puberty [9]. Regular clinical monitoring is often all that is needed. However, decision to perform surgical removal should be individualized taking into account worrisome clinical features, cosmetic or parental concerns, the location and ease of monitoring, the risks of the procedure, and anesthesia versus the benefits of surgical removal. Surgical excision can be performed for cosmetically disfiguring lesions to avoid the potential psychosocial impact of the nevus on the developing child.

Lifetime melanoma risk is estimated at 10–15% for large CMN especially those that are larger than 40 cm, accompanied by satellite lesions. Many of these melanomas will develop in the CNS and not the skin and usually develop in childhood [10]. Patients with large or giant CMN, especially those located on the posterior axis or those with smaller satellite nevi, and patients with multiple medium CMN should be screened for neurocutaneous melanosis with an MRI of the brain and spine ideally before 4–6 months of age. For large CMN, early and complete surgical excision is often recommended and desired by parents [9, 10].

Answer: 2

Case Presentation

You are called to examine a 3-day-old boy and parents ask about the pink red spots on his upper eyelids and his forehead (Fig. 4.7). The lesions become deeper red when he cries or strains.

What is the diagnosis?

1. Nevus simplex
2. Port-wine stain
3. Infantile hemangioma
4. Ecchymosis from birth trauma

This is a nevus simplex (syn. salmon patch, stork bite, angel's kiss), the preferred term for the most common vascular birthmark of infancy. It occurs in 30–40% of newborns. A nevus simplex is typically present at birth as an ill-defined, flat, dull pink or red, blanchable patch most commonly seen on the posterior scalp (aka "stork bite"), glabella (aka "angel's kiss"), forehead, upper eyelids, nose, and/or upper lip. Less often, a nevus simplex can have a more extensive, widespread distribution such as multiple lesions on the back and trunk.

Answer: 1

What is the typical natural history of nevus simplex?

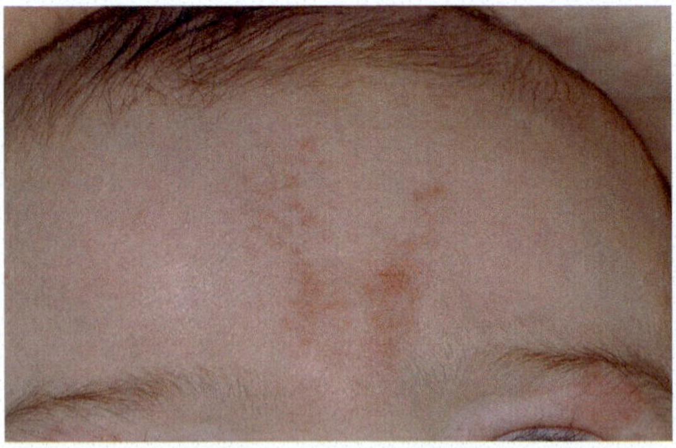

Fig. 4.7 Nevus simplex on the forehead

1. Complete resolution in the first 2 years of life
2. Darkening over time
3. Rapid growth for first year followed by involution
4. Resolution in 2–3 weeks

The etiology of nevus simplex is unknown. Some experts believe it to be a form of persistent fetal circulation rather than a true vascular malformation. Complete resolution within the first 2 years of life is expected for >95% of lesions on the face. Occipital lesions tend to persist for longer, some indefinitely. Lesions become deeper red with crying and physical exertion. No treatment is necessary as most lesions fade; in the uncommon event of persistence, treatment with the pulsed dye laser is highly effective. Port-wine stains (Fig. 4.8) darken and thicken over time; and infantile hemangiomas proliferate rapidly in the first year of life followed by gradual spontaneous involution (Table 4.3).

Answer: 1

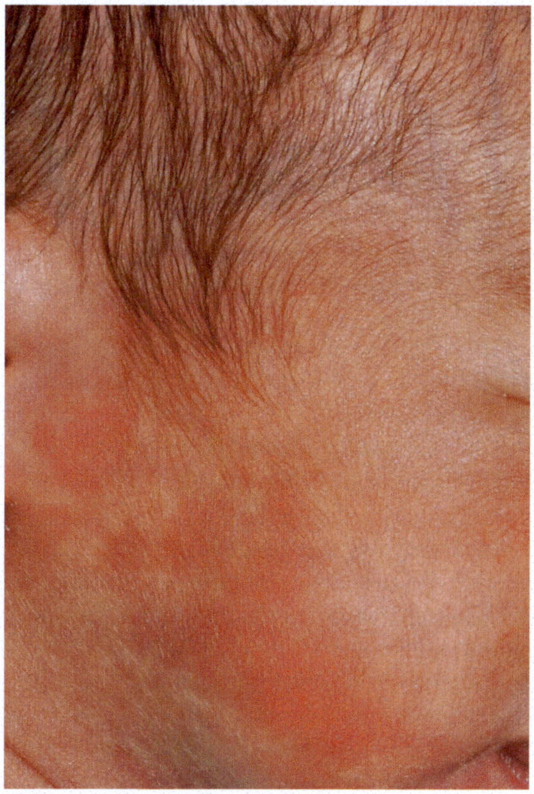

Fig. 4.8 Port-wine stain on the right cheek

Table 4.3 Key differences among the most common neonatal vascular birthmarks

	Nevus simplex	Port-wine stain (Fig. 4.8)	Infantile hemangioma
Age of onset	Birth	Birth	Absent at birth, precursor (flat pink or bruise-like patch) lesion may be present
Location	Glabella, forehead, nape of neck/posterior scalp	Head and neck most common; but can be anywhere	Head and neck most common; but can be anywhere
Clinical features	Ill-defined, light pink, blanches	Well demarcated Dark pink Darkens over time	Rapid volumetric growth in first few weeks of life
Natural history	Darkens with crying or exertion, most fade completely over first 2 years of life	Darken and thicken over time, may develop nodules at puberty	Rapid growth, plateau, and spontaneous involution
Treatment	Clinical observation	Pulsed dye laser early and often is the established treatment of choice	Localized treatments for small superficial lesions: timolol 0.5% gel forming solution Systemic treatment of choice: propranolol hydrochloride 2–3 mg/kg/day until no longer proliferating

Case Presentation

At her follow-up in the newborn clinic, a 3-week-old girl presents with the bright red, firm, warm plaque (Fig. 4.9). Her mother is alarmed because it was a small flat spot at birth that was barely visible.

How do you explain the diagnosis and natural history of this lesion to this concerned mother?

1. This is a tumor and needs an immediate biopsy
2. This is a benign birthmark that is expected to grow in infancy
3. This is a result of trauma during delivery
4. This is a hereditary birthmark

The lesion described above is an infantile hemangioma (IH), the most common benign tumor of infancy, and while the exact etiology and pathogenesis of IH is unknown. Infantile hemangiomas more common in female infants and low birth weight newborns. Several theories, including a placental embolus, a somatic mutation in a gene-mediating endothelial cell proliferation, or origination from an endothelial progenitor cell (CD34+, CD133+), have been proposed [11].

As seen in the newborn, IH are either not present at birth or a "precursor" lesion that can appear as a bluish bruise-like patch, telangiectasias with a rim of pallor, or a red flat stain. IH have a characteristic natural history consisting of three phases:

1. The rapid proliferation phase. IH experience rapid volumetric growth and are red, firm, and rubbery. This usually begins at 3 weeks of age and lasts until 6–7 months of age depending on the IH. IH with a deep component will proliferate for longer period of time. The most rapid rate of growth is thought to occur between 5 and 8 weeks of age.
2. The plateau (or late proliferative) phase. IH have a slower rate of growth and color changes to dull red or gray and begins to break apart. IH feel soft and spongy. The length of this phase is variable and can begin as early as 7 months and typically lasts until 12 months of age.
3. The involution phase. Involution of IH is a slow gradual process that usually starts at 1 year of age. In this phase, the color continues to fade and lesions flatten. Some lesions involute completely while others leave fibrofatty residua and skin texture changes (Table 4.3).

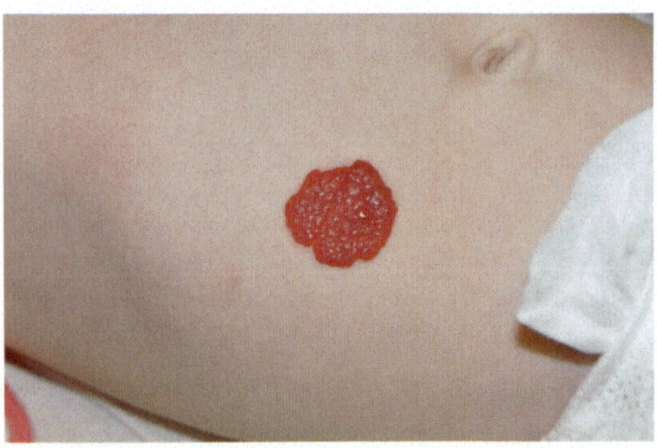

Fig. 4.9 Infantile hemangioma in the early proliferative phase on the right lower abdomen

Answer: 2

Which infantile hemangiomas require treatment?

1. Large function threatening lesions
2. Ulcerated hemangiomas
3. Infantile hemangioma at high risk for cosmetic disfigurement
4. All of the above

The vast majority of IH will proliferate and involute with minimal consequences. In these cases, active nonintervention is the treatment of choice and consists of education on the natural history of IH, close monitoring, and reassurance. There is a significant minority of IH that are high risk for complications and or associated anomalies. It is important to recognize these patterns early so that a work-up can be done and treatment initiated (preferably in the early proliferative phase), so that treatment can have maximal benefit. There are three generally accepted reasons for treatment: (1) ulceration or risk of ulceration, (2) disfigurement or risk of cosmetic disfigurement, and (3) functional impairment. IH at high risk for ulceration can be identified by their location and morphology.

For example, those located in the perineal, axillae, neck, or perioral areas are at higher risk for development of ulceration. Ulceration is heralded by a gray-white surface color during the proliferative phase, and when it occurs, it can be painful and will result in residual scarring.

Further evaluation for underlying anomalies or systemic associations is required for hemangiomas of the following morphologies and/or locations:

1. Large segmental IH (i.e., those with a configuration corresponding to a recognizable and/or significant portion of a developmental segment) on the face >5 cm should be evaluated with MRI/MRA of the head and neck, echocardiogram, and an ophthalmologic evaluation to assess for underlying PHACES syndrome [posterior fossa brain malformations, hemangiomas, arterial anomalies (most often cerebrovascular), cardiac anomalies, eye abnormalities, and sternal cleft or supraumbilical raphe or both].
2. Large segmental IH over the lumbosacral or perineal regions may be associated with underlying spinal dysraphism such as tethered cord and other structural abnormalities as part of the LUMBAR syndrome. This is a rare condition that presents as a hemangioma or several hemangiomas on the lower body in association with other congenital anomalies. These anomalies may include urogenital tract malformation, myelopathy (spinal cord defect), bone deformities, anorectal malformations, and arterial anomalies. Screening should include a spinal ultrasound if less than 3 months and/or an MRI/MRA of the lower back and affected lower extremity.
3. Large hemangiomas on the lower face or "beard" area can be a marker of a deeper laryngeal or airway hemangioma. Patients with IH in this area should be referred early for otolaryngology evaluation [12].
4. Patients with more than five IH are at significantly higher risk for hepatic hemangiomas and should be screened with abdominal US to assess for hepatic or other visceral IH [13]. The risk of visceral hemangiomas increases with increasing number of skin IH [14].

Oftentimes, the large segmental lesions described above that should prompt further work-up will also require systemic treatment because they are at high risk for hemangioma-related complications (disfigurement, ulceration, or visual compromise).

Answer: 4

What is the treatment of choice for infantile hemangioma that requires systemic treatment?

1. Oral corticosteroids
2. Oral propranolol
3. Vincristine
4. Pulsed dye laser

The vast majority of IH do not require active intervention. For small superficial hemangiomas in cosmetically sensitive areas or in an area at high risk for ulceration (perineal, axillae, neck, or perioral), the treatment of choice is timolol 0.5% gel forming solution. Timolol is a nonselective beta-blocker that is highly effective for ulcerated and superficial hemangiomas. The recommended dose of timolol 0.5% gel forming solution is 1 drop twice daily on the IH for at least 3 months for best response.

Other local therapies include intralesional triamcinolone (5–10 mg/mL), a useful option for bulky, localized lesions, and pulsed dye laser (PDL) treatment. This approach is useful for small flat lesions in the early proliferative phase or for residual telangiectasias after most of the IH has involuted.

Systemic therapy is reserved for larger IH with more aggressive growth characteristics that pose a high threat to a vital function, for cosmetic disfigurement, or for those IH not responding to local therapy. The first-line systemic treatment option is propranolol, a nonselective beta-blocker, that has demonstrated superior efficacy and safety compared to systemic corticosteroids. The recommended generic formulation to use is propranolol hydrochloride oral solution 20 mg/5 mL. The branded, infant friendly formulation, Hemangeol™ (propranolol hydrochloride 4.28 mg/mL) was used in several large international multicenter randomized controlled trials and is FDA approved and indicated for the treatment of IH in patients 5 weeks and older [15].

Practices for propranolol initiation vary. Guidelines published in 2013 recommended a baseline cardiopulmonary assessment with electrocardiogram (ECG) prior to starting propranolol in certain situations (baseline HR low for age; family history of congenital heart disease or arrhythmia; history or presence of arrhythmia) [16]. Monitoring heart rate and blood pressure at baseline and after initiation was also recommended [16]. Since the consensus guidelines were published, large safety studies have shown very low incidence of symptomatic bradycardia and/or hypotension, and thus most practitioners will start propranolol in healthy full-term infants that have a normal clinical cardiac exam (performed by either the prescribing practitioner or pediatrician) and no family history of heart disease [17]. In addition, monitoring HR and BP after initiation or dose escalation is no longer a common practice. However continued anticipatory guidance of potential side effects is imperative [18].

Optimal dosing is based on weight with a goal therapeutic dose of ~2.2 mg/kg/day (range 1–3 mg/kg/day) divided 2–3 times daily with a minimum of 6 hours between doses. Propranolol should be given during the day, with or shortly after a feeding. The most common reported side effects include sleep disturbance, intermittent acrocyanosis, cold hands and feet, gastrointestinal symptoms, and/or respiratory symptoms. Serious side effects are rare and include hypotension, bradycardia, and hypoglycemia. Parents should be educated regarding the symptoms of hypoglycemia and instructed to ensure regular feeding times, avoid prolonged fasts, and discontinue propranolol during times of decreased oral intake or if there is wheezing. Propranolol is usually continued through the growth phase of the IH and then tapered off.

When there is a contraindication to the use of propranolol and the IH requires systemic treatment, oral corticosteroids (prednisone or prednisolone; 2–4 mg/kg/day divided twice daily until growth has stopped) and/or surgical excision are used. Oral corticosteroids must be tapered slowly to avoid rebound growth and adrenal suppression.

Answer: 2

Clinical Pearls

- Most skin lesions and skin eruptions present in the first few weeks of life are benign and self- limited.
- Erythema toxicum neonatorum is a common and self-limited skin condition that can mimic other pustular neonatal skin conditions.
- Transient neonatal pustular melanosis progresses through three characteristic phases and then self-resolves without sequelae.
- Congenital cutaneous candidiasis can present with yellowing of the nail plates as the sole manifestation.
- Miliaria rubra improves spontaneously with cooling.
- Close inspection and visualization of yellow color or yellow dots can help distinguish a nevus sebaceous from aplasia cutis.
- Congenital melanocytic nevi should be classified by size and monitored clinically.
- Nevus simplex should be distinguished from a port-wine stain and an infantile hemangioma early, so parents can be reassured of their eventual resolution.
- Infantile hemangioma may resemble port-wine stains initially, but close monitoring in the first month of life will demonstrate the characteristic growth pattern of an IH.
- Most infantile hemangiomas require no treatment; for those requiring treatment, topical and systemic beta-blockers are offered first.

References

1. Rayala BZ, Morrell DS. Common skin conditions in children: neonatal skin lesions. FP Essent. 2017;453:11–7.
2. Hussain S, Venepally M, Treat JR. Vesicles and pustules in the neonate. Semin Perinatol. 2013;37(1):8–15. https://doi.org/10.1053/j.semperi.2012.11.005.
3. Oza V, Asch S, Mathes EF. Three day old with palmar pustules. JAMA Pediatr. 2016;170(2):171–2. https://doi.org/10.1001/jamapediatrics.2015.1996.
4. Darmstadt GL, Dinulos JG, Miller Z. Congenital cutaneous candidiasis: clinical presentation, pathogenesis and management guidelines. Pediatrics. 2000;105(2):438–44.
5. Kaufman DA, Coggins SA, ZanelliJörn-Hendrik Weitkamp SA. Congenital cutaneous candidiasis: prompt systemic treatment is associated with improved outcomes in neonates. Clin Infect Dis. 2017;64(10):1387–95. https://doi.org/10.1093/cid/cix119.
6. Patel DP, Castelo-Soccio L, Yan AC. Aplasia cutis congenita: evaluation of signs suggesting extracutaneous involvement. Pediatr Dermatol. 2017:27. https://doi.org/10.1111/pde.13340.
7. Idriss MH, Elston DM. Secondary neoplasms associated with nevus sebaceous of Jadassohn: a study of 707 cases. J Am Acad Dermatol. 2014;70(2):332–7.
8. Krengel S, Scope A, Dusza SW, et al. New recommendations for the categorization of cutaneous features of congenital melanocytic nevi. J Am Acad Dermatol. 2013;68:441–51.
9. Schaffer JV. Update on melanocytic nevi in children. Clin Dermatol. 2015;33(3):368–86.
10. Kinsler VA, O'Hare P, Bulstrode N, et al. Melanoma in congenital melanocytic naevi. Br J Dermatol. 2017;176(5):1131–43.
11. Rosenblatt A, Mathes EF, Rosbe KW. Infantile hemangiomas: from pathogenesis to clinical features. Res Rep Neonatol. 2012;2:55–65.
12. Piram M, Hadj-Rabia S, Boccara O, et al. Beard infantile hemangioma and subglottic involvement: are median pattern and telangiectatic aspect the clue? J Eur Acad Dermatol Venereol. 2016;30(12):2056–9.
13. Rialon KL, Murillo R, Fevurly RD, et al. Impact of screening for hepatic hemangiomas in patients with multiple cutaneous infantile hemangiomas. Pediatr Dermatol. 2015;32(6):808–12.
14. Horii KA, Drolet BA, Frieden IJ, et al. Prospective study of the frequency of hepatic hemangiomas in infants with multiple cutaneous infantile hemangiomas. Pediatr Dermatol. 2011;28(3):245–53.
15. Léauté-Labrèze C, Hoeger P, Mazereeuw-Hautier J, et al. A randomized, controlled trial of oral propranolol in infantile hemangioma. N Engl J Med. 2015;372(8):735–46.
16. Drolet BA, Frommelt PC, Chamlin SL, et al. Initiation and use of propranolol for infantile hemangioma: report of a consensus conference. Pediatrics. 2013;131(1):128–40. https://www-ncbi-nlm-nih-gov.access.library.miami.edu/pubmed/23266923.
17. Léaute-Labrèze C, Boccara O, Degrugillier-Chopinet C, et al. Safety of oral propranolol for the treatment of infantile hemangioma: a systematic review. Pediatrics. 2016;138(4):e20160353.
18. Martin K, Blei F, Chamlin SL, et al. Propranolol treatment of infantile hemangiomas: anticipatory guidance for parents and caretakers. Pediatr Dermatol. 2013;30(1):155–9.

5 Evaluation and Management of the Late Preterm Infant

Stephen A. Pearlman and Kaitlin Kenaley

Introduction

Late preterm infants are most commonly defined as those born between 34 0/7 and 36 6/7 weeks of gestation [1]. However, literature from more than 10 years ago referred to these infants as "near term" [1, 2]. This terminology was abandoned because it gave the false impression that these infants are equivalent to term. The current phrase "late preterm" more accurately conveys the sense that these infants are more vulnerable for short- and long-term complications [3].

For many years, late preterm infants were largely ignored because they were not as sick as babies born at earlier gestational ages [1]. There was an underappreciation of their underlying pathophysiology and hence their increased risk for significant morbidities and mortality. They were not well studied until the past decade when there has been increased recognition of this "at-risk" population, leading to the publication of over 500 articles on the subject of late preterm infants [2].

Demographically, late preterm infants represent 74% of all preterm deliveries [2]. In fact, data shows that between 1992 and 2007, the rate of preterm births has increased from 7.3% to 10.4% of all births [2]. This rise is likely multifactorial, but certainly the increasing rates of preeclampsia and multifetal gestations have contributed. There also was a more permissive attitude toward the elective delivery of late preterm infants. Since 2007, the incidence of late preterm births has decreased to 9.6% in 2014 which represents an 8% drop [2]. This change is likely a reflection of changes to the ACOG guidelines regarding elective preterm delivery, as well as an increased awareness of the risks of poor neonatal outcomes in this population of infants.

Through several case examples, this chapter will discuss potential etiologies, complications, and recommendations for management of the late preterm infant.

Case Presentation

A 33-year-old G1P0 presents to her obstetrician's office at 36 3/7 weeks. She developed preeclampsia in the third trimester. She also developed gestational diabetes which is diet controlled. Her fetus has no congenital anomalies by ultrasound, but growth is poor with the weight

S. A. Pearlman, MD, MSHQS (✉)
Division of Neonatology, Christiana Care Health System, Newark, DE, USA

Sidney Kimmel College of Medicine of Thomas Jefferson University, Philadelphia, PA, USA
e-mail: spearlman@christianacare.org

K. Kenaley, MD
Division of Neonatology, Christiana Care Health System, Newark, DE, USA

G. I. Martin, W. Rosenfeld (eds.), *Common Problems in the Newborn Nursery*,
https://doi.org/10.1007/978-3-319-95672-5_5

less than the third percentile. There has been no interval growth since her last ultrasound 2 weeks ago. Her obstetrician decides to induce labor, and she delivers a healthy male infant who weighs 1750 g.

How many risk factors for late preterm delivery does this patient have?

1. 1
2. 2
3. 3
4. None

Preeclampsia is a leading cause of late preterm delivery. Hypertensive disorders have become more prevalent in women of childbearing age, affecting as many as 10% of pregnancies [4]. Obstetrical surveillance of fetal well-being has also improved, leading to a higher number of medically indicated preterm deliveries. Thus, the intrauterine growth restriction noted in our example is the second risk factor for late preterm delivery. Gestational diabetes is usually not considered an etiology for late preterm delivery. Several other risk factors may precipitate delivery between 34 0/7 and 36 6/7 weeks of gestation including spontaneous rupture of membranes, preterm labor, antepartum hemorrhage, or multifetal gestation [5]. Advances in the field reproductive endocrinology have yielded higher numbers of twins, triplets, and higher-order multiples which often lead to preterm delivery. Data from the March of Dimes published in 2015 shows that late preterm delivery is almost five times more common in multiple births when compared to singletons (Fig. 5.1).

In summary, there are many risk factors that necessitate preterm delivery. Fortunately, the American College of Obstetrics and Gynecology has recent recommendations that strongly discourage induction or elective repeat cesarean section deliveries prior to 39 weeks unless specific criteria are met [6]. Many hospitals have created policies to reflect the current recommendations.

Answer: 2

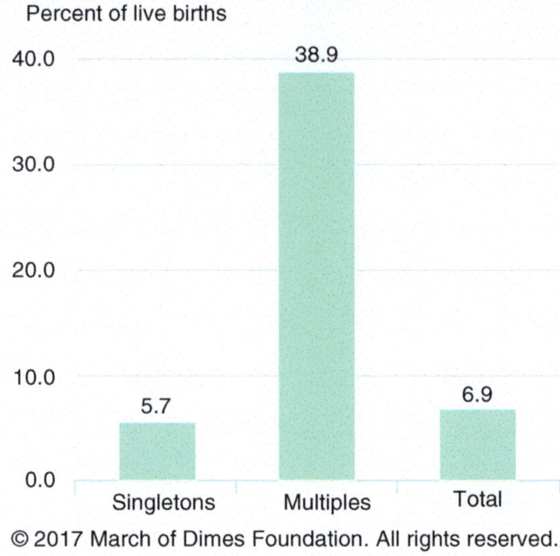

Fig. 5.1 Incidence of late preterm births by plurality 2015. (With permission from March of Dimes. Source: National Center for Health Statistics, final natality data. Retrieved December 14, 2017, from www.marchofdimes.org/peristats; Multiple deliveries include twin, triplet and higher order deliveries. Late preterm is between 34 and 36 weeks gestation)

Case Presentation

A late preterm infant is born vaginally at 36 weeks weighing 2200 g. At 42 h of life, the baby's weight is 2000 g representing a 9% weight loss. The mother wants to exclusively breastfeed and has demonstrated good milk production that day by performing hand expression. The baby is latching but sometimes falls asleep during the feeding. The baby is mildly jaundiced, and the transcutaneous bilirubin level is 7.2 mg/dl. The infant is maintaining a normal temperature in an open crib. The mother expresses her strong opinion of wanting to take the baby home as she has a 3 year old to care for. The best management of this baby is:

1. Keep the baby in the hospital, start phototherapy, and consider supplementation with formula.
2. Discharge the baby, and follow up in your office in 48–72 h.
3. Discharge the baby with formula supplementation, and follow up in your office in 24 h.

4. Keep the baby in the hospital, monitor intake closely, and if continues to lose weight, consider gavage feeds versus formula supplementation.

Studies have shown that poor feeding and jaundice are the most common reasons for delayed discharge of late preterm infants. This increases their length of stay and triples the cost of their initial hospitalization [3, 7]. With regard to the weight loss this baby experienced, the American Academy of Pediatrics recommends considering supplementation once the weight loss exceeds 7% of the birth weight [8]. Considering this mother's wishes to exclusively breastfeed and her adequate supply, gavage feeding may be a better option than formula supplementation. Late preterm infants are also twice as likely to require readmission into the hospital compared to term infants. To address specifics of this case, this baby does not require phototherapy because it is below the threshold recommended to begin phototherapy (AAP Guidelines for Phototherapy. See Chap. 5). However, it would be prudent to continue to monitor the bilirubin level in this infant. Late preterm infants are five times as likely to develop prolonged jaundice that requires phototherapy when compared to term infants.

Answer: 4

The likely etiologies of hyperbilirubinemia in this population are:

1. A relative deficiency of glucuronyl transferase
2. Feeding difficulties
3. Alpha-1-antitrypsin deficiency
4. 1 and 2

Late preterms may also be at greater risk for BIND (bilirubin-induced neurologic dysfunction) because of a diminished capacity to bind bilirubin and an immaturity of the blood-brain barrier [9]. Jaundice is the most common cause for readmission of the late preterm infant [10].

Answer: 3

Respiratory distress in the late preterm infant is often due to all of the following *except*:

1. Surfactant deficiency
2. Immature lung structure
3. Structural lung deformities (e.g. cystic adenomatoid malformation)
4. Retained lung fluid

The first three all contribute to respiratory distress in this population. There is no increased risk of congenital lung malformations. Respiratory distress syndrome (RDS) due to surfactant deficiency is 17.3 times more likely in late preterms compared to term neonates [11]. The relative risk is inversely proportional to the gestational age. At 36 weeks, infants are 10.9 times as likely to develop RDS compared to term infants. This risk of RDS increases to 28.6 times at 35 weeks of gestation and 48.4 times at 34 weeks of gestation [11]. This is due to the combination of surfactant deficiency, immature lung structure, and retained lung fluid. The results are also striking regarding the need for support. Compared to term infants, late preterm infants are 4.9 times more likely to need intubation and ventilation, 9.8 times more likely to require CPAP, and 24.4 times as likely to require supplemental oxygen by nasal cannula [11]. The respiratory distress can be quite severe resulting in bronchopulmonary dysplasia in 11% and death in 5% of late preterms with RDS. Overall, the absolute risk for death in the late preterm population is quite low. However, when compared to term infants, late preterm infants are 5.9 times more likely to die during the first month of life [11].

Obstetrical management issues that may decrease the frequency of late preterm delivery include the prevention of iatrogenic prematurity which have been addressed in the recent ACOG guidelines [6]. For those deliveries that are not preventable during the late preterm period, treatment of women with threatened preterm delivery with antenatal steroids reduces respiratory morbidity [5].

Answer: 3

Case Presentation

A nurse calls you from the well-baby nursery about one of your patients. The baby was born at 35 weeks and has a core temperature of 35.8 °C. She has put the baby under a radiant warmer, and the temperature is now 36.6. Factors contributing to this baby's temperature instability include:

1. Immature epidermal barrier
2. Decrease of brown fat
3. High surface area to body weight ratio
4. All of the above

All of those factors are contributory. In addition, more frequent interventions in the delivery room play a role in early hypothermia. Late preterm infants are 10.8 times more likely to experience hypothermia when compared to term newborns [11].

Answer: 4

The nurse has an additional concern about this same infant. As per your hospital's protocol for the late preterm infant, she is measuring the baby's blood sugar every 8 h, which is now 35. Factors affecting glucose homeostasis in the late preterm infant include all of the following *except*:

1. High activity of hepatic glucose phosphate
2. Poor feeding
3. Low glycogen stores
4. Decreased body weight

Late preterm infants have a low level of activity of the hepatic glucose phosphatase, which is an important enzyme in the last step of gluconeogenesis. This enzyme deficiency together with the other factors mentioned above leads to a 7.4-fold increase in hypoglycemia seen in the late preterm population [12].

Answer: 1

Case Presentation

A mother brings her 1-month-old baby, who was born at 34 weeks, to your office stating that she has a runny nose for the past few days. The mother also thinks she may have stopped breathing and looked a little "blue" around the lips. Your exam shows an active healthy appearing baby who is wheezing. The most likely diagnosis is:

1. Apnea of prematurity
2. RSV bronchiolitis
3. Sepsis
4. Meningitis

RSV bronchiolitis is just as common in late preterm infants as it is in infants born before 32 weeks. A late preterm baby is twice as likely as a term infant to require hospitalization for RSV bronchiolitis [13]. It is possible that reducing exposure to people who are sick and good hand hygiene may decrease a baby's chance of contracting RSV. Late preterm infants are at increased risk of apnea, as well as SIDS. Late preterms also have an increased relative risk (RR) of pneumonia (RR = 3.5), sepsis (RR = 5.6), and meningitis (RR = 21) [11].

Answer: 2

Case Presentation

You are getting ready to discharge a late preterm infant to home. According to AAP recommendation for discharge criteria of this population, you should ensure the following:

1. Physiologic stability
2. A good home environment
3. Follow-up in your office in 24–48 h
4. All of the above

The AAP and the National Perinatal Association have published guidelines containing specific recommendations for discharge of the late preterm infant [1, 14]. First, one has to ensure that the gestational age was assessed properly. A late preterm infant should be free of any medical conditions that would require ongoing hospitalization such as jaundice or hypoglycemia. Physiologic stability includes stable vital signs including temperature, adequate feeding, and passing a car seat test. Assessing the home situation is also valuable as is close follow-up after discharge.

Answer: 4

Case Presentation

A mother calls you because she doesn't think that her late preterm infant who is now 6 months old is developing as well as her previous child. She is requesting a formal developmental assessment. Your justification to the insurance company for performing this evaluation is that late preterm infants are at increased risk of each of the following *except*:

1. Cerebral palsy
2. Autism
3. Mental retardation
4. Learning disabilities

Of note, the late preterm infant is at risk for long-term adverse neurodevelopmental outcomes compared to term infants, including cerebral palsy (RR = 3) and mental retardation (RR = 1.5), and is less likely to complete high school [15, 16]. They also experience an increased burden of chronic illness leading to greater healthcare utilization [7].

Answer: 2

This chapter has focused on the reasons for short- and long-term complications of being born between 34 0/7 and 36 6/7 weeks of gestation. It is clear that this population is vulnerable for increased mortality and morbidities such as respiratory distress, jaundice, hypoglycemia, poor feeding, temperature instability, and infections. These medical complications lead to a longer initial length of hospital stay and an increased risk of hospital readmission. Additionally, late preterm infants have an increased burden of chronic illness and neurodevelopmental delays. In order to optimize their outcomes, it behooves pediatricians and hospitals to develop specific management strategies to monitor late preterm infants during their initial hospital stay as well as after discharge home.

Clinical Pearls

1. Late preterm infants, when compared to term infants, have significant short- and long-term complications.
2. Preeclampsia and other hypertensive disorders of pregnancy are the leading causes of preterm delivery.
3. Poor feeding and jaundice are common reasons for delayed discharge and readmissions of late preterm infants.
4. Late preterm infants are at a higher risk of respiratory distress that may be serious enough to lead to chronic lung disease or death.
5. Hypoglycemia and thermoregulation issues are common problems for the late preterm infant.
6. RSV bronchiolitis is just as common in the late preterm infant as in earlier preterm infants.
7. To safely discharge a late preterm infant, one should look for physiologic stability, a good home environment, and follow-up in your office within 48 h.
8. Neurodevelopmental delay is more common in the late preterm infant than in term infants.

References

1. Engle WA, Tomashek KM, Wallman C. "Late-preterm" infants: a population at risk. Pediatrics. 2007;120:1390–401.
2. Raju TNK. The "late preterm" birth – ten years later. Pediatrics. 2017;139:1–4.
3. Leone A, Ersfeld P, Adams M, Meyer Schiffer P, Bucher HO, Arlettaz R. Neonatal morbidity in singleton late preterm infants compared with full-term infants. Acta Pediatr. 2012;101:e6–10.
4. Chi C. Hypertensive disorders of pregnancy. In: Singh K, editor. Integrated approach to obstetrics and gynecology. World Scientific, New Jersey; 2016. p. 317–328.
5. Gyamfi-Bannerman C, Thom EA, Blackwell SC, Tita ATN, Reddy UM, Saade GR, et al. Antenatal betamethasone for women at risk for late preterm delivery. N Engl J Med. 2016;374:1311–20.
6. The American College of Obstetrics and Gynecology Committee on Obstetric Practice. Medically indicated late preterm and early-term deliveries. Committee opinion 560. Washington, DC: ACOG; 2013 (reaffirmed 2017). p. 1–3.
7. Mac Bird T, Bronstein JM, Hall RW, Lowery CL, Nugent R, Mays GP. Late preterm infants: birth outcomes and health care utilization in the first year. Pediatrics. 2010;126:e311–9.
8. Eidelman AI, Schanler RJ. Breastfeeding and the use of human milk. Pediatrics. 2012;129(3):e827–41.
9. Watchko JW. Hyperbilirubinemia and bilirubin toxicity in the late preterm infant. Clin Perinatol. 2006;33:839–52.
10. Kuzniewicz MW, Parker SJ, Schnake-Mahl A, Escobar GJ. Hospital readmissions and emergency department visits in moderate preterm, late preterm, and early term infants. Clin Perinatol. 2013;40:753–75.
11. Teune MJ, Bakhuizen S, Gyamfi-Bannerman C, Opmeer BG, vanKaam AH, van Wassenaer AG, et al. A systematic review of severe morbidity in infants born late preterm. Am J Obstet Gynecol. 2011;205:374.e1–9.
12. Adamkin DH. Clinical report – postnatal glucose homeostasis in late-preterm and term infants. Pediatrics. 2011;127:575–9.
13. Coffman S. Late preterm infants and risk for RSV. MCN. 2009;34:378–84.
14. Phillips RM, Goldstein M, Hougland K, Nandyal R, Pizzica A, Santo-Donato A, et al. Multidisciplinary guidelines for the care of late preterm infants. J Perinatol. 2013;33:S5–S22.
15. McGowan JE, Alderice FA, Holmes VA, Johnston L. Early childhood development of late-preterm infants: a systematic review. Pediatrics. 2011;127:1111–24.
16. Woythaler MA, McCormick MG, Smith VG. Late preterm infants have worse 24-month neurodevelopmental outcomes than term infants. Pediatrics. 2011;127:e622–9.

6 Jaundice in the Newborn

Warren Rosenfeld

Introduction

Jaundice, the clinical presentation of hyperbilirubinemia, remains one of the most common clinical problems in all of pediatrics. Nearly every baby has a rise in bilirubin, and in 60–84% of all babies [1, 2], it becomes clinically apparent so that the baby appears jaundiced to the observer. Jaundice is a normal physiologic event in the newborn, but the elevated bilirubin is almost always indirect (unconjugated) bilirubin which at high levels can enter into tissues (i.e., the brain). This rarely occurs, but if it does, serious complications with lifelong consequences (e.g., VIII nerve deafness, kernicterus) may result [3].

In the nursery, the provider is faced with a common occurrence, jaundice, which will usually not peak until after discharge and outside the hospital setting but which in rare circumstances may have a devastating effect on the baby. How to anticipate and manage jaundice and to provide a measured plan that will not lead to overtreatment but also prevent serious damage is a daily nursery dilemma. Anticipating that jaundice in some degree may appear in every baby, and having a designed approach to jaundice is basic to newborn care management.

W. Rosenfeld, MD
Department of Pediatrics, SUNY/Stony Brook School of Medicine, Stony Brook, NY, USA

Department of Pediatrics, Mount Sinai - South Nassau Medical Center, Oceanside, NY, USA
e-mail: warren.rosenfeld@snch.org

Case Presentation

It's Friday morning, and you are examining a 36-h-old neonate whose parents are anxious to go home. The baby is a male, 6 lb, 6 oz, 37 2/7 weeks of gestational age (accurate artificial insemination). The mother is 35 years old, G1P0, B+, and of Korean ethnicity with gestational diabetes.

There was prolonged rupture of the membranes for 37 h. She was induced with Pitocin and was delivered by vacuum extraction. Apgar score was 9/10.

The baby has been doing well. The weight is stable, and he is taking breast milk with supplementation. The exam is unremarkable except for a caput and ecchymosis on the scalp. The head and chest examinations are normal. The abdomen is soft, and there is no palpable liver or spleen. The baby has jaundice which covers the head, shoulders, and chest.

At this time you:

1. Order a transcutaneous bilirubin.
2. Order a total serum bilirubin.
3. Discharge the patient with follow-up within 24 h.
4. Place the baby under phototherapy.

G. I. Martin, W. Rosenfeld (eds.), *Common Problems in the Newborn Nursery*,
https://doi.org/10.1007/978-3-319-95672-5_6

Many nurseries have instituted universal screening for bilirubin prior to discharge. Babies may be screened by either transcutaneous bilirubin readings or by a heel stick serum bilirubin. (All published guidelines citing bilirubin values are based on heel stick determinations of bilirubin). If your nursery has a screening policy, then you would already have a pre-discharge value for bilirubin. If universal screening is not in place in your nursery, then as the provider you must have a systematic approach to assessing the level of jaundice and how to manage this issue during the nursery stay, at the time of discharge, and following discharge.

Visible jaundice to the chest at 36 h of life would warrant an assessment of bilirubin levels [4]. While clinical assessment of skin color can be an indicator of hyperbilirubinemia, accurate clinical assessment has wide variance and has been documented to have inconsistent correlation with laboratory values [5, 6]. Therefore performing a transcutaneous bilirubin [1] or drawing a serum bilirubin [2] would be the proper response.

Answer: (1 or 2)

In this case a transcutaneous bilirubin was done and was reported as 12.5 mg/dL.

At this time you:

1. Order a total serum bilirubin.
2. Hold discharge and order a follow-up transcutaneous bilirubin in 4 h.
3. Discharge the patient with a follow-up within 24 h.
4. Place the baby under phototherapy.

Transcutaneous measurement of bilirubin is a screening test [7–9]. Correlation with serum bilirubin is accurate at lower levels but is less accurate at levels as they approach 15 mg/dL. The exact value for bilirubin is important, and clinical decisions may be very different over a narrow range of values. Therefore a total serum bilirubin [1] should be drawn at this time to be able to make the proper clinical decision.

Answer: 1

You order a serum bilirubin, and results return an hour later. The bilirubin is 10.4 mg/dL (indirect 9.9, direct 0.5). How would you manage this patient?

1. Discharge with a follow-up on Monday (108 h of age).
2. Discharge and follow up on Saturday (60 h of age).
3. Follow in hospital with further serum bilirubin testing.
4. Place under phototherapy.

There are a number of tools available to help make your decision. The first is the Bhutani nomogram (Fig. 6.1) for the designation of risk for future hyperbilirubinemia [10]. As with all the nomograms and graphs used to manage neonatal jaundice, it is imperative that values are plotted on the graphs on an hour-to-hour basis. Bilirubin rises rapidly in the first 72 h of life, and what is considered normal at one time may be abnormal at another. A bilirubin of 10 mg/dL during the second day of life may be worrisome at 25 h of age and much less concerning at 47 h of age.

Using the Bhutani nomogram, this baby with a bilirubin of 10.4 mg/dL plots out in the top of the high-intermediate zone.

The Bhutani nomogram is an indicator of risk and does not determine what treatment a baby should receive. The majority of babies (60%) who originally plot out in the high-risk zone will fall below the 95th percentile on future bilirubin measurements, while 79% of the high-intermediate group will have their bilirubin decrease on subsequent bilirubin determinations [10]. In the publication presenting the nomogram, it was reported that there was a little risk for subsequent hyperbilirubinemia for babies who were in the low-intermediate and low zones. Several subsequent reports have shown that these babies may also be at risk for hyperbilirubinemia requiring phototherapy [11, 12]. As emphasized in Dr. Bhutani's original paper, the provider must not only determine the risk zone but also determine what risk factors are present and their potential effect on bilirubin metabolism (Table 6.1).

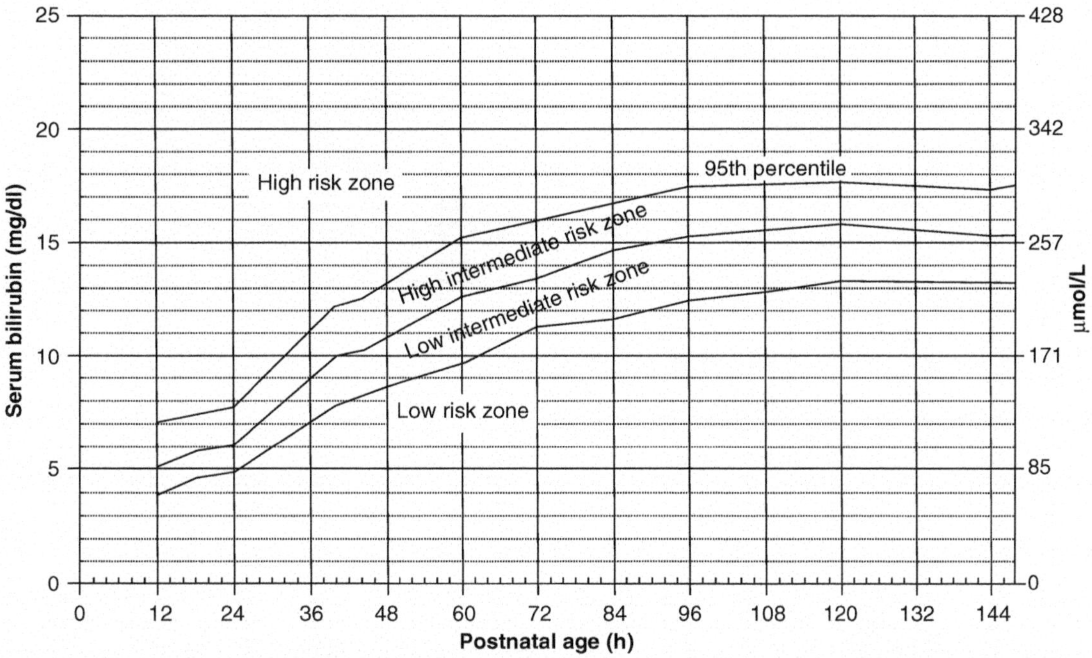

Fig. 6.1 Estimation of risk for hyperbilirubinemia. *Bilirubin values defining risk zones*. The Bhutani nomogram delineates the risk zones (low, low intermediate, high intermediate, and high) for developing clinically significant hyperbilirubinemia (≥95th percentile for age) in term and late pre-term well neonates based on hour-specific serum bilirubin values. In addition to the risk zone, the clinician must consider risk factors present at the time of discharge. If risk factor(s) are present, the baby may still be at risk even if they fall in a lower risk factor zone [10]

Table 6.1 Risk factors for development of severe hyperbilirubinemia in infants of 35 or more weeks of gestation

Major risk factors
Pre-discharge TSB or TcB level in the high-risk zone
Jaundice observed in the first 24 h
Blood group incompatibility with positive direct antiglobulin test, other known hemolytic disease (e.g., G6PD deficiency)
Gestational age of 35–36 weeks
Previous sibling received phototherapy
Cephalohematoma or significant bruising
Exclusive breastfeeding
East Asian race
Minor risk factors
Pre-discharge TSB or TcB level in the high-intermediate-risk zone
Early discharge
Gestational age of 37–38 weeks
Jaundice observed before discharge
Previous sibling with jaundice
Macrosomic infant of a diabetic mother
Maternal age ≥25 years
Male gender

Adapted from Ref. [13]
Risk factors for the development of significant hyperbilirubinemia (≥95th percentile)

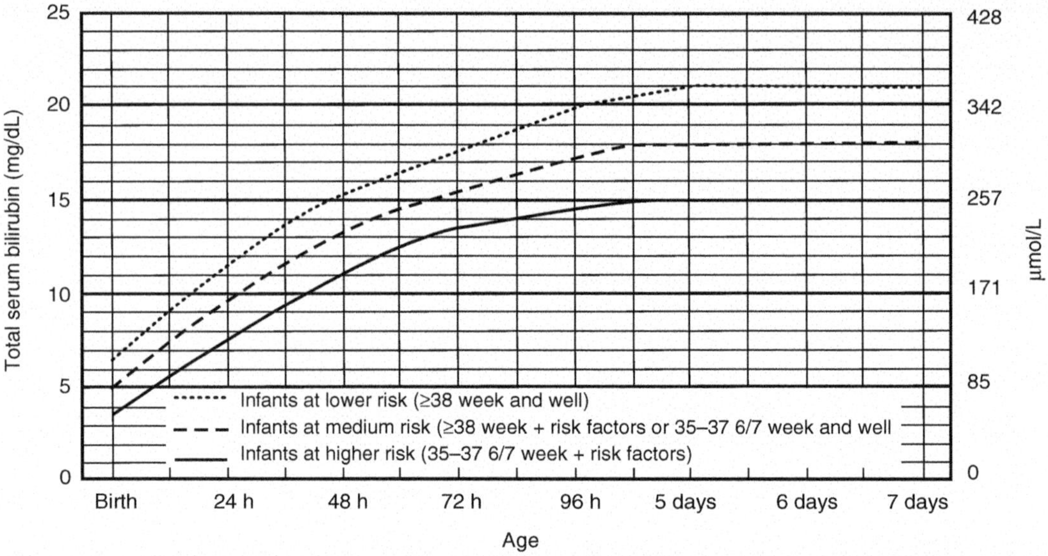

Fig. 6.2 Guideline for bilirubin threshold for initiation of phototherapy in hospitalized term and late preterm neonates. Graphic presentation of the guideline for the bilirubin level at which phototherapy should be initiated. At any given hour, the level to start phototherapy will vary depending on gestational age and presence of risk factors. Risk factors include ABO incompatibility, Rh incompatibility, other isoimmune hemolytic diseases, G-6-P-D (G6PD deficiency), asphyxia, lethargy, temperature instability, sepsis, acidosis, and albumin <3.0 m/dL (if measured) and differ from the risk factors for the development of hyperbilirubinemia [13]. Use total bilirubin. Do not subtract direct reacting or conjugated bilirubin; For well infants 35–37 6/7 week the clinician can adjust TSB levels for intervention around the medium risk line. It is an option to intervene at lower TSB levels for infants closer to 35 weeks and at higher TSB levels for those closer to 37 6/7 week; It is an option to provide conventional phototherapy in hospital or at home at TSB levels 2–3 mg/dL (35–50 mmol/L) below those shown but home phototherapy should not be used in any infant with risk factors

Without knowing the risk factors, a follow-up within 24 h of discharge (60 h of age) or keeping in the hospital for further observation is an acceptable choice. Discharge with a follow-up in 3 additional days might allow time for bilirubin to rise to critical levels. Placing a baby under phototherapy should be determined by the graphs contained in the phototherapy guidelines (Fig. 6.2).

Answer: 2 or 3

How many risk factors were present in this patient?

1. None
2. 2–5
3. 6–9
4. ≥10

Answer: 3

This patient had a large number of risk factors for subsequent hyperbilirubinemia, and this must be considered in decision-making. It should also be remembered that these are risk factors for developing hyperbilirubinemia and are different than those used when determining whether phototherapy and/or exchange transfusion are necessary [13, 14]. In the above case, many of the risk factors for subsequent hyperbilirubinemia were present and even the bilirubin was in the high-intermediate zone. Further observation in the hospital could certainly be an appropriate course of action. Discharge with close follow-up could also be considered. One risk factor not noted in the criteria below is a Friday discharge. You, as the responsible health-care provider, must be certain that there will be follow-up at the appropriate time. A follow-up bilirubin within 24 h is necessary in this case and might be determined with a transcutaneous reading (which would need a serum bilirubin done if in the high range) of serum bilirubin. A mechanism for bilirubin measurements on weekends should be in place if at risk newborns are to be discharged on Thursdays and Fridays.

The AAP guideline for hyperbilirubinemia [13, 14] makes recommendations for follow-up. Discharged newborns should be examined by a qualified health-care professional in the first few days after discharge to assess infant well-being and the presence or absence of jaundice. It is also helpful for other issues including the adequacy of feedings.

Infant discharged	Should be seen by age
Before age 24 h	72 h
Between 24 and 47.9 h	96 h
Between 48 and 72 h	120 h

When and where this assessment will occur are determined by the age (in hours) at discharge, presence or absence of risk factors for hyperbilirubinemia (as above), and risk of other neonatal problems. For some newborns discharged before 48 h, two follow-up visits may be required. The first visit is between 24 and 72 h, and the second visit is between 72 and 120 h. Clinical judgment should be used in determining a follow-up. Earlier or more frequent follow-up should be provided for those who have risk factors for hyperbilirubinemia. Those discharged with few or no risk factors can be seen after longer intervals.

If appropriate follow-up cannot be ensured in the presence of elevated risk for developing hyperbilirubinemia, it may be necessary to delay discharge either until appropriate follow-up can be ensured or the period of greatest risk has passed (72–96 h).

The patient had a 10.4 bilirubin at 36 h of life. Is he a candidate for phototherapy?

1. Yes
2. No

Although this baby was only in the high-intermediate zone for risk, he is between 36 and 38 weeks. Whether or not to start phototherapy is not based on the risk zones from the Bhutani nomogram but from the criteria for the initiation of phototherapy published in the AAP guideline for hyperbilirubinemia [13].

Phototherapy would be considered at a lower level in a baby who is 35–37 6/7 weeks compared to a ≥38 week's baby without risk. Another useful guide for determining the need for phototherapy is the application, BiliTool. This application incorporates the criteria from the AAP guidelines and is used by many clinicians [15].

As mentioned previously, the risk factors that are considered in the decision to start phototherapy differ from those for the risk of hyperbilirubinemia. These include the gestational age of the baby. The less mature the baby, the lower the threshold for initiation of phototherapy. Also the presence of hemolytic disease, including isoimmune hemolytic disease and G6PD deficiency, asphyxia, significant lethargy, temperature instability, sepsis, acidosis, or low albumin <3.0 mg/dL (if measured), would require starting phototherapy at a lower bilirubin level than in a baby with no risk factors.

Answer: 2

At this time the bilirubin level of 10.4 mg/dL is below the phototherapy value to initiate phototherapy in a neonate with medium risk (12.6 mg/dL).

An appropriate course of treatment might be:

1. Start a non-intensive phototherapy.
2. Start an intensive phototherapy.
3. Continue to observe, and repeat bilirubin in 6–8 h.
4. Discharge patient with follow-up in 24 h.

While some clinicians adjust the medium risk line on the phototherapy graph, starting phototherapy below the line for newborns closer to 35 weeks, the patient in this case is 37 2/7 weeks. It should also be remembered that the phototherapy graphs were designed to prevent kernicterus and have latitude in protecting the patient from developing complications of hyperbilirubinemia. In addition phototherapy is an intervention which for many years has been thought to be totally safe. However, new concerns are being raised. While phototherapy has been utilized for over 40 years in the United States, when originally introduced, the energy of the phototherapy lights was between 5 and 10 μw/cm²/nm. As the intensity of the lights has increased, their energy output (30–40 μw/cm²/nm) has increased as well. Will the increased intensity of the phototherapy lights utilized in the last several years lead to complications not seen previously? Recent reports of DNA breakage [16], precancerous skin lesions [17], and an increased risk of childhood cancer [18] should make clinicians aware that long-term complications may potentially be present and may now only begin to appear. Phototherapy also has several immediate side effects. It may interfere with maternal bonding, decrease the success of breastfeeding, and increase hospital length of stay [19]. With these factors in mind, phototherapy should not be started until the criteria for treatment are met. Continuing to observe and repeat bilirubin in 6–8 h is a prudent course of management.

Answer: 3

Following this treatment choice, two scenarios are possible.

Scenario 1: A repeat serum bilirubin 8 h later (44 h of life) is repeated and is reported as 10.5 mg/dL.

1. You are surprised because patients in the high-intermediate risk zone usually continue to increase and require phototherapy.
2. You expected this result because the majority of patients in the high-intermediate zone infrequently cross the 95th percentile and don't require phototherapy.

In Bhutani's study on the experience with his nomogram, only 21% of babies in the high-intermediate group crossed over the 95th percentile on a subsequent bilirubin determination, and only 40% in the high-risk zone had a similar rise [10]. It should again be emphasized that the Bhutani nomogram is a measure of risk not a guide to therapy. While high risk in the nomogram is >95th percentile, the phototherapy graph (13) does not initiate phototherapy in a full-term baby without risk factors until the 99th percentile.

At this time the bilirubin level of 10.5 mg/dL is below the medium risk line for the initiation of phototherapy (at 44 h ta level of 12.6 mg/dL would require phototherapy).

Answer: 2

An appropriate course of treatment might be:

1. Start a non-intensive phototherapy.
2. Start an intensive phototherapy.
3. Continue to observe and repeat bilirubin in 6–8 h.
4. Discharge patient with follow-up in 24 h.

This baby's levels have now remained stable over the last 8 h and are well below the levels would have needed to institute phototherapy. The clinical decision is to determine if levels have peaked and will remain stable or decrease or is there a risk of further significant increases will occur warranting phototherapy. If the baby is eating well, is not a setup for or at risk of hemolysis and the baby can be followed within the next 24 h, discharge is an appropriate choice. It should also be remembered that this patient is still being discharged at <48 h of age, making a visit necessary by 96 h. It would be appropriate for this baby to be seen the day following discharge.

Answer: 4

Scenario 2: A repeat serum bilirubin 8 h later (44 h of life) is repeated and is reported as 14.5 mg/dL.

1. Start a non-intensive phototherapy.
2. Start an intensive phototherapy.
3. Continue to observe and repeat bilirubin in 6–8 h.
4. Discharge patient with follow-up in 24 h.

The baby has now crossed the threshold (12.6 mg/dL) for a baby at medium risk (35–37

6/7 weeks of gestation) for the start of phototherapy. When phototherapy is initiated in the hospital, it should be “intensive phototherapy.” Standard phototherapy delivers an intensity of light in the range of 5–10 mw/cm^2/nm, while intensive phototherapy delivers an intensity of >30 mw/cm^2/nm.

Answer: 2

The intensity of the phototherapy equipment depends on several factors.

1. Type of light
2. Number of lights
3. Area covered by the lights
4. Distance of the baby from the light

Every hospital should have a protocol as to what is meant by intensive phototherapy [13]. Is it double lights (which may be delivered by one device)? Is it light above and below the baby? Is it done in an Isolette or in a bassinet? All these factors will determine the dose of light the baby receives.

1. Type of lights. A number of devices are effective in delivering light in the range of 430–490 nm. Special blue fluorescent tubes are the most efficient for use in traditional phototherapy units. Light-emitting diode (LED) lights are also in common use. Fiber-optic blankets and specially designed units for placement under the baby are also available.
2. Numbers of lights. Several of the LED lights can deliver a single or double dose of light. Intensive phototherapy would usually require the double mode. Placing banks of fluorescent (special blue) lights can increase dosing, but surrounding the baby with banks of lights is often cumbersome. Systems that deliver light from below the baby can also increase the dosing of light. This may include placing the baby on a biliblanket or in a specially designed bassinet that can deliver light from below.
3. Area covered by the lights can be increased by surrounding the baby with light as mentioned previously and assuring that the baby is centered in the field of light. Irradiance at the periphery is of the field of light which is far less than in the center.
4. Distance from the light source to the baby. The further the light from the baby, the less the dose of light. While many hospitals place babies in an Isolette for phototherapy and an intensive dose of light can be delivered (>30 mw/cm^2/nm), if necessary babies can be treated in an open bassinet and the lights brought closer to the baby to increase the intensity.

Intensive phototherapy with lights delivering a double dose of light from above and light from below is usually very effective in decreasing the bilirubin level. The effect is greater at the higher bilirubin levels when therapy is started and rates of decline of 0.5–1.0 mg/dL/h are not uncommon when the lights are first started.

Answer: 1, 2, 3, 4

The baby has been placed under the phototherapy lights. Which of the following should be done?

1. Stop breastfeeding.
2. Repeat bilirubin measurement in 2 h.
3. Repeat bilirubin measurement in 4 h.
4. Repeat bilirubin measurement in 6 h.
5. Repeat bilirubin measurement in 8 h.

Breastfeeding should not be stopped but rather encouraged. In fact, increasing the frequency of feedings may be helpful in decreasing bilirubin levels. Other strategies may include taking the baby out from under the lights to allow for breastfeeding, using a biliblanket to wrap the baby during time-out from under the lights, and pumping the mother’s breast for milk to be bottle or spoon-fed (considered as a last alternative by some). Unless the baby is dehydrated, supplementing the baby with water, formula, or glucose water has no effect on unconjugated bilirubin levels because it is not water soluble [20].

The frequency of reassessing bilirubin levels is a clinical decision that involves several factors.

If the level was approaching the value that would require exchange transfusion, more frequent evaluation might be considered. It would be unusual for bilirubin to continue to rise unless there is a hemolytic process as the underlying cause of the hyperbilirubinemia. In most cases intensive phototherapy can reduce bilirubin by 0.5–1.0 mg/dL/h. The higher the bilirubin at the initiation of phototherapy, the faster the decline.

Repeat levels, except in the situation cited above, do not need to be repeated for 6–8 h, giving the phototherapy an opportunity to have an effect.

Answer: 4 or 5

What laboratory test(s) would be ordered when a patient is placed under phototherapy?

1. CBC with differential
2. Reticulocytes
3. Sepsis workup
4. G6PD analysis
5. Liver enzymes
6. Direct bilirubin
7. Coombs' test
8. Blood type
9. Urine for reducing substance

Discussion: [13]

1. CBC with differential: to determine if a hemolytic process is occurring and if sepsis might be a possibility.
2. Reticulocytes: to determine if a hemolytic process is occurring.
3. Sepsis workup: may be considered if suggested by history and physical exam.
4. G6PD analysis: If family history ethnic or geographic origin suggest. Also if a poor response to phototherapy or unexplained hemolysis.
5. Liver enzymes: not for indirect hyperbilirubinemia.
6. Direct bilirubin: At this time total serum bilirubin should be fractionated (direct and indirect).
7. Coombs' test: If not previously done.
8. Blood type: If not previously done.
9. Urine for reducing substance: Galactosemia would be a rare cause of neonatal jaundice, and reducing substances in the urine could be an early indicator (most cases are now identified on newborn screening).

The level at initiation of phototherapy was 14.5 mg/dL. You would stop phototherapy at:

1. 14.5 mg/dL
2. 13.5 mg/dL
3. 12.5 mg/dL
4. 11.5 mg/dL
5. 10.5 mg/dL

The decision to decide when to stop phototherapy in a baby who is readmitted for hyperbilirubinemia is relatively straightforward. The decision to stop phototherapy in a baby who has been started during the original hospital stay is less clear. Most babies who are readmitted for hyperbilirubinemia are ≥72 h of age, and bilirubin levels are >18 mg/dL at the time of admission. Usually bilirubin conjugation has been established at this age, and the combination of light and maturation will result in a decrease of bilirubin to a safe and usually stable level. In cases of a readmitted baby, a level less than 13–14 mg/dL would be an appropriate level at which to discontinue phototherapy. It would also be appropriate to discharge the patient without a rebound bilirubin level (unless hemolysis is suspected) [13].

In the patient presented above and in whom phototherapy was initiated at 44 h of life during the initial hospital stay for a bilirubin of 14.5 mg/dL, would a subsequent decrease in bilirubin reflect the effect of the lights and/or the maturation of the liver?

If the repeat bilirubin remained at 14.5 mg/dL at 52 h, it would appear that the bilirubin levels would have continued to rise without phototherapy and are still above the line for phototherapy. The lights should be continued.

If at 52 h, bilirubin was 13.5 mg/dL, it would now be just below the threshold for phototherapy treatment. However after 8 h of phototherapy, the bilirubin level would have been expected to fall further, and the concern that the lights are just keeping up with jaundice levels should be considered. Phototherapy should be continued.

If the level fell to 12.5 mg/dL, this is more in line with the effect of phototherapy. The provider may feel both the lights and maturation of the liver have played a role. Discontinuation might be considered by some [21].

A decrease in the bilirubin to 11.5 mg/dL or below is certainly more reassuring and may indicate that both the lights and the maturation of liver conjugation may have had an effect. This level is well below the line for phototherapy. This level of jaundice would permit discontinuation of the lights [20].

Providers should remember that the proper graphs to use in making clinical decisions after phototherapy has been initiated or completed are the graphs for phototherapy and exchange transfusion. The Bhutani nomogram is used to assess risk for future jaundice and cannot be used after the use of phototherapy.

Answer: 3 or 4

Would you now order a rebound bilirubin?

1. Yes
2. No

If you are suspicious or knew that hemolysis was the cause of the jaundice, a rebound bilirubin level is indicated. Providers should also be aware that when phototherapy has been initiated early on in the nursery course, phototherapy may prevent increases in bilirubin. In babies with hemolysis, clinicians are comforted by bilirubin levels that fall below the line for phototherapy but need a rebound level to see if levels without lights will again start to increase. Since the phototherapy graph reflects the natural increase of bilirubin levels in the first days of life, a steady or decreasing level below the line for treatment may not reflect that hemolysis is continuing. The baby may not be able to keep levels in the safe zone without phototherapy. Even with a safe rebound level, these babies should be seen and evaluated within 24 h of discharge [13].

In babies where hemolysis is not the underlying cause for hyperbilirubinemia but who had phototherapy in the first 72–96 h of life during the birth admission, a bilirubin level should be measured within 24 h of discontinuing phototherapy. As mentioned above in babies readmitted for hyperbilirubinemia and in whom hemolysis is not thought to be the underlying cause of the hyperbilirubinemia, no rebound value is necessary.

Answer: 1

Clinical Pearls

1. Follow the guidelines for follow-up even if a discharge bilirubin is done and may be considered safe.
2. Use the Bhutani nomogram to assess risk, not treatment.
3. Remember risk factors for the development of hyperbilirubinemia. Even babies in the low and low-intermediate zones with risk factors may develop hyperbilirubinemia. Late preterm and breast-fed babies are certainly among this group.
4. Remember risk factors for initiation of phototherapy. They differ from those that put a baby at risk for hyperbilirubinemia.
5. Use phototherapy graphs and their risk stratification to determine if phototherapy is necessary.
6. Encourage breastfeeding. More frequent feedings and supporting the mother are vital to the success of breastfeeding and decreasing the incidence of jaundice.
7. Don't use phototherapy unless it is indicated (don't treat prophylactically).

References

1. Keren R, Tremont K, Luan X, Cnaan A. Visual assessment of jaundice in term and late preterm infants. Arch Dis Child Fetal Neonatal El. 2009;94: F317–22.
2. Bhutani VK, Stark AR, Lazzeroni LC, Poland R, Gourly GR, Kazmierczak S, et al. Predischarge screening for severe hyperbilirubinemia identifies infants who need phototherapy. J Pediatr. 2013;162:477–82.e1.
3. Watchko JF, Tiribelli C. Bilirubin induced neurologic damage: mechanisms and management approaches. N Engl J Med. 2013;369:2021.
4. Kramer LI. Advancement of dermal icterus in the jaundiced newborn. Amer J Dis Child. 1969;118:454.
5. Moyer VA, Ahn C, Sneed S. Accuracy of clinical judgment in neonatal jaundice. Arch Pediatr Adolesc Med. 2000;154:391.
6. Tayaba R, Gribetz D, Gribetz D, Holzman IR. Noninvasive estimation of serum bilirubin. Pediatrics. 1998;102:E28.
7. Engle W, Jackson GL, Engle NG. Transcutaneous bilirubinometry. Semin Perinat. 2014;38:438.
8. Rubaltelli FF, Gourley GR, Loskamp N, Modi N, Roth-Kleiner M, Sender A, Vert P. Transcutaneous bilirubin measurement: a multicenter evaluation of a new device. Pediatrics. 2001;107:1264.
9. Taylor JA, Burgos AE, Flaherman V, Chung E, Simpson EA, Goyal NK, Von Kohorn I, Dhepyasuwan N, The Better Outcomes Through Research Network. Discrepancies between transcutaneous and serum bilirubin measurements. Pediatrics. 2015;135:224. https://doi.org/10.1542/peds.2014-1919.
10. Bhutani VK, Johnson L, Sivieri MS. Predictive ability of a pre-discharge serum bilirubin for subsequent significant hyperbilirubinemia in healthy term and near-term newborns. Pediatrics. 1999;103:6.
11. Bromiker R, Bin-Nun A, Schimmel MS, Hammerman C, Kaplan M. Neonatal hyperbilirubinemia in the low-intermediate-risk category on the bilirubin nomogram. Pediatrics. 2012;130:e470. https://doi.org/10.1542/peds.2012-0005.
12. Slaughter J, Annibale D, Suresh G. False-negative results of pre-discharge bilirubin screening to predict severe hyperbilirubinemia: a need for caution. Eur J Pediatr. 2009;168:1461.
13. American Academy of Pediatrics Subcommittee on Hyperbilirubinemia. Management of hyperbilirubinemia in the newborn infant 35 or more weeks of gestation. Pediatrics. 2004;114:297. https://doi.org/10.1542/peds.114.1.297.
14. Maisels MJ, Bhutani VK, Bogen D, Newman TB, Ar S, Watchko JF. Hyperbilirubinemia in the newborn infant ≥35 weeks' gestation: an update with clarification. Pediatrics. 2009;124:1193. https://doi.org/10.1542/peds.2009-0329.
15. Longhurst C, Turner S, Burgos AE. Development of a web-based decision support tool to increase use of neonatal hyperbilirubinemia guidelines. Jt Comm J Qual Patient Saf. 2009;35:256.
16. Christensen T, Reitan JB, Kinn G. Single-strand breaks in the DNA of human cells exposed to visible light from phototherapy lamps in the presence and absence of bilirubin. J Photochem Photobiol B. 1990;7:337.
17. Csoma Z, Toth-Molnar E, Balogh K, et al. Neonatal blue light phototherapy and melanocytic nevi: a twin study. Pediatrics. 2011;128:e856.
18. Newman TB, Wickeremasinghe C, Walsh EM, Grimes BA, McCulloch CE, Kuzniewicz MW. Retrospective cohort study of phototherapy and childhood cancer in Northern California. Pediatrics. 2016;137:1.
19. Maisels MJ. Managing the jaundiced newborn. A persistent challenge. CMAJ. 2015;187:335.
20. Martinez JC, Otheguy L, Garcia H, Savorani M, Mogni B, Martinez JC Jr, Maisels MJ. Hyperbilirubinemia in the breast-fed newborn: a control trial of four interventions. Pediatrics. 1993;91:470.
21. Barak M, Berger I, Dollberg S, Mimouni FB, Mandel D. When should phototherapy be stopped? A pilot study comparing two targets of serum bilirubin concentrations. Acta Paediatri. 2009;98:277.

Neonatal Bacterial Infections

7

Thomas A. Hooven and Richard A. Polin

Introduction

The perinatal period is a time of increased susceptibility to bacterial infections. While recent literature has shown that the amnioplacental unit has a distinct and likely adaptive microbiome [1], the fact remains that during birth the newborn transitions from a nearly sterile milieu into an extrauterine environment teeming with bacteria. Exposure to potentially pathogenic species can occur prenatally, during passage through the birth canal, or from environmental sources after birth.

Furthermore, the neonatal immune system has key limitations that render it vulnerable to invasion by bacteria that pose little threat later in childhood (e.g., group B *Streptococcus*). Adaptive immunity—which depends on a diverse repertoire of antibodies against foreign antigens—is rudimentary at birth, consisting mainly of maternal IgG transferred across the placenta during pregnancy.

Neonatal innate immunity is also relatively weak compared with later in childhood. Neutrophils, the first responders to developing infection, are less abundant and less effective during the newborn period [2, 3]. Newborn skin and mucosal barriers are more permeable to bacteria [4]. Finally, the baby's own colonizing microbiome, which primes the immune system and excludes potential pathogens, takes months to become established and stabilized [5, 6]. Underdevelopment of these protective systems leaves the newborn at high risk of infection.

Many newborn bacterial infections present with non-specific signs, which can be subtle in the early stages. For the practitioner in the nursery, the challenge is maintaining a high level of suspicion and readiness to act with appropriate urgency if there is persuasive evidence of infection while simultaneously recognizing that the majority of babies with mild symptoms early in life are not actually infected.

T. A. Hooven · R. A. Polin (✉)
Department of Pediatrics, Vagelos College of Physicians and Surgeons, Columbia University, New York, NY, USA
e-mail: rap32@columbia.edu

Case Presentation

You arrive at the nursery, where a 3-h-old, ex-39-week gestation, 4.1 kg boy awaits your assessment. His primiparous mother is a healthy 32-year-old. Delivery was by Cesarean section following arrest of descent, 22 h after spontaneous rupture of the membranes. The amniotic fluid

G. I. Martin, W. Rosenfeld (eds.), *Common Problems in the Newborn Nursery*,
https://doi.org/10.1007/978-3-319-95672-5_7

was clear. A maternal temperature of 101.5 °C was recorded 60 min before delivery, which her obstetrician attributed to her epidural anesthesia. There was fetal tachycardia to 190 beats per minute coincident with the fever. Maternal GBS screening at 35 weeks was negative, and she received no intrapartum antibiotics. Her CBC and differential, drawn an hour before delivery, were unremarkable.

The baby is pink and comfortably sleeping. You note a respiratory rate of 70 breaths per minute, with no retractions. Other vital signs are normal for a newborn. During your examination, he wakes briefly and cries but otherwise remains asleep. There are no other significant examination findings. The nurse says that he has breastfed once since birth. His blood glucose level was 53 mmol/L before feeding and rose to 65 mmol/L after feeding.

What risk factor for early-onset sepsis is present in this case?

1. Chorioamnionitis.
2. Prolonged rupture of membranes.
3. Male gender.
4. Hypoglycemia.

Prolonged rupture of membranes ($\geq$18 h) is a risk factor for early-onset sepsis (sepsis that develops within the first 72 h of life). Shorter durations of rupture are also associated with sepsis risk that increases over time [7]. The chorioamniotic membranes and the amniotic fluid together provide an important physical and immunologic barrier against bacterial infection of the fetus. Ex vivo studies of intact membrane samples have shown that they are impermeable to GBS, even at high inoculum densities [8]. Amniotic fluid is rich in antimicrobial peptides (AMPs), and bacterial exposure increases AMP expression by the membranes [9].

When these integrated protective barriers are compromised for a prolonged period, bacteria that have ascended from the lower reproductive tract are able to multiply in the uterine cavity, colonize the fetus, and potentially invade the bloodstream before or shortly after birth, leading to early-onset sepsis.

Chorioamnionitis, meaning invasion of the membranes and amniotic fluid by a pathogenic microorganism, is an independent risk factor for early-onset sepsis [10], but was not diagnosed in this case. The diagnosis of chorioamnionitis is typically made based on clinical criteria of maternal fever plus two of the five additional signs: maternal leukocytosis, maternal tachycardia, fetal tachycardia, uterine tenderness, and purulent amniotic fluid. The diagnosis can also be made based on histological identification of placental infection.

In reality, however, studies have shown that formal criteria for diagnosing maternal chorioamnionitis are frequently bypassed by practitioners, who make the diagnosis of chorioamnionitis on the basis of maternal fever alone [11]. This can put the provider in a difficult position: caring for a newborn whose mother was diagnosed with chorioamnionitis on the basis of a single criterion that may have other potential causes (such as epidural anesthesia).

While the most recent versions of official guidelines for managing newborns with risk factors for sepsis recommend a conservative approach—with automatic empiric antibiotic administration—to babies whose mothers were diagnosed with chorioamnionitis [12–14], a consensus among neonatologists has been shifting toward a more nuanced approach. Many believe that, when the only risk factor is maternal chorioamnionitis (regardless of how it was diagnosed), term or late-preterm newborns without symptoms can be safely managed with regularly scheduled serial examinations rather than a laboratory workup and empiric antibiotics [15]. Strong evidence is accruing for this approach [16–18], and updated guidelines with a greater degree of flexibility are likely forthcoming.

Hypoglycemia is a non-specific sign of early-onset sepsis, but is not an independent risk factor, and the blood glucose measurements reported in this case are normal for a newborn. Male gender is not an independent risk factor for early-onset sepsis.

Answer: 2

Case Presentation (Continued)

Over the next 2 h, the baby's condition deteriorates. By 5 h of age, he is tachypneic to 100 breaths per minute, and his tone is decreased.

Your next step should be to obtain:

1. Blood culture.
2. Surface cultures of the axilla and ear canal.
3. Head ultrasound.
4. Urine culture.

Signs of early-onset sepsis are variable and often non-specific. A previously well-appearing newborn who develops abnormal vital signs and a concerning physical examination should always prompt consideration of infection. In these circumstances, multiple steps should be taken: blood should be drawn for culture, a complete blood count, and C-reactive protein or procalcitonin measurement. A repeat blood glucose evaluation would also be prudent. At least one chest X-ray should be obtained as part of an evaluation for early-onset sepsis, which often develops from an underlying pneumonia.

Urinary tract infection, though a common infection in older infants, is extremely unusual in the immediate newborn period (unless there is an underlying genitourinary malformation). Urine culture should therefore not be part of routine evaluations for early-onset sepsis. If surface cultures are positive, they represent colonization and not infection. They add expense to the sepsis workup and provide very little information.

Answer: 1

Although central nervous system injury could present with tachypnea and hypotonia, there was no suggestion of hypoxic/ischemic injury during birth, and a sudden deterioration at 3–5 h of life should prompt assessment for infection before brain imaging.

Although not among the answer choices, a lumbar puncture might also be reasonably performed along with the blood culture at this time. Lumbar puncture is appropriate for babies with signs highly suggestive of sepsis, regardless of the blood culture status. Obtaining a cerebrospinal fluid sample prior to initiating antibiotics increases the odds of growing the causative organism. However, in cases where the diagnosis of sepsis is less clear but still necessary to exclude with a blood culture, it is acceptable to proceed without a lumbar puncture. If the blood culture does grow a pathogen, a lumbar puncture can be performed after antibiotics are initiated, often permitting meningitis to be diagnosed or excluded based on spinal fluid glucose, protein concentrations, and cell counts.

Case Presentation (Continued)

The baby is started on ampicillin and gentamicin and transferred to the neonatal ICU. Twenty-two hours after the blood culture is drawn, the laboratory confirms that it grew group B *Streptococcus*. A subsequent lumbar puncture yields CSF with glucose 15 mmol/L, protein 730 mg/dL, 10,000 RBC/μL, and 95 nucleated cells/μL with 90% PMNs and 10% lymphocytes.

Antibiotics should be started at anti-meningitis dosages when ruling out early-onset sepsis.

1. True
2. False

Multiple factors, including the dose, affect an antibiotic's ability to cross the blood-brain barrier [19]. Inflammation disrupts intercellular tight junctions, improving the penetrance of hydrophilic antibiotics (e.g., β-lactams and vancomycin) but not lipophilic antibiotics (e.g., fluoroquinolones and rifampin). Low molecular weight drugs penetrate more easily than those with higher molecular weight. Other factors include the degree of protein binding (antibiotics which are more tightly bound to serum proteins are less penetrant), presence of active transport systems, and specific etiology of the infection (*L. monocytogenes* causes more permeability than *E. coli*, for instance).

Ampicillin and gentamicin provide reasonably broad coverage against Gram-positive and Gram-negative bacteria in the cerebrospinal fluid and have synergistic effects for group B *Streptococcus*, *Listeria*, and *Enterococcus* that promote rapid sterilization of the central nervous system.

Adequate meningitis treatment consists of intravenous ampicillin 150 mg/kg per dose every 12 h and gentamicin 4 mg/kg per dose every 24 h. These doses are recommended regardless of whether a lumbar puncture has been performed. As mentioned above, in the case that the blood culture turns positive, a lumbar puncture can still provide significant diagnostic value even if the cerebrospinal fluid is already sterile.

Proven group B *Streptococcus* meningitis can be treated with ampicillin monotherapy for 14 days following the first negative blood culture. Combination of ampicillin and cefotaxime (75 mg/kg every 12 h) therapy is a good choice for early-onset meningitis without a definite organism (e.g., based on cerebrospinal fluid leukocytosis and elevated protein) in the setting of negative blood cultures.

Answer: 1

Approximately what percent of infants with early-onset sepsis due to group B *Streptococcus* are born to mothers with negative colonization screens?

1. 5%.
2. 20%.
3. 40%.
4. 70%.

Antenatal screening for maternal colonization with GBS and administration of intrapartum antibiotics have reduced the incidence of early-onset GBS sepsis from 1.7/1000 to 0.28/1000 live births [20, 21]. Screening has had no effect on the incidence of late-onset GBS sepsis. The majority of early-onset group B *Streptococcus* sepsis (between 60% and 75%) occurs in babies whose mother's antenatal colonization screen was negative [21]. Negative colonization screens in mothers whose babies develop group B *Streptococcus* early-onset sepsis may reflect improper testing procedures, maternal factors that decrease test sensitivity (such as undisclosed antibiotic use), or late colonization in the intervening weeks between the negative screen and delivery.

Answer: 4

What is the upper limit of acceptable CSF leukocytosis in a term neonate on day of life 1?

1. Any leukocytes in the CSF are indicative of meningitis
2. 8 cells/μL.
3. 14 cells/μL.
4. 40 cells/μL.

The normal CSF leukocyte count decreases during the first 7–10 days of life, eventually stabilizing at a mean count of 5 cells/μL [22]. A 2012 prospective study examined CSF indices in hospitalized babies undergoing lumbar puncture as part of sepsis evaluations that were ultimately negative (i.e., no definitive evidence of meningitis or bacteremia, Table 7.1) [23].

Among 130 term babies whose lumbar puncture was performed during the first week of life, the upper limit of normal CSF leukocytosis was 14 cells/μL (the upper limit was defined as the 75th percentile plus 1.5 × the interquartile range).

Answer: 3

Table 7.1 Normal CSF values from term infants

CSF index[a]	≤7 days (n = 130)	>7 days (n = 40)[b]
Median leukocytes (IQR)	3 (1–6)	2 (1–4)
Leukocyte upper limit	14	9
Median protein (IQR)	74 (54–96)	78 (60–100)
Protein upper limit	159	160
Median glucose (IQR)	50 (44–56)	52 (45–64)
Glucose lower limit	26	17

IQR interquartile range
[a]Upper/lower limit = upper/lower IQR bound +/− 1.5 × IQR
[b]Postnatal age range = 7–83 days
Srinivasan et al. [23]

The resident on service asks about correcting the number of WBCs in the CSF for the number of RBCs because the lumbar puncture was traumatic.

What is the best way to correct the CSF leukocyte count for blood contamination in a traumatic lumbar puncture?

1. Set the acceptable leukocyte threshold at 0.002 × CSF RBC.
2. Set the acceptable leukocyte threshold at (blood WBC × CSF RBC)/(blood RBC × 1000,000).
3. For every 1000 RBC/μL CSF, add 2 to the upper limit of normal CSF leukocytes.
4. Do not make any correction for the blood contamination.

Variants of the first three corrections have been used over the years, but have not held up under systematic scrutiny. Specifically, several groups have examined records from traumatic lumbar punctures in children ultimately found not to have meningitis (based on clinical course and culture results). Comparisons between measured CSF leukocyte counts from these traumatic lumbar punctures and predicted counts based on proposed correction factors have shown a poor correlation [24].

While it can be tempting to allow a higher CSF leukocyte count in babies whose CSF is contaminated with blood, the prudent approach is to retain standard test limits. Babies with true bacterial meningitis usually exhibit other abnormal CSF values (such as low CSF glucose concentrations) and clinical signs. This fact can be helpful when deciding how to proceed in a case where the CSF leukocyte count is slightly elevated and blood contamination is present.

Answer: 4

Case Presentation

You are caring for a 3-day-old, ex-38-week gestation boy whose mother had postpartum hemorrhage, complicating her discharge home. The pregnancy was uncomplicated. Maternal antenatal laboratory studies were normal except for a positive screen for group B *Streptococcus*, for which she received appropriate intrapartum antibiotic prophylaxis.

Until today, the baby has had an uneventful course, rooming in with the mother. This is her second child, and breastfeeding was established smoothly. Serial physical examinations have been unremarkable except for a mild pectus excavatum and a Mongolian spot.

Today the mother reports that the baby has been much more irritable and difficult to console. He has been feeding poorly since early morning, pulling off the breast and crying for up to 15 min at a time. He had a stool at midnight and a wet diaper at 8 AM, but no urine for the past 5 h. No fever has been recorded.

On examination, he is awake and crying loudly. When briefly calmed with a pacifier, his respiratory rate is 85 breaths per minute with mild retractions that are accentuated by his pectus. You note mild clear rhinorrhea. Lung auscultation is clear bilaterally. The cardiac exam is normal. The abdomen is soft and non-tender, with normal bowel sounds. His extremities are warm and well-perfused. Tone is normal.

You tell the mother that you will closely observe the baby. You also plan to send several laboratory studies.

Which sepsis screening laboratory result provides the most reassurance that the baby is uninfected?

1. White blood cell count under 10,000 cells/μL.
2. A normal absolute neutrophil count (ANC).
3. C-reactive protein (CRP) <10 mg/L.
4. Serum procalcitonin concentration > 0.2 ng/mL.

The white blood cell count is a poor predictor of sepsis unless very low (<5000/μL) or very high (>40,000/μL), in which case it has a better predictive value. A normal white blood cell count in a newborn should not be reassuring (i.e., the baby may still have sepsis). The same is true for a normal ANC.

CRP and procalcitonin are two well-studied infectious biomarkers [25, 26]. Procalcitonin levels start to rise 2–3 h after onset of a bacterial infection, peak at around 12 h, and then gradually normalize over the following 48–72 h. A normal procalcitonin (less than 0.2 ng/mL) is reassuring the baby is not infected. An elevated procalcitonin level is not predictive of infection, because inflammation from any etiology can elevate procalcitonin levels.

CRP follows a similar response curve, but the initial rise is slightly delayed (6–8 h after infection), and the peak is also reached later (between 24 and 48 h) than procalcitonin. Like procalcitonin, a persistently normal CRP value (<10 mg/L) is a good evidence the baby is uninfected, while CRP elevation can result from other forms of inflammation and therefore is not a strong predictor of sepsis.

Answer: 3

Case Presentation (Continued)

The CBC returns with a normal white blood cell count and ANC. The CRP is modestly elevated at 15.5 mg/L. The baby remains fussy and has had two dry diapers in a row. You decide to initiate an evaluation for sepsis by drawing a blood culture.

What is an appropriate volume of blood to draw to optimize culture sensitivity?

1. >0.5 mL.
2. >1 mL.
3. 2–3 mL.
4. Because symptomatic sepsis requires a bacterial concentration of at least 1×10^6 bacteria/mL blood, the volume doesn't matter; if the baby has sepsis, the culture will grow.

Several clinical and laboratory studies have shown that symptomatic sepsis can occur in the setting of bacterial burdens low enough that blood culture volumes <1 mL might not grow [27, 28]. Sensitivity is improved significantly if an adequate volume is obtained. Since a volume > 1 mL will grow—even in the setting of very low bacterial burden—there is no advantage to drawing 2–3 mL of blood. The size of the blood culture bottle itself (adult vs. pediatric) does not impact the sensitivity.

Answer: 2

Case Presentation (Continued)

You are preparing to draw the culture when the baby's 3-year-old brother enters the room with his father. Both appear tired. The 3-year-old has rhinorrhea, and the father speaks with a hoarse voice before pausing for a coughing fit.

The best test to identify the likely cause of the infant's symptoms is:

1. A tracheal aspirate to check for growth of *Streptococcus pneumoniae.*
2. Urine culture for cytomegalovirus.
3. A viral PCR panel from a nasotracheal aspirate sample.
4. A rapid screen for group A *Streptococcus* pharyngitis.

Common respiratory viruses are a frequent (and often overlooked) cause of fussiness and poor feeding in neonates. A recent prospective study found that, out of 137 infants with suspected late-onset sepsis, 7% had a viral infection [29]. A variety of high-sensitivity, high-specificity PCR- and ELISA-based assays are now widely available and should be strongly considered when evaluating a symptomatic infant with any potential respiratory viral exposures.

Answer: 3

Importantly, just because a newborn has a viral infection rather than bacterial sepsis does not mean that he or she does not need medical attention. Viruses that rarely cause severe illness in older children and adults, such as rhinovirus, can lead to significant dehydration, hyperbilirubinemia, and poor weight gain in a newborn who cannot feed adequately. Adenovirus, which is rarely serious in older patients, can cause life-threatening multiorgan system failure in newborns. The baby in the scenario should be closely observed. Laboratory testing to track electrolytes and serum bilirubin would be appropriate, and he may need transfer to the NICU for respiratory support, fluid replacement, or both. The time required to receive viral testing results varies between hospitals. Empiric antibiotics should not be withheld while awaiting viral testing results, since there is substantial overlap between the presentations of viral and bacterial infections in the newborn.

Tracheal aspirate Gram stain and culture studies are sometimes used when diagnosing ventilator-associated pneumonia, but are not useful in babies with mild, non-specific symptoms. The trachea is not a sterile site, and colonization by a variety of microorganisms occurs quickly during and after birth [6]. Bacteria that grow from a suctioned tracheal sputum sample are likely harmless commensals.

Perinatal transmission of cytomegalovirus (not to be confused with congenital cytomegalovirus, which implies vertical transmission earlier in pregnancy) is usually asymptomatic but in a subset of babies can cause pneumonitis that presents with tachypnea, retractions, wheezing, and poor feeding. The family history in this case is more suggestive of a respiratory virus.

"Strep throat" from group A *Streptococcus* infection does not occur during the neonatal period (group A *Streptococcus* can cause neonatal sepsis, however).

Case Presentation

You attend the Cesarean section delivery of a 38-week gestation baby girl. The mother is a 32-year-old primigravida whose pregnancy has been complicated by gestational diabetes, group B *Streptococcus* urinary tract infection at 20 weeks' gestation, and persistent breech positioning of the fetus. The Cesarean delivery, performed because of the fetal position, occurs 3 h after the onset of spontaneous labor. One dose of penicillin was administered an hour before delivery. The membranes are ruptured in the operating room just prior to delivery. The amniotic fluid is clear. The highest maternal temperature recorded was 99.1°F. The baby emerges pink, cries vigorously, and is dried under radiant warmth. The Apgar scores are 9 and 9 at 1 and 5 min, respectively.

At 30 min of life, she has a respiratory rate of 70 breaths per minute with expiratory grunting and symmetric intercostal and subcostal retractions. Her oxygen saturation is 98%. Her lungs are mildly coarse to auscultation bilaterally, with decent aeration. You provide nasotracheal suctioning and gentle chest percussion.

At 2 h of life, the baby is still grunting. Her blood glucose is normal, and she has made one attempt at breastfeeding. Her vital signs are essentially unchanged, and her oxygen saturation remains >95%.

At this point, you should:

1. Allow the infant to room in with the mother.
2. Draw a blood culture and start ampicillin and gentamicin.
3. Transfer the baby to the NICU for CPAP.
4. Continue close observation.

The physiologic transition to extrauterine life can be marked by a period of mild respiratory distress, sometimes lasting up to 6 h. It is important that the newborn not be simply left to her mother's care. In this case, incomplete administration of intrapartum antibiotic prophylaxis for maternal GBS colonization represents a risk factor for sepsis. However, decisions about whether to perform a workup should ultimately be driven by the newborn's clinical status and should take into consideration that the transition to extrauterine life is not instantaneous. While the risk of sepsis in this case is low, close monitoring for resolution or worsening of symptoms remains essential. Observations should be at least hourly until symptoms resolve.

Answer: 4

While talking with the mother, she asks you, "What are the odds that my baby has a bacterial infection"?

What tool or measure can you use to establish an estimate of the sepsis risk in this case?

1. Gastric aspirate analysis.
2. A sepsis screen using neutrophil indices and CRP.
3. An online sepsis risk calculator.
4. Histopathological examination of the placenta.

A 2011 study by Puopolo et al. used records from over 600,000 mother-infant pairs to establish an online, publically accessible, data-driven algorithm for determining the risk of early-onset sepsis in babies ≥34 weeks' gestation based on maternal risk factors [30].

An updated version of the online sepsis calculator, released in 2014, stratifies neonatal risk based on postnatal physical exam findings [31]. The calculator is available online at https://neonatalsepsiscalculator.kaiserpermanente.org. Entering this baby's data reveals a risk of early-onset sepsis of 0.08 per 1000 live births, but taking into consideration the mild respiratory symptoms (which place the baby in the "equivocal" exam category) increases the risk to 0.38 per 1000 live births. The calculator makes management recommendations, suggesting empiric treatment for well-appearing patients whose risk factors alone place the chances of early-onset sepsis at >1.54/1000 live births and for those with equivocal clinical presentations whose risk at birth is >0.65/1000 live births. As with all recommendations, these must be viewed in the context of the complete history and clinical scenario.

Gastric aspirates contain bacteria and white blood cells found in the amniotic fluid. They are poor predictors of infection. Histopathological examination of the placenta may reveal inflammation; however, it has a poor correlation with early-onset neonatal sepsis.

Answer: 3

Case Presentation (Continued)

At 5 h of life, the baby is still mildly retracting and intermittently tachypneic, but the symptoms are improving. She is no longer grunting. Her oxygen saturation remains 98–100%. A nurse is concerned that the presentation is consistent with early-onset sepsis partially masked by the single perinatal maternal dose of penicillin.

Among babies with culture-positive early-onset sepsis, the main effect of perinatal maternal antibiotics is:

1. Increased time to positivity for the infant's blood culture.
2. Need for two blood cultures in the infant.
3. Increased risk of infection by resistant Gram-negative bacteria.
4. No proven effect.

Although clinicians often worry about maternal antibiotics causing a false-negative infant blood culture by transiently decreasing the bacterial burden, there is no evidence that maternal antibiotics systematically alter the clinical course for septic infants [32].

Babies with signs consistent with sepsis should be managed the same way regardless of maternal antibiotic history. There is no need to draw multiple blood cultures and no data showing that maternal antibiotics increase the time required for an initial blood culture to turn positive.

While it is true that widespread use of broad-spectrum antibiotics promotes infection by resistant bacteria, there is no evidence that a single course of maternal antibiotics increases the risk of early-onset sepsis with an organism resistant to that specific antibiotic.

Answer: 4

In the case of the baby in the example, her improving symptoms within 6 h of birth are consistent with the physiologic transition to extra-uterine life. Over the next 2 h, her breathing pattern normalized, and she had an uneventful course in the newborn nursery.

Clinical Pearls

1. In deciding whether to perform a laboratory evaluation and treat for neonatal sepsis, one must consider historical risk factors, the infant's clinical appearance, and the time since delivery. Remember that the postnatal transition may take up to 6 h.
2. In the absence of significant risk factors for sepsis, a term or late-preterm newborn with mild or moderate respiratory signs—which are improving over the first 6 h of life—can usually be observed for resolution of the physiologic transition.
3. The majority of group B *Streptococcus* early-onset sepsis affects infants whose mothers had negative screens for GBS colonization.
4. Serial normal C-reactive protein or procalcitonin values provide a high degree of reassurance the baby is uninfected. Elevations in either measure can result from noninfectious causes.
5. An adequate blood culture is >1 mL.
6. There is no evidence to support algorithmic "correction" of blood contamination in CSF following a traumatic lumbar puncture.
7. When assessing a newborn with signs consistent with sepsis, consider potential viral exposures.
8. Urinary tract infection is uncommon in the immediate newborn period.
9. Maternal antibiotic exposure will not obscure symptoms or systematically alter laboratory results in a baby with early-onset sepsis.

References

1. Aagaard K, Ma J, Antony KM, Ganu R, Petrosino J, Versalovic J. The placenta harbors a unique microbiome. Sci Transl Med. 2014;6(237):237ra65.
2. Schmutz N, Henry E, Jopling J, Christensen RD. Expected ranges for blood neutrophil concentrations of neonates: the Manroe and Mouzinho charts revisited. J Perinatol. 2008;28(4):275–81.
3. Birle A, Nebe CT, Hill S, Hartmann K, Poeschl J, Koch L. Neutrophil chemotaxis in cord blood of term and preterm neonates is reduced in preterm neonates and influenced by the mode of delivery and anaesthesia. PLoS One. 2015;10(4):e0120341.
4. Levy O. Innate immunity of the newborn: basic mechanisms and clinical correlates. Nat Rev Immunol. 2007;7(5):379–90.
5. Murgas Torrazza R, Neu J. The developing intestinal microbiome and its relationship to health and disease in the neonate. J Perinatol. 2011;31(Suppl 1): S29–34.
6. Lal CV, Travers C, Aghai ZH, Eipers P, Jilling T, Halloran B, et al. The airway microbiome at birth. Sci Rep Nat Pub Group. 2016;6(1):31023.
7. Jackson GL, Rawiki P, Sendelbach D, Manning MD, Engle WD. Hospital course and short-term outcomes of term and late preterm neonates following exposure to prolonged rupture of membranes and/or chorioamnionitis. Pediatr Infect Dis J. 2012;31(1):89–90.
8. Kjaergaard N, Helmig RB, Schønheyder HC, Uldbjerg N, Hansen ES, Madsen H. Chorioamniotic membranes constitute a competent barrier to group b streptococcus in vitro. Eur J Obstet Gynecol Reprod Biol. 1999;83(2):165–9.
9. Boldenow E, Jones S, Lieberman RW, Chames MC, Aronoff DM, Xi C, et al. Antimicrobial peptide response to group B Streptococcus in human extraplacental membranes in culture. Placenta. 2013;34(6):480–5.
10. Wortham JM, Hansen NI, Schrag SJ, Hale E, Van Meurs K, Sánchez PJ, et al. Chorioamnionitis and culture-confirmed, early-onset neonatal infections. Pediatr Am Acad Pediatr. 2016;137(1):e20152323.
11. Greenberg MB, Anderson BL, Schulkin J, Norton ME, Aziz N. A first look at chorioamnionitis management practice variation among US obstetricians. Infect Dis Obstet Gynecol. 2012;2012(2):628362–9.
12. Verani JR, McGee L, Schrag SJ. Division of Bacterial Diseases, National Center for Immunization and Respiratory Diseases, Centers for Disease Control and Prevention (CDC). Prevention of perinatal group B streptococcal disease--revised guidelines from CDC. MMWR. Recommendations and reports : Morbidity and mortality weekly report. Recommendations and reports. 2010;59:1–36.
13. National Collaborating Centre for Women's and Children's Health (UK). Antibiotics for Early-Onset Neonatal Infection. Antibiotics for the prevention and treatment of early-onset neonatal infection. London: RCOG Press; 2012.
14. Polin RA. Committee on fetus and newborn. Management of neonates with suspected or proven early-onset bacterial sepsis. Pediatrics. 2012;129(5):1006–15.
15. Benitz WE, Wynn JL, Polin RA. Reappraisal of guidelines for management of neonates with suspected early-onset sepsis. J Pediatr. 2015;166(4):1070–4.

16. Berardi A, Buffagni AM, Rossi C, Vaccina E, Cattelani C, Gambini L, et al. Serial physical examinations, a simple and reliable tool for managing neonates at risk for early-onset sepsis. World J Clin Pediatr. 2016;5(4):358–64.
17. Berardi A, Fornaciari S, Rossi C, Patianna V, Bacchi Reggiani ML, Ferrari F, et al. Safety of physical examination alone for managing well-appearing neonates ≥ 35 weeks' gestation at risk for early-onset sepsis. J Matern Fetal Neonatal Med Informa Healthcare. 2015;28(10):1123–7.
18. Jan AI, Ramanathan R, Chorioamnionitis CRG. Management of Asymptomatic Infants ≥35 weeks without empiric antibiotics. Pediatrics. 2017;140(1):e20162744.
19. Sullins AK, Abdel-Rahman SM. Pharmacokinetics of antibacterial agents in the CSF of children and adolescents. Paediatr Drugs. 2013;15(2):93–117.
20. Hamada S, Vearncombe M, McGeer A, Shah PS. Neonatal group B streptococcal disease: incidence, presentation, and mortality. J Matern Fetal Neonatal Med. 2008;21(1):53–7.
21. Stoll BJ, Hansen NI, Sánchez PJ, Faix RG, Poindexter BB, Van Meurs KP, et al. Early onset neonatal sepsis: the burden of group B streptococcal and E. coli disease continues. Pediatr Am Acad Pediatr. 2011;127(5):817–26.
22. Martin-Ancel A, García-Alix A, Salas S, Del Castillo F, Cabañas F, Quero J. Cerebrospinal fluid leucocyte counts in healthy neonates. Arch Dis Child Fetal Neonatal Ed. 2006;91(5):F357–8.
23. Srinivasan L, Shah SS, Padula MA, Abbasi S, McGowan KL, Harris MC. Cerebrospinal fluid reference ranges in term and preterm infants in the neonatal intensive care unit. J Pediatr. 2012;161(4):729–34.
24. Bonsu BK, Harper MB. Corrections for leukocytes and percent of neutrophils do not match observations in blood-contaminated cerebrospinal fluid and have no value over uncorrected cells for diagnosis. Pediatr Infect Dis J. 2006;25(1):8–11.
25. Benitz WE, Han MY, Madan A, Ramachandra P. Serial serum C-reactive protein levels in the diagnosis of neonatal infection. Pediatrics. 1998;102(4):E41.
26. Lam HS, Ng PC. Biochemical markers of neonatal sepsis. Pathology. 2008;40(2):141–8.
27. Schelonka RL, Chai MK, Yoder BA, Hensley D, Brockett RM, Ascher DP. Volume of blood required to detect common neonatal pathogens. J Pediatr. 1996;129(2):275–8.
28. Connell TG, Rele M, Cowley D, Buttery JP, Curtis N. How reliable is a negative blood culture result? Volume of blood submitted for culture in routine practice in a children's hospital. Pediatrics. 2007;119(5):891–6.
29. Kidszun A, Klein L, Winter J, Schmeh I, Gröndahl B, Gehring S, et al. Viral infections in neonates with suspected late-onset bacterial sepsis-a prospective cohort study. Am J Perinatol. 2017;34(1):1–7.
30. Puopolo KM, Draper D, Wi S, Newman TB, Zupancic J, Lieberman E, et al. Estimating the probability of neonatal early-onset infection on the basis of maternal risk factors. Pediatrics. 2011;128(5):e1155–63.
31. Escobar GJ, Puopolo KM, Wi S, Turk BJ, Kuzniewicz MW, Walsh EM, et al. Stratification of risk of early-onset sepsis in newborns >= 34 Weeks' gestation. Pediatrics. Am Acad Pediatr. 2014;133(1):30–6.
32. Sarkar SS, Bhagat I, Bhatt-Mehta V, Sarkar S. Does maternal intrapartum antibiotic treatment prolong the incubation time required for blood cultures to become positive for infants with early-onset sepsis? Am J Perinatol. 2015;32(4):357–62.

Viral Infections in the Nursery

8

Asif Noor, Theresa M. Fiorito, and Leonard R. Krilov

Introduction

Viral infections seen in the newborn nursery may be acquired in utero or during delivery. Human immunodeficiency virus (HIV), hepatitis B virus, cytomegalovirus (CMV), Zika virus, herpes simplex virus (HSV), and parvovirus B19 are examples of congenital infections that may be encountered in the nursery. The spectrum of these infections ranges from asymptomatic to severe multi-system organ involvement. Issues for the clinician include aspects of diagnosis and treatment.

Through a series of case vignettes, we will overview a number of these conditions and present an approach for the clinician faced with one of these scenarios.

A. Noor, MD (✉) · T. M. Fiorito, MD
Department of Pediatrics, Children's Medical Center at NYU Winthrop Hospital, Mineola, NY, USA
e-mail: anoor@nyuwinthrop.org

L. R. Krilov, MD
Department of Pediatrics, Children's Medical Center at NYU Winthrop Hospital, Mineola, NY, USA

Department of Pediatrics State University of New York at Stony Brook School of Medicine, Stony Brook, NY, USA

Case Presentation

You are examining a 24-h-old female infant born at 38 weeks who failed her newborn hearing screen. Her mother works as a teacher's aide in a child care program. The infant's weight and head circumference are both within the 95th percentile. Physical examination is normal, without any evidence of hepatosplenomegaly, rashes, or jaundice. You order a urine CMV PCR, which returns positive. At this time, you:

1. Confirm CMV testing with a urine viral culture and CMV IgM.
2. Discharge the patient with pediatrician follow-up within 24 h.
3. Schedule outpatient audiology follow-up for sequential hearing tests.
4. Start the patient on antiviral therapy (valganciclovir).

Cytomegalovirus (CMV) infection is the most common congenital viral infection in the United States. Asymptomatic infection is the most common presentation at birth; only 10% exhibit clinical findings. Primary infection in pregnant women is often more severe and may present as a "mono-like" illness during pregnancy. Those with prior immunity to CMV may be asymptomatic. CMV infection acquired in the first half of gestation is associated with more severe sequelae in the neonate [1, 2].

G. I. Martin, W. Rosenfeld (eds.), *Common Problems in the Newborn Nursery*,
https://doi.org/10.1007/978-3-319-95672-5_8

The most common sequela of congenital CMV infection is sensorineural hearing loss, higher in symptomatic infections (50%), but occurring in up to 15% of asymptomatic infections. All children found to have congenital CMV infection must be evaluated with sequential hearing tests. A normal newborn hearing screen in a CMV+, asymptomatic infant does not rule out CMV-related hearing loss; 55% of symptomatic and 75% of asymptomatic children who develop CMV-associated hearing loss have a normal hearing test at birth. Hearing loss can be delayed for years, which is why sequential testing is so important [1].

Proof of congenital CMV infection *must be obtained within 3 weeks of birth*. Otherwise, it is impossible to differentiate perinatal/postnatally acquired infection from congenitally acquired asymptomatic infection. Diagnosis of congenital CMV includes real-time PCR of saliva, urine, or both (saliva is preferred). CMV culture has equal specificity but is less sensitive than PCR. A CMV-specific IgM, though suggestive of congenital infection, has lower specificity and a higher false-positive rate, making use of this test problematic [1].

Valganciclovir is an oral antiviral with activity against CMV. Valganciclovir is *not* recommended for asymptomatic neonates with isolated hearing loss or mild congenital infection (defined as mild hepatomegaly, single low platelet count, single raised ALT, and/or 1–2 isolated manifestations) [3]. Antiviral therapy is only recommended for neonates with moderate-severe symptomatic disease. Neonates with moderate-severe symptomatic congenital CMV with or without CNS involvement have improved neurodevelopmental and audiologic outcomes at age 2 when treated with valganciclovir for 6 months [4]. Moderate-severe disease is defined as *multiple* manifestations attributable to CMV, including hepatosplenomegaly, intrauterine growth restriction, hepatitis, thrombocytopenia, and petechiae/purpura, and CNS involvement may be present (ventriculomegaly, periventricular echogenicity, calcifications, cortical/cerebellar malformations, chorioretinitis, hearing loss).

Significant neutropenia occurs in 20% of infants treated with valganciclovir. Absolute neutrophil counts should be checked weekly for the first 6 weeks, at 8 weeks, and then monthly for the remainder of the treatment [4].

Answer: 3

Case Presentation

A healthy 38-week-old male was born abruptly via NSVD to a mother with a history of HIV infection. Maternal viral load was >1000 copies/ml throughout pregnancy, and she reports non-compliance with her antiretroviral therapy. For the infant, the next best step is to:

1. Start zidovudine (AZT).
2. Obtain an HIV genotype.
3. Start nevirapine and zidovudine.
4. Obtain an HIV DNA PCR to assess viral load.

Mother-to-child HIV transmission can occur in utero, during labor and delivery, or postnatally through breastfeeding [5]. Since the 1990s, a sharp decrease in rates of mother-to-child HIV transmission has been observed in the United States due to antenatal HIV testing, antiretroviral (ARV) prophylaxis, combination ARV during pregnancy, cesarean delivery before labor (when indicated), and avoidance of breastfeeding and pre-mastication of food [6].

Most transmission occurs during the intrapartum period. Risk factors include elevated maternal viral load and duration of exposure (e.g., prolonged ruptured membranes, breastfeeding). Without any intervention, the risk of transmission from an HIV-infected mother to her infant is 22.6–25.5% [7].

In infants, a DNA PCR is the preferred diagnostic test for HIV. RNA assays have similar specificity and sensitivity, but there is greater clinical experience with DNA assays. False-negative RNA assays may occur in infants receiving ARV prophylaxis. Serology is not helpful in diagnosing children under 18–24 months of age, as infants born to HIV-infected mothers acquire maternal antibodies passively.

To reduce the risk of perinatal transmission, all HIV-exposed infants should receive ARV prophylaxis as close to birth as possible (within 6–12 h of delivery). If infected, 95% of infants will have positive results by 1 month. Infants should be tested sequentially in follow-up with an infectious diseases specialist [5].

A combination prophylaxis regimen (zidovudine and nevirapine) should be considered in HIV-exposed infants whose mothers are "high risk": those who have not received antepartum or intrapartum ARV, have only received intrapartum ARV, or have not achieved viral suppression near delivery [6].

Infants of mothers who report compliance with their medications throughout pregnancy, or whose viral loads are undetectable, are considered "low risk" and should be started solely on zidovudine (AZT) [6, 7]. Both the infant and mother should have prescriptions for ARV before leaving the hospital. A 4-week regimen can be used for full-term infants when the mother has been adherent to a standard ARV regimen during pregnancy with sustained viral suppression. The most common side effect of AZT is bone marrow suppression. A CBC and differential should be performed on newborns as a baseline evaluation [5].

For infants born to mothers with unknown HIV status, expedited HIV testing of mothers and infants is recommended, with immediate initiation of infant ARV prophylaxis *if* the initial test is positive [6].

Answer: 3

Case Presentation

You are seeing a full-term 24-h-old male whose mother traveled to Ecuador 2 months prior to delivery. She recalls fever, rash, and fatigue 2 weeks post-travel. She has been tested for Zika virus and reports "Zika RNA detected." After a thorough physical exam of the infant, you find no abnormalities.

At this time, you:

1. Order a neurology consult for evaluation of sequelae of Zika.
2. Refer the baby for outpatient infectious disease follow-up in 1–2 months.
3. Provide reassurance, and discharge the infant with close follow-up with his pediatrician.
4. Perform hearing testing, ophthalmology exam, Zika laboratory testing, and head ultrasound.

Zika virus infection during pregnancy can cause severe fetal brain defects. Congenital Zika syndrome is characterized by microcephaly, intracranial calcifications and other brain anomalies, eye anomalies, tremors, seizures, and/or irritability. Clubfoot and joint contractures (arthrogryposis) have also been observed [8].

Practitioners should ask about potential congenital Zika exposure for every newborn, including travel/residence in an area with risk of Zika during pregnancy or 8-week preconception and/or unprotected sex during pregnancy/preconception with a partner with this exposure (who did not receive testing) [8]. See the CDC website (as referenced) for a full list of countries with Zika risk.

For infants without evidence of birth defects consistent with congenital Zika syndrome born to mothers *without* laboratory evidence of Zika virus infection during pregnancy, further evaluation and testing for Zika virus are not recommended unless abnormalities are noted on physical exam [8]. A full, detailed algorithm of testing and follow-up can be found on the CDC website.

For infants without evidence of birth defects consistent with congenital Zika syndrome born to mothers *with* laboratory evidence of Zika virus infection during pregnancy, Zika virus testing and a comprehensive physical exam (including growth parameters and repeated, consistent head circumference measurements) should be performed. A head ultrasound, ABR (automated auditory brain stem response), and ophthalmology exam should be performed within 1 month of birth [8].

For infants *with* evidence of birth defects consistent with congenital Zika syndrome born to mothers with possible exposure to Zika virus during pregnancy (*regardless of mother's Zika test results*), the above testing should be performed with additional referrals to early intervention services and a developmental specialist. Consultation with infectious diseases, genetics, and neurology should also be considered. Family support should be made available, and infants should be continually monitored for additional clinical findings of congenital Zika syndrome, including increased intracranial pressure, dysphagia, or respiratory distress [8].

Recommended laboratory testing for congenital Zika syndrome includes Zika virus RNA in blood and urine and Zika virus IgM antibodies in blood. If CSF is obtained for other purposes, RNA and IgM antibody testing should be performed. Testing of cord blood is not recommended, as false-positive and false-negative results have been reported. If infant's Zika virus RNA testing is positive, this represents a confirmed congenital Zika virus infection, regardless of IgM results. If infant's Zika virus RNA testing is negative, but IgM is positive/equivocal, this indicates probable congenital Zika virus infection. If confirmatory testing with plaque neutralization testing (PRNT) is negative, this suggests that the infant's IgM test is a false positive. If both Zika RNA and IgM are negative, congenital Zika virus infection is unlikely [8].

Answer: 4

Case Presentation

A call comes from the labor and delivery room. The OB/GYN resident informs you of a 20-year-old female in active labor with painful genital ulcers. They have high suspicion for genital herpes simplex infection and have sent an HSV PCR from a genital lesion as well as maternal serology for HSV-1, HSV-2 IgG, and IgM. Later in the day, you examine the baby. His weight is 6 lbs (2700 grams), and physical exam is normal with no rashes. At this time, the next best step is:

1. Reassure the mother as the baby is completely asymptomatic.
2. Obtain HSV surface cultures now.
3. Obtain HSV surface cultures at 24 hours of life.
4. Obtain HSV surface cultures if lesions develop.

Neonatal herpes simplex virus (HSV) infection has an estimated incidence of 1 in 3000 to 1 in 20,000 live births in the United States. HSV is a DNA virus capable of establishing latency after primary infection. There are two types, HSV -1 and HSV-2, both of which can cause neonatal disease. The management of an asymptomatic neonate born to a mother with active genital herpes simplex virus infection poses a challenge. HSV is an uncommon infection in neonates, despite a 20% rate of genital herpes among adults in the United States, and signs of neonatal infection are often not apparent until the second to third week of life.

As delineated in the report of the Committee on Infectious Diseases and Committee on Fetus and Newborn of American Academy of Pediatrics [9], the risk of neonatal HSV infection depends upon five factors:

(a) Type of maternal infection (primary versus recurrent): The risk of neonatal HSV is 57% in primary infection and 2% in recurrent infection.
(b) Maternal HSV antibody status: The risk is lower with preexisting maternal antibodies.
(c) Duration of rupture of membranes (increased risk if $\geq$4 h).
(d) Integrity of mucocutaneous barrier (e.g., use of a fetal scalp monitoring device increases risk).
(e) Mode of delivery (increased risk with vaginal delivery).

After obtaining maternal information as listed above, a through physical examination should be performed. If a skin lesion is seen, the base of the vesicle or ulcer should be scraped and sent for HSV culture in viral transport medium. The sensitivity of HSV PCR on surface specimens has not been studied; therefore if used, it should be sent in addition to HSV cultures.

If the baby is asymptomatic with a normal exam, surface cultures and HSV DNA blood PCR should be obtained at 24 h of life. Surface cultures are obtained from the conjunctivae, mouth, nasopharynx, and rectum. The rationale for waiting for 24 h is detection of a virus at that time represents viral replication at infant's mucosal membrane, rather than contamination from maternal lesions.

After 3 days, the parents are anxious to go home. The baby is still asymptomatic, but the HSV culture comes back positive. At this time, the next best step is to:

1. Reassure the parents as the baby is still asymptomatic and discharge home.
2. Obtain CSF for HSV PCR and start PO acyclovir.
3. Obtain CSF for HSV PCR and start IV acyclovir.
4. Repeat surface cultures and observe.

If the baby remains asymptomatic and 48-h HSV surface cultures and serum PCR are negative, then the baby can safely go home, provided other parameters of discharge are met.

If the baby remains asymptomatic but HSV surface cultures and/or serum PCR return positive, the neonate should undergo a complete evaluation, including CSF for HSV PCR as well as serum alanine aminotransferase to determine the extent of infection. The neonate should be started on intravenous acyclovir at a dose of 60 mg/kg/day divided every 8 h [10].

If this evaluation is normal, it will imply that the baby acquired HSV infection but did not develop HSV disease. In this situation the duration of acyclovir is 10 days. In terms of symptomatic neonatal HSV infection, about 45% of cases present with skin eye mouth (SEM) disease, 30% present with CNS disease (with or without skin involvement), and 25% develop disseminated disease.

Answer: 3

Case Presentation

You are seeing a newborn girl at 37 weeks of gestation born to a 35-year-old Chinese mother. While reviewing the prenatal laboratory testing, you notice the hepatitis screen is not available. The baby received hepatitis B vaccination in the delivery room. The baby is 5 lb and 5 ounces (2500 grams) and appropriate for gestational age. Physical examination is normal with no hepatomegaly. The next best step in this baby's management would be to:

1. Administer hepatitis B immunoglobulin at a dose of 0.5 ml within 12 h.
2. Administer hepatitis B immunoglobulin at a dose of 0.5 ml within 7 days.
3. Obtain maternal hepatitis B surface antibody and antigen.
4. Reassure the mother as the baby is asymptomatic.

Hepatitis B virus (HBV) is a DNA virus transmitted through blood or other bodily fluids. Perinatal transmission of HBV is highly efficient and usually occurs via blood exposure during labor and delivery. All pregnant women should be screened for hepatitis B surface antigen (HBsAg) at the first prenatal visit.

In the United States, a comprehensive immunization strategy to eliminate perinatal HBV transmission has been implemented [11]. The core elements of this program include (a) universal immunization of all infants beginning at birth and (b) postexposure prophylaxis with hepatitis B immunoglobulin in neonates born to mothers with a positive HBsAg or unknown hepatitis B status.

Hepatitis B vaccine is >90% effective in preventing infection. Without postexposure hepatitis B immunoglobulin (HBIG) prophylaxis, the risk of an infant acquiring HBV from a HBsAg+, HBeAg+ mother is 70–90%. The risk is 5–20% for infants born to HBsAg+, HBeAg− mothers.

Recommendations are provided by the Centers of Disease Control and Prevention based on risk of infection [12] (Table 8.1).

Table 8.1 Recommendations for care of the newborn based on newborn's weight and maternal hepatitis status. Recommendations are provided by the Centers of Disease Control and Prevention based on risk of infection [12]

Infant's birth weight	Maternal hepatitis B status		
	HB surface Ag Negative	HB surface Ag Positive	HB surface Ag unknown
> *2000 g*	HBV vaccine at birth	HBV vaccine at birth *plus* HBIG within 12 h of birth	Test mother for HBsAg immediately after delivery HBV vaccine at birth HBIG *within 7 days* (if mothers HBsAg positive or unknown)
< *2000 g*	Until age 1 month or nursery discharge	HBV vaccine at birth *plus* HBIG within 12 h of birth	Test mother for HBsAg immediately after delivery HBV vaccine at birth HBIG *within 12 h* (if mothers HBsAg positive or unknown

Other hepatitis B serological and nucleic acid testing classifies maternal infection as either acute or chronic infection, as well as predicts infectivity to the baby. The presence of hepatitis B DNA and hepatitis B e-antigen infers high infectivity. A positive HB core antibody (anti-HBc) may represent chronic HBV infection. Pediatricians should be aware that passively transferred maternal anti-HBc is detectable for as long as 24 months among infants born to HBsAg-positive women.

Answer: 3

Clinical Pearls

- Testing for CMV in newborns *must* be performed within the first 3 weeks if congenital infection is suspected, using a real-time PCR on a specimen of urine or saliva.
- Valganciclovir antiviral therapy is *not* recommended for asymptomatic neonates with isolated hearing loss or mild congenital infection, only those with moderate-severe symptomatic infections.
- Only 30–40% of HIV-infected infants will have positive DNA PCR assay results before 48 h of life. All HIV-exposed infants should receive ARV therapy as close to birth as possible (within 6–12 h).
- Laboratory testing for Zika virus is recommended for infants with birth defects consistent with congenital Zika syndrome (regardless of mother's Zika test results) and infants without birth defects consistent with congenital Zika syndrome whose mothers have laboratory evidence of Zika virus infection during pregnancy. See CDC algorithm for full details.
- Most cases of neonatal HSV occur in infants born to mothers whom are unaware they are infected. The risk of neonatal infection is 57% in primary infection, as opposed 2% in recurrent infection.
- All infants should receive hepatitis B vaccination within 24 h of birth, and infants born to mothers with positive hepatitis B surface antigen should receive hepatitis B immunoglobulin as well within 12 h.

References

1. American Academy of Pediatrics. Cytomegalovirus. In: Kimberlin DW, editor. Red book: 2015 report of the committee on infectious diseases. 30th ed. Elk Grove: American Academy of Pediatrics; 2015.
2. CDC: Congenital CMV Infection. https://www.cdc.gov/cmv/congenital-infection.html. Accessed August, 2017.

3. Rawlinson WD, Boppana SB, Fowler KB, et al. Congenital CMV infection in pregnancy and the neonate: consensus recommendations for prevention, diagnosis, and therapy. Lancet Infect Dis. 2017;17(6):e177–88.
4. Kimberlin DW, Jester PM, Sanchez PJ, et al. Valganciclovir for symptomatic congenital CMV disease. N Engl J Med. 2015;372(10):933–43.
5. Postpartum Care Recommendations for Use of Antiretroviral Drugs in Pregnant HIV-1-Infected Women for Maternal Health and Interventions to Reduce Perinatal HIV Transmission in the United States: Initial Postnatal Management of the HIV-Exposed Neonate. https://aidsinfo.nih.gov/guidelines/html/3/perinatal-guidelines/188/initial-postnatal-management-of-the-hiv-exposed-neonate. Accessed August, 2017.
6. CDC: HIV Infection. https://www.cdc.gov/globalaids/Resources/pmtct-care/docs/%20Complete_Presentation_Bklt.pdf. Accessed August, 2017.
7. American Academy of Pediatrics. HIV infection. In: Kimberlin DW, editor. Red Book: 2015 report of the committee on infectious diseases. 30th ed. Elk Grove: American Academy of Pediatrics; 2015.
8. CDC: Zika virus: Healthcare Providers Caring for Infants and Children. https://www.cdc.gov/zika/hc-providers/infants-children.html. Accessed August, 2017.
9. Kimberlin DW, Baley J. Committee on infectious diseases; committee on fetus and newborn. Guidance on management of asymptomatic neonates born to women with active genital herpes lesions. Pediatrics. 2013;131(2):e635–46.
10. American Academy of Pediatrics. Herpes simplex. In: Kimberlin DW, editor. Red Book: 2015 report of the committee on infectious diseases. 30th ed. Elk Grove: American Academy of Pediatrics; 2015.
11. American Academy of Pediatrics. Hepatitis B. In: Kimberlin DW, editor. Red Book: 2015 report of the committee on infectious diseases. 30th ed. Elk Grove: American Academy of Pediatrics; 2015.
12. Centers for Disease Control and Prevention. A comprehensive immunization strategy to eliminate transmission of hepatitis B virus infection in the United States: recommendations of the Advisory Committee on Immunization Practices (ACIP); Part 1 : immunizatoion of infants, children and adolescents. MMWR. 2005;54(RR–16).

9 Anemia in the Nursery: When to Observe, When to Treat, and When to Refer

Emily A. Morris and Ann R. Stark

Introduction

Anemia is an uncommon problem in the newborn nursery but, when it occurs, may have serious consequences. All infants experience a physiologic nadir in hemoglobin level that typically occurs after they leave the nursery. This nadir occurs at about 8 to 12 weeks of age in term infants and earlier in preterm infants, at approximately 6 weeks of age. Although infants with anemia may appear pale on exam, they are usually asymptomatic. In contrast, when anemia occurs at or soon after birth signs may range from mild to severe. As a result, the provider must know how to recognize the signs and symptoms of anemia, plan an evaluation to detect the etiology, anticipate the clinical course, and know when to consult a subspecialist and/or refer the infant to a higher level of care.

E. A. Morris, MD (✉) · A. R. Stark, MD
Neonatal-Perinatal Medicine, Vanderbilt University School of Medicine, Mildred Stahlman Division of Neonatology, Monroe Carell Jr. Children's Hospital, Nashville, TN, USA
e-mail: emily.a.morris@vanderbilt.edu; ann.r.stark@vanderbilt.edu

Case Presentation

You are caring for a 48-hour-old infant boy with hyperbilirubinemia who is being treated with intensive phototherapy. Because his mother's blood type is O positive and her antibody screen was positive, cord blood was sent for blood type and Coombs test. Results showed that the infant's blood type was A positive and the Coombs test was positive. On exam, the infant appears well with no palpable hepatosplenomegaly and no skin lesions.

Which laboratory tests should you obtain at this point?

1. Hemoglobin/hematocrit.
2. Reticulocyte count.
3. Indirect antiglobulin test.
4. Peripheral blood smear for RBC morphology.

Anemia is defined by a hemoglobin or hematocrit value less than the reference range for the infant's gestational or postnatal age. Hemoglobin and hematocrit vary by gestational and postnatal age. Because blood samples for routine hemoglobin and hematocrit testing are not obtained from healthy term infants, "normal" values are unavailable. However, reference ranges have been established from newborns with minimal pathology with the assumption that these hematologic values are near normal [1].

G. I. Martin, W. Rosenfeld (eds.), *Common Problems in the Newborn Nursery*,
https://doi.org/10.1007/978-3-319-95672-5_9

Table 9.1 Reference range of common red cell indices

	Term (39–40 weeks)	Early term (37–38 weeks)	Late preterm (35–36 weeks)
Hematocrit (%)[a]	42–65	42–65	40–60
Hemoglobin gm/dL[a]	14–22	14–22	13.5–21
MCV (fl)[a]	97–115	97–117	98–118
MCH(pg)[a]	32.5–39.5	33–40	33–41
Reticulocytes (%)[b]	0.4–6	0.6–7.8	0.7–7.1

Values are reported as 5th–95th percentile for gestational age

Adapted from Refs. [1–4] [a] and Ref. [5][b]

Table 9.1 shows reference ranges in the newborn period by gestational age.

Answer: 1 and 2

A short while later, you receive the report of this infant's laboratory values with hemoglobin 15.1 gm/dL, hematocrit 45%, and reticulocyte count of 9%.

Given these values, what is the most likely cause of this infant's condition?

1. Acute blood loss.
2. ABO Incompatibility.
3. Congenital Infection.

When you compare these values to reference values, you note that the infant does not have anemia but does have an elevated reticulocyte count. An elevated reticulocyte count can be a marker of ongoing red blood cell destruction or hemolysis. When maternal antibodies result in hemolysis of red blood cells, the infant's bone marrow responds by increasing the production of red blood cells, resulting in increased immature red blood cells known as reticulocytes. Though this newborn does not have anemia now, he is at risk for anemia later due to ongoing hemolysis.

Answer: 2

Hemolytic disease is the most common cause of anemia in the nursery, and almost any hemolytic disease can lead to anemia. However, the expected time course for hemolytic anemia differs according to its etiology. The most common forms of hemolytic disease in the newborn are ABO incompatibility and Rh incompatibility; less common forms include incompatibilities of other minor blood groups (anti-Kell, anti-Kidd, anti-Duffy).

Approximately 15% of all mother/fetal pairs are ABO incompatible. What percent of infants from ABO incompatible maternal/fetal pairs have clinical signs of hemolysis?

1. 15%
2. 10%
3. 5%
4. 3%

Hemolytic disease from ABO incompatibility can occur during the first pregnancy; however, this occurs in only 1–3% of these pairs. Severe hemolytic disease due to Rh D incompatibility affects approximately 1 in 1200 pregnancies and only when the mother is sensitized [5, 6]. Blood group type and antibody status are tested with routine prenatal care, so this information is usually available to the pediatrician. Hyperbilirubinemia is a hallmark of hemolytic disease of the newborn, but anemia can follow the onset of hyperbilirubinemia. Anemia tends to be more severe in Rh D disease than in ABO incompatibility [6].

ABO incompatibility rarely results in clinically significant anemia in the early newborn period. However, ongoing hemolysis may sometimes result in late-onset anemia at 1–3 weeks of age [7]. Sensitized infants who need phototherapy should have at least one hemoglobin/hematocrit level checked during their hospitalization. If prolonged phototherapy is required, serial hemoglobin/hematocrit levels may be warranted for monitoring and to guide follow-up.

Rh D disease can present with profound anemia, hydrops fetalis, and shock at delivery in an infant born to a sensitized mother. These infants should be referred to the NICU and may require an exchange transfusion for management of anemia and hyperbilirubinemia. They are also at risk for ongoing anemia in the weeks to months after discharge and need close follow-up [8, 9].

Understanding the underlying pathophysiology will help the provider to both anticipate the projected clinical course and manage the ongoing anemia. The etiologies of neonatal anemia fall into three categories: (1) blood loss, (2) increased red cell destruction, and (3) decreased red cell production (Table 9.2). Figure 9.1 shows a suggested general framework for approaching the differential diagnosis and evaluation of anemia in the nursery.

Answer: 4

Table 9.2 Etiologies of neonatal anemia

Blood loss	Increased destruction	Reduced production
Fetomaternal	ABO or minor blood group incompatibility	Diamond-Blackfan anemia
Twin-twin	Rh incompatibility	Fanconi anemia
Trauma	Maternal autoimmune disorders	Sepsis
Internal bleeding	Drug induced (penicillin, valproic acid)	Congenital infection (parvovirus, HIV, syphilis, rubella)
Obstetrical[a]	Red cell enzyme deficiencies (G-6-PD deficiency)	Nutritional deficiencies (iron, folate, B12)
	Red cell membrane defects (hereditary spherocytosis)	Congenital leukemia
	Thalassemia syndromes	Congenital dyserythropoietic anemia
	Metabolic syndromes (galactosemia)	

Adapted from Refs. [5, 10]

[a]Examples of obstetrical bleeding include placental abruption, placental previa, and abnormal placental insertion/invasion

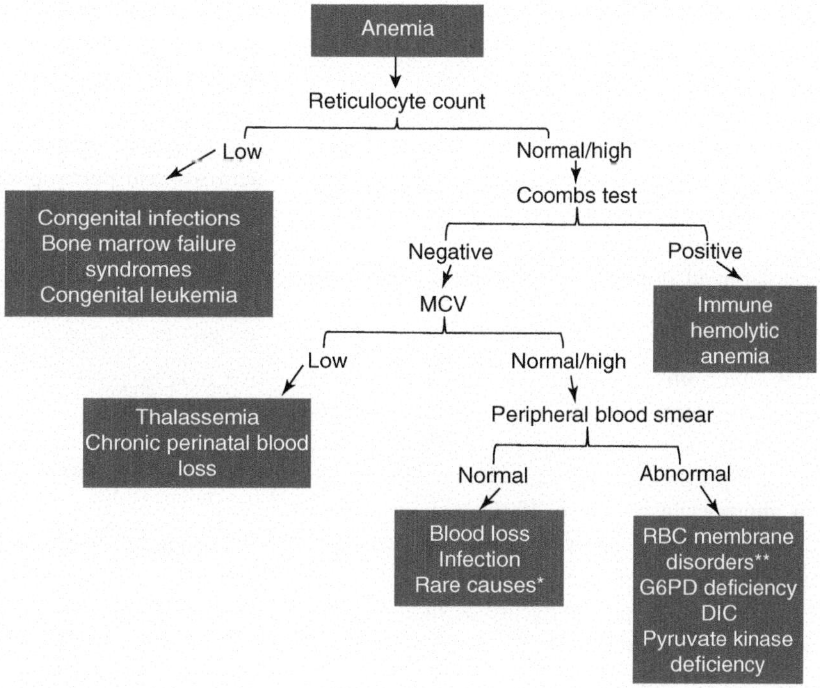

Fig. 9.1 Suggested general framework for approaching the differential diagnosis and evaluation of anemia in the nursery

Case Presentation

It is Thursday morning and you are examining a 6-hour-old newborn. The newborn is a female, 7 lbs 2 oz birth weight, and at 38 1/7-week gestation according to last menstrual period. The mother is a 26-year-old G2P2002 with gestational hypertension. Her laboratory results include blood type A+ and negative antibody screen. Her serologies for infection are unremarkable.

The mother's membranes were ruptured for 10 h. The infant was delivered by vacuum-assisted vaginal delivery. Apgar scores were 8 and 9 at 1 and 5 min, respectively. At present, the infant is doing well and has breastfed three times. On your exam, the infant appears pale but otherwise well. She is afebrile with heart rate 130–140 beats per minute and respiratory rate 40 breaths per minute. The abdomen is benign, with no hepatomegaly and no palpable spleen. She is alert and responsive. You note a large cephalohematoma over the posterior occiput.

At this time you:

1. Continue to observe the infant with vital signs per nursery protocol.
2. Obtain a hemoglobin/hematocrit level.
3. Order a total serum bilirubin.
4. Obtain a transcutaneous bilirubin.

Routine evaluation of the term newborn's hemoglobin and hematocrit levels is not recommended as a part of well-baby care unless the history and/or presentation raise a clinical suspicion [11]. Therefore, most nurseries do not have a standardized protocol for evaluation and assessment of anemia.

In this case, the infant appears well with normal vital signs, adequate feeding, and no clinically apparent jaundice. Continuing to observe the infant with vital signs per nursery protocol and for progression of the cephalohematoma is an appropriate response. If the patient were to develop pallor or tachycardia, a CBC would be indicated as part of an extended workup for other causes of pallor and tachycardia, such as sepsis or congenital heart disease.

Answer: 1

In vacuum-assisted deliveries, what is the risk of complications?

1. 0.5%
2. 3%
3. 5%
4. 10%

In 2015, operative (vacuum or forceps assisted) vaginal deliveries accounted for 3.1% of all deliveries in the United States. The absolute number of operative deliveries varies by geographic region [12]. Operative vaginal deliveries can cause significant morbidity including cephalohematoma, subgaleal hematoma, laceration, and intracranial hemorrhage. The risk of neonatal complications with vacuum-assisted deliveries is approximately 5% [13]. In both vacuum and forceps deliveries, the rate of neonatal death due to intracranial hemorrhage is 3–4 per 10,000 deliveries [14].

Answer: 3

Cephalohematoma and subgaleal hemorrhage are the most common type of cranial hemorrhage in the term newborn [15]. Cephalohematomas are typically localized to the subperiosteal space and thus confined by suture lines. Most cephalohematomas resolve spontaneously. However, subgaleal hemorrhages can lead to substantial accumulation of a large volume of blood between the aponeurosis and periosteum, resulting in significant blood loss that may lead to hemorrhagic shock or death [16]. When subgaleal hemorrhage is suspected, serial measurements of head circumference may be helpful, but intensive monitoring in the NICU to detect early signs of decompensation may be prudent.

Case Presentation

One evening, the on-call obstetrician calls you to attend a Cesarean delivery on a G1 mother. The obstetrician reports the following indications for this delivery: fetal tachycardia, decreased fetal heart rate variability, and failure to progress. The mother's prenatal laboratory evaluation is notable for blood type B+, antibody screen negative, hematocrit 31%, and negative serologies for infection.

Membranes are ruptured at delivery and the amniotic fluid is bloody. The infant is apneic and is given positive pressure ventilation (PPV) by bag and mask for 60 s. After PPV, the infant initiates appropriate and sustained respiratory effort but is mildly hypotonic and appears pale. The infant's heart rate is approximately 190 beats per minute; the remainder of a brief assessment in the delivery room reveals decreased perfusion with delayed capillary refill of 3–4 s. Apgar scores are 6 and 7 at 1 and 5 min, respectively. Umbilical cord blood gases are reassuring.

Based on the clinical information provided, is this infant's presentation more consistent with:

1. Acute blood loss
2. Chronic blood loss

An infant with anemia can be asymptomatic or present with a range of signs and symptoms. Anemia becomes clinically significant when the blood's oxygen carrying capacity no longer meets the demands of the body's tissues. Common clinical signs of anemia include pallor, tachycardia, prolonged capillary refill, lethargy, and poor feeding.

In an infant with acute blood loss, the hematocrit is often normal early in the clinical course and spleen and liver size will also be normal. If blood loss is substantial, the infant may present with hypovolemic shock. Signs of hypovolemic shock may include tachycardia, delayed capillary refill, respiratory distress, hypotonia, acidosis, and decreased level of alertness.

In presentations of chronic blood loss, the infant typically appears pale and may have hepatosplenomegaly. If the chronic blood loss is mild, the infant will likely be hemodynamically stable; however, infants with severe chronic blood loss may present with heart failure and hydrops fetalis. Causes of acute and chronic causes of blood loss are listed in Table 9.3.

Table 9.3 Causes of acute and chronic blood loss in newborn infants

Acute blood loss	Chronic blood loss
Cord prolapse	Chronic obstetrical bleeding (placental previa)
Placental abruption	Maternal-fetal hemorrhage
Acute obstetrical bleeding (vaginal delivery through placental previa, trauma to the placenta during delivery)	Twin-twin transfusion syndrome
Birth trauma: subgaleal, subdural, epidural, intraventricular (preterm infants) bleeding	
Other internal bleeding (subcapsular liver hemorrhage, adrenal hemorrhage, renal vein thrombosis, gastrointestinal)	
Bleeding due to coagulation disorders including galactosemia, other liver dysfunction, vitamin K deficiency, hemophilias, von Willebrand disease	

Adapted from [5, 7, 10, 15, 17]

In this case, presentation with bloody amniotic fluid at delivery and the findings on physical exam of pallor, delayed capillary refill, and tachycardia should cause the provider to worry about acute blood loss.

Answer: 1

At this time you:

1. Admit infant to the nursery for observation.
2. Obtain a hemoglobin/hematocrit.
3. Obtain a blood culture and start antibiotics.
4. Obtain vascular access and give a 10 mL/kg normal saline bolus infusion.

The next steps should include obtaining a CBC, fluid resuscitation with a normal saline bolus infusion of 10 mL/kg, and continued observation for vital sign abnormalities. All of these steps should happen simultaneously. The fluid resuscitation should be prioritized and should not be delayed to obtain blood for laboratory testing. In infants who require fluid resuscitation, transfer of care to a NICU is usually indicated for continued monitoring, stabilization, and treatment.

Answer: 1, 2, 4

What method of vascular access is preferred for a stable infant? What about for a critically ill infant?

1. Peripheral intravenous catheter (PIV)
2. Umbilical venous catheter (UVC)
3. Intraosseous catheter (IO)

In stable infants, a peripheral intravenous line may be placed for volume resuscitation. However, in emergent situations, umbilical venous catheterization is the preferred mode of vascular access [18]. A secondary option is placement of an intraosseous line. Blood products can be transfused through all three vascular access options (PIV, UVC, IO). If the infant's exam remains abnormal after one or two saline bolus infusions, evaluation for sepsis should also be considered.

Answer: 2

When anemia is suspected either in the delivery room or in the nursery, the provider should perform a detailed history (maternal, obstetric, and family) and physical exam and obtain initial laboratory studies to help guide the workup. Table 9.4 shows the recommended initial laboratory assessment.

These laboratory data will help the clinician establish the likely source of anemia by following the diagnostic algorithm in Fig. 9.1.

A pediatrician who attends deliveries should know the signs of fetal anemia as well as signs of anemia in the newborn. Signs of fetal anemia include elevated middle cerebral artery peak systolic velocity obtained by Doppler assessment, fetal growth restriction, fetal distress, and hydrops. When fetal anemia is suspected, the laboratory data listed in Table 10.4 should be ordered, and the bilirubin level should be measured in the cord blood.

Table 9.4 Recommended initial laboratory assessment in suspected anemia

Initial laboratory assessment in suspected anemia
Complete blood count (CBC)
Reticulocyte count
Blood type/Rh status
Direct Coombs test (DAT)
Peripheral smear

Adapted from [5, 7, 10, 17]

In our case, the infant is given a 10 mL/kg saline bolus infusion through a peripheral intravenous catheter at 1 h of age but continues to have tachycardia with heart rate in the 190 s and delayed capillary refill. Laboratory results reveal hemoglobin 8 g/dL, hematocrit 24%, blood type B+, direct Coombs test negative, and reticulocyte count 2%. It is important to remember that a subsequent hematocrit value may be even lower after postnatal fluid equilibration occurs. With confirmation of anemia, you reexamine the infant for ongoing sources of blood loss including detailed assessment of the head, fontanelles, neck, heart and lungs, abdomen, and extremities. You find no apparent source for an acute bleed or evidence of active ongoing bleeding. You suspect the source of blood loss may be abruption, cord injury at the time of delivery, or maternal-fetal hemorrhage.

At this time you:

1. Administer a second 10 mL/kg saline bolus infusion.
2. Order a packed red blood cell transfusion.
3. Repeat a CBC in 4–6 h.
4. Call your affiliated higher level NICU for a transfer.

This infant remains symptomatic from anemia and volume depletion. At this time, a packed red blood cell transfusion is indicated. If the provider does not have quick access to a packed red blood cell transfusion, a second 10 mL/kg saline bolus infusion is warranted to improve circulation. The infant will also need a follow-up CBC to monitor for continuing losses. Given the ongoing need for resuscitation, this infant should be transferred to higher level of care.

Answer: 1, 2, 3, 4

Nearly every pregnancy has some bleeding from the fetal to the maternal circulation [19]. However, the rate of significant transplacental hemorrhage is variable and, unless very large, rarely presents with hemodynamic instability at the time of birth [20]. The diagnosis of fetal-maternal hemorrhage is made on a sample of the mother's blood using either the Kleihauer-Betke test or flow cytometry. The Kleihauer-Betke test is done by exposing a slide with a smear of mother's blood to an acidic solution. The acid differentiates fetal from maternal red blood cells because fetal hemoglobin is stable at low pH and adult hemoglobin is not. Calculating the percent of fetal cells in the sample allows an estimate of the volume of fetal blood in the mother's circulation [7, 21]. Flow cytometry uses a monoclonal antibody to detect fetal hemoglobin in the mother's blood. The flow cytometry method is more accurate and reproducible than the Kleihauer-Betke method [22, 23]. The mother's obstetrician typically orders these tests unless the pediatrician is able to place orders for the mother.

Does this infant need a red blood cell transfusion:

1. Blood transfusion as an emergency (within 15–30 min).
2. Blood transfusion as a nonemergency (2–4 h).
3. Does not need a transfusion.

Blood transfusion therapy and policies have been actively studied in the premature neonatal population. Transfusion thresholds for premature infants have evolved over the past 20 years and are still an active area of research [24–27]. However, blood transfusions in term infants are rare and have not been extensively studied [28]. As a result, blood transfusion guidelines for term newborns are largely based on expert opinion and extrapolated from the work in premature infants. See Table 9.5 for suggested transfusion guidelines.

In this case, the infant is symptomatic with a hematocrit of 24% and would meet criteria for a blood transfusion. At this time, the infant is hemodynamically stable and does not need emergent blood (within 15 min) but would optimally be given a blood transfusion within the next 2–4 h. Whether the infant can remain in the nursery or be transferred to a NICU for the transfusion will depend on the institution's policies.

Answer: 2

Table 9.5 Suggested indications for blood transfusion for late preterm and term newborns in the first few days of life

Hematocrit	Clinical setting
Any	Acute blood loss resulting in hypovolemic shock
≤20%	Well appearing
20–30%	Signs of mild to moderate illness including but not limited to oxygen requirement, tachycardia, respiratory distress, or other clinical illnesses
30–35%	Extreme illness including but not limited to hypoxemia, need for mechanical ventilation, sepsis, and/or shock

These guidelines are based on [24–27, 29, 30]

Table 9.6 Suggested provider checklist prior to administration of packed red blood cells in newborns

Checklist prior to administering blood
Type and screen
State screen
Vascular access (preferably PIV in a stable infant). UVC or IO in unstable infant.
Parental consent in non-emergent cases

PIV peripheral intravenous line

Blood transfusions require special monitoring, including frequent assessment of vital signs and the infusion site. Most nurseries do not have sufficient equipment or staff to administer a blood transfusion, in which case the infant should be transferred to a higher level of care.

If a nursery is capable of performing a blood transfusion, a type and screen should be sent on the infant's blood (if not done already). Additionally, the *state/newborn screen should be performed on all infants prior to receiving blood products*. Every institution's blood bank will have a set of blood product regulations and guidelines for blood administration. Below are some recommendations and reminders that are unique to the neonatal population (Tables 9.6 and 9.7).

Providers should be aware that blood transfusions have risks and potential complications including both infectious and noninfectious etiologies. The primary noninfectious complications involve the following: acute immune-mediated, febrile non-hemolytic transfusion reactions, transfusion-related acute lung injury (TRALI), transfusion-related graft-versus-host disease,

Table 9.7 Reminders for packed red blood cell (pRBC) administration in newborns

Emergent situations	Non-emergent/urgent situations
Blood bank will usually provide emergency type O negative non-cross-matched blood	Blood bank will send a unit typed and cross-matched to mother's blood
15 mL/kg of pRBCs given over 15–30 min	15 mL/kg of pRBCs given over 3–4 h
	Neonatal blood products may be irradiated to help prevent graft-versus-host disease and leuko-reduced to minimize exposure to cytomegalovirus

Adapted from [30] and [31]

fluid overload, hyperkalemia, and hypocalcemia. These are quite rare in newborns. The infectious risks associated with blood transfusion are HIV, hepatitis C, hepatitis B, and bacterial contamination. All blood products in the United States undergo rigorous screening and the rates of viral transmission through blood products are exceedingly low [31].

Case Presentation

You are caring for a 1-day-old female infant who appeared to be 38-week gestational age by Ballard assessment; ultrasound data and date of last menstrual period were not available. The infant's mother immigrated to the United States from Central Africa when she was about 4 months pregnant. She received no prenatal care until the week before delivery. Maternal blood type is O positive and antibody screen negative. Screening tests for hepatitis B surface antigen and HIV are negative. The remainder of her serologies are pending at this time, and no family history is available.

The infant was born by vaginal delivery the preceding day. The mother was diagnosed with chorioamnionitis based on fever and tachycardia during labor. There was no report of a difficult extraction and the infant did well after delivery. Apgar scores were 8 and 9 at 1 and 5 min, respectively. On your daily rounds, the infant appears well perfused and active and has been feeding well. Vital signs and physical exam are within normal limits.

Although the infant is asymptomatic, you obtain a CBC as part of a sepsis evaluation due to maternal chorioamnionitis. The white blood cell count, differential, and platelet count are all within the reference range for gestational age. The hemoglobin is 9.3 gm/dL, and hematocrit is 28%. Mean corpuscular volume (MCV) is within the reference range for age. The infant's blood type is O positive and direct Coombs negative.

What do you do next?

1. Repeat the CBC in 24 h.
2. Obtain a reticulocyte count.
3. Obtain a peripheral blood smear.
4. Continue to observe with no additional laboratory data.

In this case, a reticulocyte count and peripheral smear would be the next steps in evaluating this patient. These tests (reticulocyte count and peripheral smear) are important for determining the cause of anemia. (See Fig. 9.1 for a general diagnostic approach to anemia.) After a short while, the reticulocyte count returns with a value of 0.02% (very low for age).

Answer: 2, 3

Of the following, which infection is ***least likely to*** cause of anemia in the newborn period?

1. Parvovirus
2. HIV
3. Rubella
4. Rhinovirus

When you question the mother again, she mentions that she had a cold-like illness in the days and weeks before delivery. You suspect a transient effect on red blood cell production from a maternal infection. The mother's obstetrician obtains a viral panel that returns positive for acute parvovirus infection. Other common infections that can present as anemia in the nursery include HIV, rubella, and syphilis [5]. Rhinovirus does not typically cause anemia in the newborn period.

Answer: 4

If the reticulocyte count is normal to high, other considerations would include hemoglobinopathies such sickle cell disease or thalassemia or RBC structural abnormalities (hereditary spherocytosis, hereditary elliptocytosis, and spectrin deficiency). Hemoglobinopathies can be divided into two categories based on their etiology: thalassemias (alteration in the number of globin chains) and hemoglobin structural variants such as hemoglobin S and hemoglobin C. Hemoglobinopathies may be diagnosed prenatally, on the newborn screen, or later in childhood if clinical manifestations are mild [32]. The newborn screen is state specific, so it is important to know whether your state screen includes testing for hemoglobinopathies.

If the family history is positive, peripheral smear is abnormal, and/or the infant has a nonhemolytic (Coombs negative) anemia, you would need to consider RBC structural abnormalities. The two most common types of RBC membrane abnormalities include hereditary spherocytosis and hereditary elliptocytosis. With hereditary spherocytosis, anemia rarely occurs in the first few days after birth. However, the infant may have a rapid rise in bilirubin requiring intervention. Anemia may present in days to weeks and these infants will need close follow-up [5]. All patients with a suspected hemoglobinopathy or RBC membrane deficiency should be referred to a hematologist.

Unusual considerations include bone marrow failure syndromes including Diamond-Blackfan anemia, Fanconi anemia, Shwachman-Diamond syndrome, or congenital dyserythropoietic anemia [33, 34]. These conditions are rare and often have associated physical anomalies. All bone marrow failure syndromes will require subspecialty referral and follow-up.

Clinical Pearls

1. Define anemia by comparing the hemoglobin or hematocrit to the reference range for gestational or postnatal age.
2. Order a complete blood count, blood type and antibody screen, reticulocyte count, direct antiglobulin test (DAT), and peripheral smear as first-line diagnostic laboratory studies for anemia.
3. A pediatrician can manage most cases of mild to moderate anemia in the newborn nursery.
4. Closely monitor infants with subgaleal hemorrhage, as they can progress rapidly to hemorrhagic shock.
5. Recognize the indications for emergent or controlled blood transfusions.
6. Refer infants with known or suspected hemoglobinopathy, RBC membrane disorder, or bone marrow failure syndrome to a pediatric hematologist.

References

1. Christensen RD, Henry E, Jopling J, Wiedmeier SE. The CBC: reference ranges for neonates. Semin Perinatol. 2009;33(1):3–11. https://doi.org/10.1053/j.semperi.2008.10.010.
2. Jopling J, Henry E, Wiedmeier SE, Christensen RD. Reference ranges for hematocrit and blood hemoglobin concentration during the neonatal period: data from a multihospital health care system. Pediatrics. 2009;123(2):e333–7. https://doi.org/10.1542/peds.2008-2654.
3. Christensen RD, Del Vecchio A, Henry E. Expected erythrocyte, platelet and neutrophil values for term and preterm neonates. The journal of maternal-fetal & neonatal medicine : the official journal of the European Association of Perinatal Medicine, the Federation of Asia and Oceania Perinatal Societies, the International Society of Perinatal Obstet. 2012;25(Suppl 5):77–9. https://doi.org/10.3109/14767058.2012.715472.
4. Christensen RD, Yaish HM, Henry E, Bennett ST. Red blood cell distribution width: reference intervals for neonates. The journal of maternal-fetal & neonatal medicine : the official journal of the European Association of Perinatal Medicine, the Federation of Asia and Oceania Perinatal Societies, the International

Society of Perinatal Obstet. 2015;28(8):883-8. https://doi.org/10.3109/14767058.2014.938044.
5. Bizzarro MJ, Colson E, Ehrenkranz RA. Differential diagnosis and management of anemia in the newborn. Pediatr Clin N Am. 2004;51(4):1087–107. https://doi.org/10.1016/j.pcl.2004.03.006.
6. Murray NA, Roberts IAG. Haemolytic disease of the newborn. Arch Dis Child Fetal Neonatal Ed. 2007;92(2):F83–F8. https://doi.org/10.1136/adc.2005.076794.
7. Maheshwari A, Carlo W. Blood Disorders. In: Nelson textbook of pediatrics [internet]. 20th ed. Philadelphia: Elsevier; 2016. p. 880–9.e1.
8. Mitchell S, James A. Severe late anemia of hemolytic disease of the newborn. Paediatr Child Health. 1999;4(3):201–3.
9. Ree IMC, Smits-Wintjens V, van der Bom JG, van Klink JMM, Oepkes D, Lopriore E. Neonatal management and outcome in alloimmune hemolytic disease. Expert Rev Hematol. 2017:1–10. https://doi.org/10.1080/17474086.2017.1331124.
10. Blanchette VS, Zipursky A. Assessment of anemia in newborn infants. Clin Perinatol. 1984;11(2):489–510.
11. Hospital Stay for Healthy Term Newborns. Pediatrics. 2010;125(2):405.
12. Martin JA, Hamilton BE, Osterman MJ, Driscoll AK, Births MTJ. Final data for 2015. National vital statistics reports : from the Centers for Disease Control and Prevention, National Center for Health Statistics, National Vital Statistics System. 2017;66(1):1.
13. Ali UA, Norwitz ER. Vacuum-assisted vaginal delivery. Reviews in Obstetrics and Gynecology. 2009;2(1):5–17.
14. Walsh CA, Robson M, McAuliffe FM. Mode of delivery at term and adverse neonatal outcomes. Obstet Gynecol. 2013;121(1):122–8. https://doi.org/10.1097/AOG.0b013e3182749ac9.
15. Lubin B. Neonatal anaemia secondary to blood loss. Clin Haematol. 1978;7(1):19–34.
16. Chadwick LM, Pemberton PJ, Kurinczuk JJ. Neonatal subgaleal haematoma: associated risk factors. complications and outcome Journal of paediatrics and child health. 1996;32(3):228–32.
17. Pearson HA. Anemia in the newborn: a diagnostic approach and challenge. Seminars in Perinatology. 1991;15(3 Suppl 2):2-8.
18. Weiner GM, Zaichkin J, American Heart Association., American Academy of Pediatrics. Textbook of neonatal resuscitation. 2016. Available from: https://ebooks.aappublications.org/content/textbook-of-neonatal-resuscitation-nrp-7th-ed.
19. Wylie BJ, D'Alton ME. Fetomaternal hemorrhage. Obstet Gynecol. 2010;115(5):1039–51. https://doi.org/10.1097/AOG.0b013e3181da7929.
20. Solomonia N, Playforth K, Reynolds EW. Fetal-maternal hemorrhage: a case and literature review. AJP Reports. 2012;2(1):7–14. https://doi.org/10.1055/s-0031-1296028.
21. Kleihauer E, Braun H, Betke K. Demonstration of fetal hemoglobin in erythrocytes of a blood smear. Klin Wochenschr. 1957;35(12):637–8.
22. Bromilow IM, Duguid JK. Measurement of feto-maternal haemorrhage: a comparative study of three Kleihauer techniques and tow flow cytometry methods. Clin Lab Haematol. 1997;19(2):137–42.
23. Dziegiel MH, Nielsen LK, Berkowicz A. Detecting fetomaternal hemorrhage by flow cytometry. Curr Opin Hematol. 2006;13(6):490–5. https://doi.org/10.1097/01.moh.0000245687.09215.c4.
24. Bell EF, Strauss RG, Widness JA, Mahoney LT, Mock DM, Seward VJ, et al. Randomized trial of liberal versus restrictive guidelines for red blood cell transfusion in preterm infants. Pediatrics. 2005;115(6):1685–91. https://doi.org/10.1542/peds.2004-1884.
25. Kirpalani H, Whyte RK, Andersen C, Asztalos EV, Heddle N, Blajchman MA, et al. The premature infants in need of transfusion (PINT) study: a randomized, controlled trial of a restrictive (low) versus liberal (high) transfusion threshold for extremely low birth weight infants. J Pediatr. 2006;149(3):301–7. https://doi.org/10.1016/j.jpeds.2006.05.011.
26. Whyte R, Kirpalani H. Low versus high haemoglobin concentration threshold for blood transfusion for preventing morbidity and mortality in very low birth weight infants. Cochrane Database Syst Rev. 2011;11:CD000512. https://doi.org/10.1002/14651858.CD000512.pub2.
27. Red blood cell transfusions in newborn infants. Revised guidelines. Paediatr Child Health. 2002;7(8):553–8.
28. Alverson DC. The physiologic impact of anemia in the neonate. Clin Perinatol. 1995;22(3):609–25.
29. Venkatesh V, Khan R, Curley A, New H, Stanworth S. How we decide when a neonate needs a transfusion. Br J Haematol. 2013;160(4):421–33. https://doi.org/10.1111/bjh.12095.
30. Girelli G, Antoncecchi S, Casadei AM, Del Vecchio A, Isernia P, Motta M, et al. Recommendations for transfusion therapy in neonatology. Blood Transfus. 2015;13(3):484–97. https://doi.org/10.2450/2015.0113-15.
31. Galel SA, Fontaine MJ. Hazards of neonatal blood transfusion. NeoReviews. 2006;7(2):e69.
32. Ryan K, Bain BJ, Worthington D, James J, Plews D, Mason A, et al. Significant haemoglobinopathies: guidelines for screening and diagnosis. Br J Haematol. 2010;149(1):35–49. https://doi.org/10.1111/j.1365-2141.2009.08054.x.
33. Shalev H, Moser A, Kapelushnik J, Karplus M, Zucker N, Yaniv I, et al. Congenital dyserythropoietic anemia type I presenting as persistent pulmonary hypertension of the newborn. J Pediatr. 2000;136(4):553–5.
34. Sieff CA, Nisbet-Brown E, Nathan DG. Congenital bone marrow failure syndromes. Br J Haematol. 2000;111(1):30–42. https://doi.org/10.1111/j.1365-2141.2000.02263.x.

Neonatal Hypoglycemia

10

David H. Adamkin

Introduction

The management of low blood glucose concentrations in the first 48 h of life is one of the most frequently encountered issues the healthcare provider faces in the newborn nursery. The blood levels of glucose upon which we base our decision-making remain more a matter of expert opinion rather than being evidence-based. The data needed to establish a consensus opinion on blood glucose levels that should be treated in the newborn are still not definitive enough.

In fact, the lack of consensus has led to further confusion for the clinician as two pediatric organizations, the Committee on the Fetus and Newborn from the American Academy of Pediatrics (AAP) and the Pediatric Endocrine Society (PES), have recently provided expert opinions on the management of neonatal hypoglycemia that suggested different ranges of actionable blood glucose levels [1, 2]. The AAP guidance applies only to the first 24 h of life, and the PES strategy focuses on infants beyond 48 h of life with the emphasis on making certain we identify cases of persistent hypoglycemia before these infants are discharged. The two organizations used different approaches to suggest the different ranges of glucose to act upon in the first 48 h of life.

In a recent editorial entitled "Imperfect Advice," Adamkin and Polin contrast the approaches of the two organizations and offer suggestions on how to merge their advice for management [3]. The AAP statement addressed only the first 24 h of life [1]. This editorial recommended a glucose level > 45 mg/dL for 24–48 h, which was not covered in the AAP algorithm. This allows transition to the PES recommendations for blood glucose >60 mg /dL after 72–96 h of age [3]. In addition, the editorial addressed the main PES concern of not missing cases of persistent neonatal hypoglycemia, whereby infants with low blood glucose levels are either missed or infants treated for hypoglycemia the first day or two are discharged before they demonstrate levels >60 to 70 mg/dL through several normal feed-fast cycles before being discharged [3].

Management of glucose in the neonate involves management of several different and at times opposing, clinical issues. The clinician must diagnose and manage hypoglycemia, promote successful breastfeeding, avoid unnecessary admissions to the neonatal intensive care unit, and also prevent infants from reaching higher blood glucose levels that reflect glucose instability and untoward neurodevelopmental outcome [4].

D. H. Adamkin, MD
Division of Neonatal Medicine, Department of Pediatrics, University of Louisville, Louisville, KY, USA
e-mail: David.Adamkin@louisville.edu

G. I. Martin, W. Rosenfeld (eds.), *Common Problems in the Newborn Nursery*,
https://doi.org/10.1007/978-3-319-95672-5_10

Case Presentation

A 24-year-old primigravida, after an uncomplicated pregnancy, is admitted in labor at 40-week gestation. She has had perinatal screening tests including a negative screen for group B streptococcal (GBS) colonization at 36-week gestation. She also had normal screening blood glucose values early in pregnancy and no history of diabetes or abnormal glucose values at any time. Rupture of membranes occurred 2 h prior to delivery; Apgars were 8 and 9 at 1 and 5 min, respectively. The male infant is AGA, weighing 3200 g.

The mother has read about breastfeeding, spoken prenatally with a lactation consultant, and plans to exclusively breastfeed. She begins by breastfeeding the infant in the delivery room, described as "successful" in the record at 45 min of age. A point-of-care (POC) blood glucose is performed after the feeding, and it is 35 mg/dL. The nurse calls you to let you know about this level and if you want to do anything. Shortly thereafter, the mother is transferred to a postpartum room.

Should this term AGA infant with no history of maternal diabetes or other risk factors have been screened at all? Indications for screening for hypoglycemia include all of the following except:

1. Small for gestational.
2. Large for gestational age.
3. Exclusive breastfeeding.
4. Infant of a diabetic mother.
5. Late preterm infant.

You have your smartphone at your bedside and you pull up the "Glucose App, Sugar Wheel" (Fig. 10.1) [4], and you confirm what you thought: that this baby's perinatal course met none of the risk factors that would lead to a screening blood glucose. Indications include large for gestational age, small for gestational age, infant of a diabetic mother, and late preterm infants (35–37 weeks of gestation). Some authors suggest that babies with perinatal asphyxia (Apgars ≤5 at 5 min) also be screened.

Answer: 3

At this time you:

1. Discontinue breastfeeding and start formula.
2. Supplement breastfeeding with formula.
3. Order 40% oral glucose gel.
4. Give IV D10W.
5. Continue breastfeeding.

You look at the wheel, and you note that the initial feeding took place within the first hour of life and the level they obtained (which should have been 30 min after the first feed if the baby was at high risk) was at a level that is considered acceptable during the first 4 h of life. You advise continued breastfeeding and no further screens unless the infant shows signs of hypoglycemia.

Answer: 5

It is 5 am and the baby is breastfed again at 8 h of age. After the feeding, the nurse on routine assessment thinks the baby is slightly tremulous. She performs point-of-care (POC) glucose level, and it is 36 mg/dL. The nurse tells the mother that the baby should be supplemented with 1 oz of term formula to raise the blood glucose. The mother is very disappointed and asks the nurse to call you because her plan was to exclusively breastfeed the infant.

For some reason the next feeding wasn't until 8 h of age. You recommended frequent feedings to promote glucose homeostasis and an optimal initiation of breastfeeding. The nurse called again at 8 h to report a POC of 36 mg/dL. On your wheel, this POC is just above the actionable level of 35 mg/dL for intravenous glucose (35 mg/dL for 4 to 24 h of age). Your choices include refeeding or IV glucose for levels 35–45 mg/dL. You should always confirm the POC with a plasma level from the lab and can wait to see if that value aligns with the POC. However, the nurse said that the infant was slightly tremulous.

At this time you:

1. Discontinue breastfeeding and start formula.
2. Supplement breastfeeding with formula.
3. Order 40% oral glucose gel.

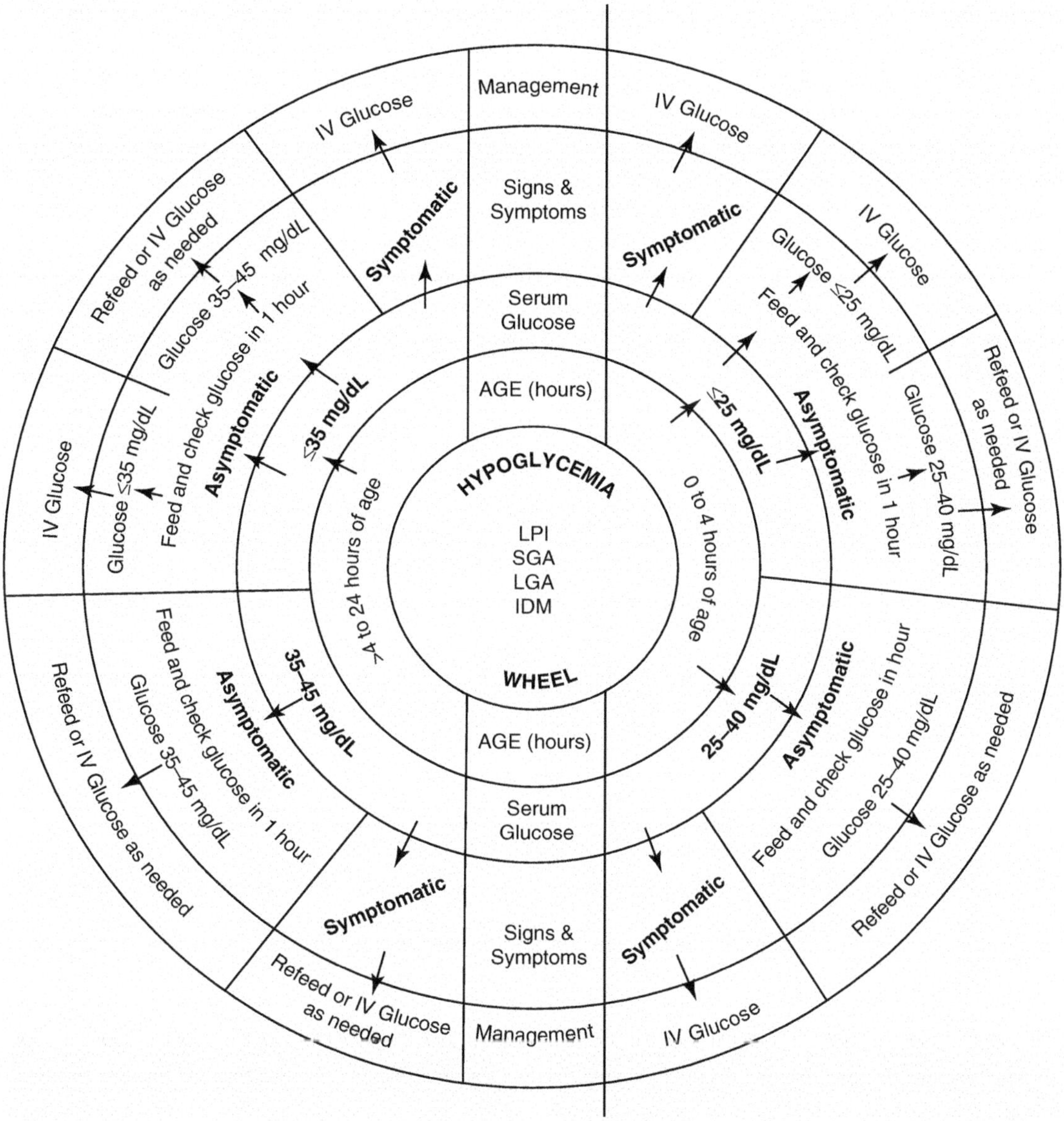

Fig. 10.1 The Sugar Wheel nomogram for the management of neonatal hypoglycemia in the first 24 h of life. Start at the center of the wheel, select the correct age and glucose level, and then determine whether the patient is symptomatic or asymptomatic. The proper treatment can then be selected. (From Polin and Yoder [4]).

4. Give IV D10W.
5. Continue breastfeeding.

If this baby is truly jittery, then everything changes because the infant is symptomatic. The recommendation for the symptomatic infant below 40 mg/dL is immediate intravenous glucose, while you wait for the confirmatory laboratory plasma glucose. The clinical signs of hypoglycemia are not specific and include a wide range of local or generalized manifestations that are common in sick neonates.

Your conundrum is whether this baby is truly symptomatic requiring IV glucose or is this normal newborn activity that would allow for feeding again and rechecking the POC glucose in 30 min? Remember this mother wanted exclusive breastfeeding for her infant. Do you have donor milk for this infant if you choose to refeed? What about using dextrose gel to treat the glucose level to avoid the use of formula? The answers to these two questions are frequently "not yet." Donor human milk as a supplement for the sluggishly feeding breastfed infant and the use of the new dextrose gel [5] may help to prevent babies with modest hypoglycemia from needing to go to the NICU for intravenous fluids. Current data suggest that the gel is safe and prevented admission to the NICU for intravenous fluids, but it did not improve neurodevelopmental outcome at 2 years of age [5, 6].

Therefore, formula might be the only choice, unless you believe the symptoms deserve intravenous treatment. If in your opinion the baby is truly "jittery," then you would order a mini-bolus of D10W at 2 mL/kg and/or IV infusion at 5 to 8 mg/k/min of D10W (80 mL/k/d) to achieve a plasma glucose of 40 to 50 mg/dL. The "Sugar Wheel" offers you all these choices, and it is based on Fig. 10.2, the algorithm from the Clinical Report, Postnatal Glucose Homeostasis in Late Preterm and Term Infants, published in Pediatrics in March 2011 from the AAP Committee on the Fetus and Newborn [1].

Could this infant simply have been left to continue breastfeeding? Yes, one of the choices was to continue simply breastfeeding this infant, monitoring POC glucose levels prior to feedings every 2 to 3 h because of the observation of this non-specific, ill-defined tremulousness that will probably resolve with further feedings and increased glucose levels. However, true jitteriness would require intravenous fluids.

Answer: 4 (If Truly Jittery); 5 (If No Clearly Defined Symptoms)

What is the value for plasma glucose at which a symptomatic infant should receive treatment?

1. 20 mg/dL.
2. 30 mg/dL.
3. 40 mg/dL.
4. 50 mg/dL.

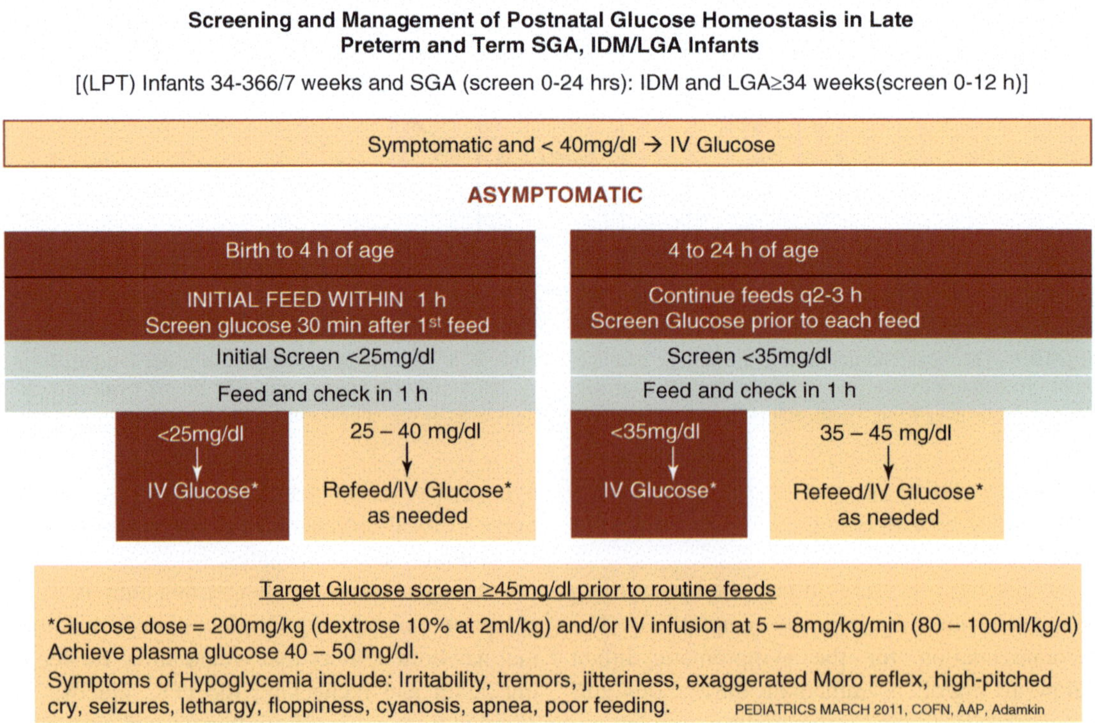

Fig. 10.2 Algorithm developed by the American Academy of Pediatrics for evaluation and treatment of neonates in the first 24 h of life. (Adamkin [1])

As alluded to above, the plasma glucose level that applies to symptomatic infants (signs included on the AAP algorithm and Sugar Wheel is <40 mg/dL [1, 4].

Answer: 3

Do infants that are exclusively breastfed have lower plasma glucose concentrations than those fed formula?

1. Yes
2. No

Infants who are exclusively breastfed tend to have lower blood glucose concentrations than those fed formula. Studies show a wide range of blood glucose values during the first 72 h of life for breastfeeding infants [7]. These same infants tend to have higher ketone levels, the principal alternate metabolic fuel for the brain. Therefore, studies indicate that breastfed term infants might have lower blood glucose concentrations and higher levels of ketone bodies than formula fed [7]. Still the same levels in the AAP algorithm should be applied to the breastfeeding infant.

Answer: 1

It is clear from this first case that the screening and management of postnatal glucose homeostasis in late preterm and term SGA, IDM/LGA infants (infant of a diabetic mother, large for gestational age) requires individual judgments and clinical choices based upon the risk and physical examination.

After birth, the normal newborn infant's plasma glucose concentration falls below levels that were prevalent in fetal life. In fact, at birth the blood glucose is about 70% of the maternal level. It falls rapidly to a nadir by 1 h of life to a value as low as 20 to 25 mg/dL [1]. These modest levels are common in healthy neonates and this fall is seen in all mammalian newborns. This is part of the normal transition to an extrauterine life. These levels are transient and the vast majority of infants are asymptomatic. Finally, the infant activates endocrine and metabolic transitions associated with successful adaptation. When this adaptation fails, perhaps secondary to immaturity or illness, there is a limitation of substrate supply, which may disturb cerebral function and potentially result in neurologic sequelae [8]. A low plasma glucose may be indicative of this process but is not per se diagnostic. What is meant by "low"? How low is "too low"? At what glucose level does hypoglycemia lead to irreversible changes in brain structure or function?

A consistent definition of hypoglycemia does not exist for the first 2 days of life. The first neonates recognized as having significant hypoglycemia 60 years ago had seizures and blood glucose levels consistently below 20 to 25 mg/dL [9]. The abnormal signs cleared quickly after increasing the blood glucose level to >40 mg/dL. This is how "40" became a classic standard for defining hypoglycemia. Despite our enhanced understanding of metabolic disturbances and genetic disorders, we still do not have a precise complete definition of hypoglycemia. Because we don't have sufficient evidence to answer "how low is too low and for how long," we continue to rely on expert opinion and best available evidence.

Case Presentation

A term AGA infant was born after negative prenatal screens and an uneventful pregnancy to a 35-year-old gravida 2 woman. The mother also had normal prenatal glucose screens and no history of diabetes. Apgar scores were 5, 7, and 8 at 1, 5, and 10 min, respectively. The baby appeared cyanotic in the delivery room and received brief blow by oxygen.

At approximately 1 h of age, a bedside glucose was performed in the nursery when it was noted the baby had received oxygen in the delivery room. A POC glucose was obtained before the infant was sent out to the mother's room. The baby had normal vital signs and exam findings, and the oxygen saturation in room air was 97%. The POC glucose was 27 mg/dL. A stat specimen was also sent to the laboratory. The infant actually received a feeding of formula after this at approximately 1.5 h of age, and another POC was done 30 min after this feeding. As the nurse is calling you about what to do with this baby, the plasma glucose from the lab is called to the nursery, and it was 37 mg/dL.

Should this baby have received the initial screening bedside POC glucose at 1 h of age before the feedings were initiated?

1. Yes
2. No

Cyanosis is a potential sign or symptom of hypoglycemia with established hypoglycemia (Refer to Signs and Symptoms of hypoglycemia in newborn infants in Hypoglycemia in Newborn Infants: Features Associated with Adverse Outcomes. Rozance PJ and Hay WH: Biol Neonate 2006;90;p 81.) [10]. However, brief cyanosis, associated with transition in the delivery room with rapid resolution, would not be. Apgar scores were not compatible with asphyxia. Therefore, this infant did not meet any of the risk factors to screen for hypoglycemia.

Answer: 2

POC screening tests are often:

1. Higher than values analyzed in the laboratory on plasma samples.
2. Lower than values analyzed in the laboratory on plasma samples.
3. The same as values analyzed in the laboratory on plasma samples.

Bedside screening values of POC glucose are not as accurate as plasma levels from the laboratory and usually are lower. This is particularly true at the lower levels of glucose where accurate data is needed the most [11]. Therefore we use the POC in order to treat glucose levels in symptomatic infants. In asymptomatic infants we can wait for the laboratory glucose for correlation with the bedside POC.

Answer: 2

What is the significance of the POC of 27 mg/dL at 1 h of age prior to feeding and the actual plasma glucose from the lab of 37 mg/dL for the same sample?

1. It was drawn appropriately and should be acted on.
2. The POC value of 27 mg/dL must be treated with an IV glucose infusion.
3. The laboratory value is 37 mg/dL and the baby requires no treatment.

The bedside screen of 27 mg/dL at 1 h of age is typical of the nadir the glucose can reach at the lower centiles during transitional hypoglycemia and may not accurately reflect the true plasma glucose level. The AAP decided that it did not want to sample the nadir value to decide on management of hypoglycemia. Therefore, the screening was inappropriate. The POC value is low but if accurate is not abnormal since it represents a physiologic nadir. The 37 mg/dL plasma value is the most accurate, is normal, and also represents a physiologic nadir. To be consistent with WHO standards, all newborns should be fed by 1 h of age, and the screen should take place 30 min after the first feed [1].

Answer: 3

The repeat bedside POC at 2 h of age is 37 mg/dL. Is that an actionable level?

1. Yes
2. No

The repeat level of 37 mg/dL at 2 h of age should again be confirmed with a lab level because it is in the actionable range of 25–40 mg/dL. However, none of these levels were necessary in this infant who had no risk factors and was asymptomatic. The treatment for this infant is to let it be treated as a normal newborn and feed frequently.

Answer: 2

The AAP and the PES have provided us with expert opinion about the management of neonatal hypoglycemia. The PES used neuroendocrine and metabolic data to demonstrate that the first 48 h can be characterized as a transitional hyperinsulinemia with low ketone levels, inappropriate preservation of glycogen, and mean glucose levels of 55–65 mg/dL. By 72 h, levels rise to those observed in older children and adults of >70 mg/dL. The 55–65 mg/dL range is the same level at which adults and older children demonstrate neurogenic symptoms, and this range defines the critical recommendation from the PES for the first 48 h of life [2].

The AAP relied on analyses of the lower range of glucose that occurs during the establishment of postnatal glucose homeostasis and advised actionable ranges of 25–40 mg/dL for the first 4 h of age and 35–45 mg /dL from 4 to 24 h of age. Adamkin and Polin, in a commentary in the *Journal of Pediatrics*, advised using a level of >45 mg/dL for infants between 24 and 48 h of age [3].

By 72 h of age, levels rise to >60–70 mg/dL, similar to older children and adults. The AAP recommendations and the Adamkin and Polin editorial for treatment below or in the actionable ranges for the first 48 h are based on the individual risk assessment and examination of the infant [1, 3]. The AAP believed that these levels provided a margin of safety and flexibility to identify those infants who require intravenous dextrose and those with borderline levels that need to be followed beyond 48 h to prevent missing cases of persistent hypoglycemia. It was thought that this approach would promote successful breastfeeding and avoid unnecessary admission to the NICU in contrast to the PES recommendation of plasma glucose >50 mg/dl for the first 48 h. However, over time the two organizations' recommendations have come closer together. The commitment to try and identify cases of persistent hypoglycemia prior to discharge has been accepted by the AAP, including the "fasting challenge" for some infants with borderline blood glucose levels after 48 h of life and who had been treated with IV dextrose or maintained lower levels of glucose over the first days of life [2].

Case Presentation

A term male infant is born to a 21-year-old primigravida who had no prenatal care. Because of failure to progress, a cesarean section was performed. Apgar scores were 6 and 7 at 1 and 5 min, respectively. The infant weighed 4200 g, and length and head circumference plotted around the 75th percentile on the growth chart. At 6 h of age, the infant appeared lethargic, feeding poorly at the breast and very jittery. A bedside POC was done and was 10 mg/dL. A laboratory specimen was also sent simultaneously.

When should this infant have been screened for hypoglycemia?

1. Immediately after birth.
2. After the first feed (within the first hour of life).
3. 2 h.
4. 4 h.
5. 6 h.

This macrosomic infant with asymmetric macrosomia (suggesting birth to a diabetic mother) should have been screened at the first sign of symptoms and, if asymptomatic, screened 30 min after the first feeding, within 1 h after delivery. Relevant conditions in the pathogenesis of neonatal hypoglycemia include those that cause excess utilization of glucose, such as hyperinsulinism in infants of diabetic mothers, LGA, SGA, islet cell, or other endocrine pathologies. Both IDM and LGA term infants are considered high risk and should be screened according to the algorithm.

Answer: 2

What is the appropriate treatment of this baby?

1. Refeed with breast milk.
2. Refeed with formula.
3. Refeed with D10W.
4. Treat with continuous IV infusion.

5. Treat with a bolus of D10W at 2 mL/kg and IV infusion at 5–8 mg/k/min of D10W (80 mL/k/d).

While the AAP algorithm states that for the asymptomatic baby with low glucose, another feeding could be attempted, this is a severely symptomatic infant that should be treated with intravenous dextrose (bolus followed by continuous infusion) and monitored closely.

Answer: 5

Case Presentation

A 32-year-old gravida 2 delivers a male infant by cesarean section because of failure to progress, a fetal heart rate tracing with fetal distress, and meconium-stained amniotic fluid. Fetal macrosomia was suspected during the pregnancy and the mother had been monitored for hyperglycemia and was treated with insulin for diabetes during the pregnancy. Apgar scores were 4, 6, and 8 at 1, 5, and 10 min, respectively. The infant's birthweight was 4.6 kg. The infant was breastfed in the delivery room and was screened with a bedside POC glucose 30 min after the completion of the breastfeeding. The baby's examination revealed macrosomia, but he was in no distress and was described as quiet but with normal reflexes, tone, and color. The first screening POC glucose was 15 mg/dL; a plasma glucose sent from the same sample was 18 mg/dL. The nurse called the pediatrician and asked what to do next. The decision was to refeed since the baby was asymptomatic, but clearly, concerns were raised about the maternal diabetes and the baby's macrosomia. The baby was refed, and 30 min later the POC was 20 mg/dL and plasma glucose from the laboratory was 23 mg/dL.

Was it the right decision to refeed this baby after the initial POC of 15 and confirmed with an 18 mg/dL from the lab?

1. Yes
2. No

It was the right decision to refeed after the initial feed when the baby had a POC of 15 mg/dL, which the lab confirmed to be low at 18 mg / dL. Despite a low blood glucose, some babies like the one presented may respond and can be managed enterally. The macrosomia suggests it is unlikely this infant will be manageable with only breastfeedings and supplements, but if the baby looks well and is asymptomatic, this approach can be attempted.

Answer: 1

What do you do next after the second phone call with the laboratory glucose of 20 mg/dL in a baby that is still described as non-distressed but sleepy?

1. Refeed with breast milk.
2. Refeed with formula.
3. Gavage with D10W.
4. Administer 40% glucose gel to the oral mucosa.
5. Treat with a bolus of D10W at 2 mL/kg and/or IV infusion at 5 to 8 mg/k/min of D10W (80 mL/k/d).

This baby needs to go to a site that can provide intravenous fluids and monitor glucose very carefully, particularly if this infant requires hypertonic dextrose for persistent hypoglycemia.

Answer: 5

The baby is transferred to the tertiary care center, and despite increasing IV rates, the infant still has glucose levels below 40 mg/dL at a glucose infusion rate of 16 mg/kg/min. Unfortunately, this infant has a difficult course attaining a normal glucose despite very high glucose infusion rates and is treated with steroids and then octreotide for persistent hypoglycemia. An endocrine work-up for severe hypoglycemia would be necessary if the hypoglycemia persists despite vigorous treatment with intravenous glucose.

Infants with persistent hypoglycemia or those with inadequate response to treatment need

Table 10.1 Causes of recurrent or persistent hypoglycemia [10]

Hormone deficiencies	
Multiple endocrine deficiency or congenital hypopituitarism	Anterior pituitary "aplasia"
	Congenital optic nerve hypoplasia
Primary endocrine deficiency	Isolated growth hormone deficiency
	Adrenogenital syndrome
	Adrenal hemorrhage
Hormone excess with hyperinsulinism	Beckwith-Wiedemann syndrome
	Hereditary defects of pancreatic islet cells
Hereditary deficits in carbohydrate metabolism	Glycogen storage disease
	Fructose intolerance
	Galactosemia
	Glycogen synthase deficiency
	Fructose, 1–6 diphosphatase deficiency
Hereditary deficits in amino acid metabolism	Maple syrup urine disease
	Propionic acidemia
	Methylmalonic acidemia
	Methylmalonic acidemia Tyrosinosis
	3-OH-3-methylglutaryl-COA lyase deficiency
Hereditary defects in fatty acid metabolism	Acyl-CoA dehydrogenase—medium, long chain
	Deficiency
	Mitochondrial β-oxidation and degradation defects

From Cornblath and Ichord [12]

further evaluation. Recurrent or persistent hypoglycemia (Table 10.1) [12] is defined as a condition that [1] requires infusions of large amounts of glucose (>12 to 16 mg/k/min) to maintain normoglycemia or [2] persists or recurs beyond the first 7 to 14 days of life. These infants require specific diagnostic determinations such as a rapid trial of therapeutic/diagnostic agents to determine the cause and therapy [2].

Hyperinsulinism, hypopituitarism, and fatty acid oxidation disorders are probably the most common of these rarer causes of neonatal hypoglycemia that should be diagnosed before discharge.

An underlying metabolic or hormonal etiology should be suspected when hypoglycemia is of unusual severity or occurs in an otherwise low-risk infant. Some clues to a possible underlying metabolic-hormonal disorder include:

- Symptomatic hypoglycemia in a healthy, well-grown term infant
- Hypoglycemia with seizures or abnormalities of consciousness
- Persistent or recurrent hypoglycemia
- Hypoglycemia with other abnormalities (midline defects, micropenis, exophthalmos, labile thermoregulation)
- Hypoglycemia requiring greater than 10 mg/kg/min of glucose
- Family history of sudden infant deaths or developmental delays

Clinical Pearls

1. Neonates at risk for hypoglycemia LGA, IDM, SGA, late preterm) should be screened in the first hour of life (after a feed) for hypoglycemia.
2. Newborns displaying symptoms that could be caused by hypoglycemia need to be responded to immediately. The correct diagnosis must be determined and treatment initiated immediately if hypoglycemia is found.
3. The American Academy of Pediatrics (AAP) algorithm can be used to monitor and treat neonatal hypoglycemia in the first 24 h of life.
4. The recommendations of the Pediatric Endocrine Society (PES) discuss glucose levels after 48 h of life and were developed to heighten awareness of persistent hypoglycemic syndromes in infants with low levels of glucose that do not normalize.
5. There is a gap (24–48 h) not covered by either the AAP guideline or PES recommendations. Maintaining a glucose level > 45 mg/dL from 24 to 48 h of life is recommended.
6. It is critical to identify those with persistent hypoglycemic syndromes to pre-

vent neurologic injury. It is possible that low glucose levels seen in the first 48 h of life may herald metabolic disorders.

7. Neonates diagnosed with hypoglycemia need to achieve a glucose level of >60 mg/dL after 48 h, and levels must be maintained through several fast-feed cycles.

References

1. Adamkin D. Committee on fetus and newborn. Postnatal glucose homeostasis in late-preterm and term infants. Pediatr. 2011;127(3):575–9.
2. Thornton PS, Stanley CA, DeLeon DD, Harris D, Haymon MW, Hussain K, et al. Recommendations from the pediatric Endocrine Society for evaluation and management of persistent hypoglycemia in neonate, infants, and children. J Pediatr. 2015;167:238–45.
3. Adamkin D, Polin R. Imperfect advice: neonatal hypoglycemia. J Pediatr. 2016;176:195–6.
4. Adamkin D. Hypoglycemia. In: Polin R, Yoder M, editors. Workbook in practical neonatology. 5th ed. New York: Saunders; 2014. p. 47.
5. Harris DL, Weston PJ, Signal M, Chase JG, Harding JE. Dextrose gel for neonatal hypoglycaemia (the sugar babies study): a randomized, double-blind, placebo-controlled trial. Lancet. 2013;382: 2077–83.
6. Harris DL, Alsweiler JM, Ansell JM, Gamble GD, Thompson B, Wouldes TA, et al. Outcome at 2 years after dextrose gel treatment for neonatal hypoglycemia: follow-up of a randomized trial. J Pediatr. 2016;170:54–9.
7. Hoseth E, Jorgensen A, Ebbesen F, Moeller M. Blood glucose levels in a population of healthy, breastfed, term infants of appropriate size foe gestational age. Arch Dis Child Fetal Neonatal Ed. 2000;83(2):F117–9.
8. Cornblath M, Hawdon JM, Willams AF, Aynsley-Green A, Ward-Platt MP, Schwartz R, et al. Controversies regarding definition of neonatal hypoglycemia: suggested operational thresholds. Pediatrics. 2000;105(5):1141–5.
9. Cornblath M. Reminiscence of a 50 year adventure. NeoReviews. 2006;90(2):74–86.
10. Rozance P, Hay W. Hypoglycemia in newborn infants: features associated with adverse outcomes. Biol Neonate. 2006;90:74–86.
11. Altimier L, Roberts W. One touch ll hospital system foe neonates: correlation with serum glucose values. Neonatal Netw. 1996;15(2):15–8.
12. Cornblath M, Ichord R. Hypoglycemia in the neonate. Semin Perinatol. 2000;24:136–49.

Disorders of Calcium, Phosphorous, and Magnesium in the Newborn

11

Arielle L. Olicker, Avroy A. Fanaroff, and Jonathan M. Fanaroff

Disorders of Calcium, Phosphorous, and Magnesium in the Newborn

Calcium, phosphorous, and magnesium are stored mainly in the bone; hence these minerals are referred to as the "bone minerals." A portion of these minerals reside in the intracellular and extracellular spaces where they have important roles in critical physiological processes, including transport across cell membranes, enzyme activation and inhibition, regulation of intracellular metabolic pathways, and secretion and activity of hormones. These minerals are also involved in protein synthesis, maintaining membrane integrity, muscle contractility, neuromuscular excitation, nerve conduction, coagulation, and energy metabolism. Additionally, phosphorous is an important constituent of nucleic acids and cell membranes.

In the normal newborn nursery, symptoms of calcium, magnesium, and phosphorous abnormalities are relatively uncommon and often nonspecific. Awareness of these disorders facilitates early recognition and the institution of appropriate therapies. Failure to recognize the significance of symptomatic infants with these disorders can have dire consequences.

Case Presentation

A female infant is born at 37 4/7-week gestational age, with a birth weight of 4320 grams (9 pounds, 8 ounces). This is the first pregnancy for a 24-year-old mother whose blood type is A+. She had good prenatal care, and screening for group B streptococcus at 35-week gestation was negative. The pregnancy was complicated by maternal obesity (BMI 37) and gestational diabetes, with an abnormal oral glucose tolerance test and hemoglobin A1C level of 8.3% (desired value <6%). Onset of labor is spontaneous but ultimately results in caesarian section

A. L. Olicker, MD (✉)
Pediatrics, Division of Neonatology, Case Western Reserve University School of Medicine, Rainbow Babies and Children's Hospital, University Hospitals Cleveland Medical Center, Cleveland, OH, USA
e-mail: arielle.olicker@uhhospitals.org

A. A. Fanaroff, MD, FRCP, FRCPCH
Pediatrics, Division of Neonatology, Case Western Reserve School of Medicine and Eliza Henry Barnes Chair in Neonatology, Rainbow Babies and Children's Hospital, University Hospitals Cleveland Medical Center, Cleveland, OH, USA
e-mail: aaf2@case.edu

J. M. Fanaroff, MD, JD
Pediatrics, Division of Neonatology, Case Western Reserve University School of Medicine, Rainbow Center for Pediatric Ethics, Neonatal Intensive Care Unit, Rainbow Babies and Children's Hospital, University Hospitals Cleveland Medical Center, Cleveland, OH, USA
e-mail: jonathan.fanaroff@uhhospitals.org

G. I. Martin, W. Rosenfeld (eds.), *Common Problems in the Newborn Nursery*,
https://doi.org/10.1007/978-3-319-95672-5_11

due to arrest of descent of the fetal head into the maternal pelvis. Rupture of membranes was 12 h prior to delivery. The infant is vigorous upon delivery, and no resuscitation is required beyond drying, bulb suction, and tactile stimulation. Apgar scores at 1 and 5 min are 9 and 9, respectively.

The infant is transferred to the newborn nursery at 1 h of life. She is doing well. She has attempted direct breastfeeding once and had a good latch and effective suck; however her mother's milk has not yet come in. At approximately 2 h of life, the infant is noted to be jittery.

What should you do?

1. Check blood glucose.
2. Check urine toxicology screen.
3. Check electrolytes including calcium and magnesium levels.
4. Draw blood culture and start antibiotics.

Given that this infant is large for gestational age, and the infant of a diabetic mother, the most likely cause of jitteriness and one that would require immediate attention, is hypoglycemia. Therefore, a reasonable first step would be to check a blood glucose level at the bedside.

Answer: 1

It would not be wrong, in the case of a jittery infant, to check a urine toxicology screen or electrolytes. However, in the case of the infant of a diabetic mother where neonatal hypoglycemia is the most common cause of jitteriness, this quick bedside point-of-care test is an appropriate first step.

Blood glucose checked and noted to be 25 mg/dL. The infant is fed, and blood glucose is checked again and is noted to be 32 mg/dL. Peripheral intravenous access is established, and the infant is given 2 ml/kg of 10% dextrose in water as an intravenous bolus, followed by the initiation of intravenous infusion of 10% dextrose in water at a glucose infusion rate (GIR) of 6 mg/kg/min. The blood glucose is checked again 10 min later and is now 70 mg/dL. On exam, however, the infant remains jittery.

Infants of diabetic mothers are at risk for hypoglycemia following delivery. This occurs as the result of fetal pancreatic islet cell hypertrophy in response to increased placental transfer of glucose from hyperglycemic mother to fetus. Maternal insulin is not transferred to the fetus across the placenta; therefore, in order to maintain euglycemia, the fetus increases endogenous production of insulin. At delivery, the placental transfer of glucose is abruptly discontinued, but the pancreatic islet cells continue to secrete insulin at the rate that was necessary for glucose metabolism during fetal life, placing the infant at risk for hyperinsulinemic hypoglycemia. Hypoglycemia is a common cause of jitteriness in an infant, but it is not the only cause.

What are your next steps?

1. Check electrolytes including calcium and magnesium.
2. EEG.
3. Give a second D10W IV bolus and recheck blood glucose level.
4. Increase GIR until jitteriness resolves.

The most recent blood glucose, taken when the infant was on a GIR of 6 mg/kg/min, is within normal limits. Since the infant remains on consistent GIR, and remains jittery, the next step is to evaluate for other causes of jitteriness, including electrolyte abnormalities.

Answer: 1

A set of electrolytes is sent to the lab for analysis and reveals the infant to have a total serum calcium level of 6.8 mg/dL with an ionized calcium level of 0.79 mmol/L.

What is/are the next step(s)?

1. Add oral calcium supplementation to enteral feeds.
2. Add calcium gluconate to IV fluid infusion.
3. Give calcium bolus.
4. Check magnesium.

Because the infant is symptomatic, IV calcium gluconate is added to continuous IV fluids with dextrose. The infant's jitteriness resolves. Upon recheck, total serum calcium concentration is 8.8 mg/dL, and ionized calcium level is 1.2 mmol/L. As the infant begins to feed, she is able to be weaned off of continuous infusion of dextrose and calcium, and neither hypoglycemia nor hypocalcemia recur.

Answer: 2

Neonatal Hypocalcemia

Neonatal hypocalcemia is defined as a serum calcium concentration of less than 2 mmol/L (8 mg/dL) or an ionized calcium concentration of less than 1.1 mmol/L (4.8 mg/dL). The interruption of the placental calcium supply at the time of birth is associated with a physiologic drop in the serum calcium concentration. The infant normally maintains serum calcium homeostasis by reabsorption of calcium stored in the bones and from enteral nutrition.

Hypocalcemia may be associated with?

1. Prematurity.
2. Maternal diabetes.
3. Perinatal asphyxia.
4. Intrauterine growth restriction.
5. All of the above.

The most common causes of hypocalcemia in the newborn (1–4 days of life) include prematurity, maternal diabetes, perinatal stress/asphyxia, and intrauterine growth restriction. Symptoms are nonspecific and may include jitteriness, apnea, cyanosis, or seizures.

Answer: 5

Infants of diabetic mothers (IDM) have an exaggerated drop in serum calcium concentration. IDMs are also at increased risk of being born prematurely and of perinatal stress/asphyxia, both of which are independent risk factors for hypocalcemia and further increase the risk for an infant of a diabetic mother. Hypocalcemia in an IDM may be related to maternal hypomagnesemia which is caused by increased urinary excretion of magnesium. This can result in fetal and neonatal hypoparathyroidism and will make it difficult to correct the serum calcium concentration until the serum magnesium concentration is replete. The degree of hypocalcemia in an IDM is correlated with the severity of maternal diabetes during the pregnancy.

When an infant has symptoms associated with hypocalcemia, it is important to determine the concentrations of total serum calcium as well as the ionized portion. It is important to consider the ionized portion in addition to the total blood calcium concentration, as calcium is highly bound to albumin. It is the ionized portion of calcium that is physiologically active. Newborns often have relatively low levels of blood albumin; therefore, their total blood calcium concentration may be proportionally lower than their ionized calcium concentration. When this is the case, the infant is generally not symptomatic, as the physiologically active ionized portion may be within normal limits. It is also important to check serum albumin, a blood gas (acidosis will displace calcium from albumin, allowing for a relatively increased ionized portion of total serum calcium), and urine concentrations of calcium, magnesium, and phosphorous. If hypocalcemia is refractory to treatment with calcium supplementation, it may be accompanied by concurrent hypomagnesemia. If the cause remains undetermined, the next steps may be to perform a thorough physical exam including a cardiac exam, check parathyroid hormone and calcitonin levels, obtain a radiograph of the chest looking for absence of the thymus, and obtain genetic studies to evaluate for DiGeorge syndrome.

The treatment for hypocalcemia is to provide supplemental calcium. In most cases, asymptomatic neonatal hypocalcemia will resolve spontaneously with enteral nutrition, and many providers will choose to monitor without treatment. Symptomatic hypocalcemia, on the other hand, is treated with administration of calcium salts, usually intravenously. In cases of hypocalcemic seizure, tetany, or apnea, an intravenous bolus of a calcium salt should be given, usually in an intensive care setting. First choice is usually calcium gluconate, but calcium chloride may be more readily available and may be used in an emergency. A bolus of 1–2 ml/kg of 10% calcium gluconate (approximately 9–18 mg/kg elemental calcium) may be administered intravenously over 10 min. This must be done while an infant is on a continuous heart rate monitor, as it can be accompanied by bradycardia. Following a bolus, or to correct more slowly in cases of lower urgency, IV calcium replacement may be given as a continuous infusion at a rate of up to 75 mg/kg/day of elemental calcium until serum calcium levels normalize and then should be weaned slowly over a period of approximately 8–24 h. Calcium levels should be monitored closely during the period of replacement and for at least 1–2 days following discontinuation of therapy. Alternatively, if an infant is tolerating oral feeds, enteral calcium preparations may be used to provide calcium supplementation, but this should also be done with caution, as all calcium preparations are hypertonic and are accompanied by a theoretical risk of necrotizing enterocolitis. Infants requiring calcium replacement for symptomatic hypocalcemia should generally be transferred to a tertiary care setting for close monitoring during replacement.

Complications of IV calcium infusions include:

1. Cardiac arrhythmias.
2. Cardiac arrest.
3. Nephrolithiasis.
4. Skin necrosis.
5. All of the above.

IV infusion of calcium has a number of potential complications. The cardiac rhythm may be affected, most commonly as bradycardia, but other arrhythmias may occur as well. For this reason, IV calcium boluses should be administered slowly in a controlled setting with continuous cardiac monitor. Nephrolithiasis is another possible complication of IV calcium administration. Additionally, intravenous calcium can extravasate from the vein into the soft tissues, causing calcium deposition into the tissues and sometimes even tissue necrosis.

Answer: 5

Neonatal Hypercalcemia

Neonatal hypercalcemia is defined as a serum calcium concentration of greater than 2.75 mmol/L (11 mg/dL) or an ionized calcium concentration of greater than 1.35 mmol/L (5.4 mg/dL). It is generally caused by excess administration of calcium or vitamin D_3, although there can be other causes. Thiazide diuretics, for example, cause the kidney to retain calcium and can lead to hypercalcemia. Other potential causes include hyperparathyroidism (maternal or neonatal), vitamin A toxicity, and hypophosphatemia. Signs are nonspecific, including poor feeding, vomiting, constipation, and hypotonia. Treatment will depend in part on the etiology but in general involves intravenous hydration and loop diuretics to increase calcium excretion.

Case Presentation

A 27-year-old G2 P1001 woman is admitted to labor and delivery at 36 6/7-week gestation for severe headaches and is found to have a blood pressure of 180/100 and proteinuria. She is diagnosed with severe preeclampsia and started on IV blood pressure medication and IV magnesium sulfate (initial loading dose of 4 g, followed by IV infusion of 1 g/h) for seizure prophylaxis. Her blood pressure proves difficult to control on IV antihypertensive medication and magnesium sulfate, and the decision is made to induce labor. Thirty six hours later, she delivers a female infant with a birth weight of 2270 grams (5 pounds). At the time of delivery, the infant has spontaneous respiratory effort and a heart rate of 130 but is noted to have low tone. Apgar scores are 6, 7, and 8 at 1, 5, and 10 min, respectively. She is transferred to the normal nursery. On your exam 2 h later, you notice significant hypotonia and decreased respiratory drive with shallow breathing.

What is the most likely cause of the infant's condition?

1. Prematurity.
2. Hypermagnesemia.

3. Spinal muscular atrophy.
4. Perinatal asphyxia.

In light of the prolonged exposure to high-dose intravenous magnesium sulfate, the most likely diagnosis for this infant is hypermagnesemia. The infant is late preterm, and this degree of hypotonia and shallow breathing is out of proportion for what would be expected of a late preterm infant. Spinal Muscular atrophy is characterized by severe hypotonia as well as tongue fasiculations, which are absent in this infant. The Apgar scores were not compatible with perinatal asphyxia. A set of electrolytes is sent, including a magnesium level, which was 3.4 mg/dL. Hypermagnesemia is defined as a serum magnesium concentration greater than 1.15 mmol/L (2.8 mg/dL).

Answer: 2

Neonatal Hypermagnesemia

Question: Neonatal hypermagnesemia is usually caused by?

1. Maternal hyperparathyroidism.
2. Hypercalcemia.
3. Renal impairment of magnesium excretion.
4. Exogenous administration of magnesium.

In the fetus and newborn, hypermagnesemia is always the result of exogenous magnesium sources, including intrapartum magnesium sulfate, gastric acid suppressive medications taken during pregnancy, neonatal parenteral nutrition, or magnesium administered to critically ill infants as therapy for such conditions as persistent pulmonary hypertension of the newborn.

Answer: 4

Magnesium sulfate is frequently given intravenously intrapartum as a prophylactic measure in women with preeclampsia to prevent the development of seizures and progression to eclampsia. In the case of threatened or impending preterm delivery, magnesium sulfate infusion is also used for prevention of cerebral palsy in the fetus. However, maternal hypermagnesemia and fetal/neonatal hypermagnesemia may be induced by the infusion. In the scenario of intrapartum magnesium exposure, the serum magnesium concentration in the neonate will usually spontaneously return to normal over a period of hours to a few days.

Hypotonia is the most common symptom seen in neonatal hypermagnesemia, but infants can also exhibit respiratory depression as seen in the vignette, neuromuscular depression, hypotension, and urinary retention.

For most infants, treatment of hypermagnesemia is simply close monitoring and supportive care, while the excess magnesium is eliminated by the body by urinary excretion. This may include support of respiration until enough excess magnesium has been eliminated to allow for resolution of CNS depression. Intravenous fluids may be given to optimize hydration and increase urinary flow rate, or loop diuretics may be given to aid in renal elimination of excess magnesium. In acute cases, intravenous calcium may be given as a direct inhibitor magnesium.

Neonatal Hypomagnesemia

While the definition of hypomagnesemia is a serum magnesium concentration below 0.66 mmol/L (1.6 mg/dL), clinical signs are not seen until the level is less than 0.49 mmol/L (1.2 mg/dL). The two main causes are decreased magnesium supply (IUGR, malabsorption syndromes, intestinal magnesium transport defects) or increased urinary magnesium losses (maternal diabetes, hypoparathyroidism, renal tubular defects). Because magnesium influences parathyroid hormone secretion, severe hypomagnesemia may lead to hypoparathyroidism and resultant hypocalcemia. Signs of hypomagnesemia include hyperexcitability, irritability, tremors, and seizures. If the neonate has hypocalcemic seizures that do not respond to calcium infusion and anti-seizure medications, hypomagnesemia should be considered. Treatment is with magnesium salts, which should be given in an intensive care unit or other location with appropriate monitoring, as intravenous magnesium infusion can lead to hypotension and arrhythmias.

Neonatal Phosphorous Metabolism

Phosphorous has an important role and is found throughout the body, as opposed to calcium which is primarily stored in the bone. Given the critical role of phosphorous in multiple areas, phosphate deficiency can lead to a number of problems, including muscle weakness, poor immune system function, and abnormal bone metabolism. Hypophosphatemia is seen with high parathyroid hormone levels leading to increased renal phosphate excretion or with poor phosphate intake. The American Academy of Pediatrics recommends 100 mg/day of phosphorous in the first 6 months of life. Hyperphosphatemia can be seen with impaired phosphate excretion by the kidneys due to renal failure or low parathyroid hormone levels (Tables 11.1, 11.2, and 11.3).

Table 11.1 Normal values of calcium, magnesium, and phosphorous in the serum

Normal concentration in serum	mmol/L	mg/dL
Total calcium	2–2.75	8–11
Ionized calcium	1.1–1.35	4.28–5.4
Magnesium	0.66–1.15	1.6–2.8
Phosphorous	1.62–2.52	4.3–7.1

Derived from Abrams and Tiosano [1]; Kubicka and Little [4]

Table 11.2 Causes, signs, and evaluation of early neonatal hypocalcemia

Early hypocalcemia	
Causes	Prematurity
	Infant of a diabetic mother
	Perinatal stress and/or asphyxia
	Intrauterine growth restriction
	Maternal medications
Signs	Jitteriness
	Apnea
	Cyanosis
	Seizures
	Tetany
Evaluation	Total and ionized serum calcium concentrations
	Serum magnesium level
	Serum phosphorous level
	Blood glucose testing
	Acid/base balance (blood gas)
	Chest radiograph (thymic shadow)
	Urine calcium, magnesium, and phosphorous levels

Derived from Abrams and Tiosano [1]

Table 11.3 Causes, signs, evaluation, and treatment of neonatal hypermagnesemia

Hypermagnesemia	
Causes	Perinatal magnesium sulfate therapy
(All relate to increased supply)	Neonatal magnesium therapy
	Parenteral nutrition
	Acid suppressive medications
	Enemas
Signs	Birth depression in infants of mothers treated with perinatal magnesium
	Hypotonia
	Neuromuscular depression
	Hypotension
	Urinary retention
	Respiratory depression
Evaluation	Serum magnesium level
Treatment	Supportive
	IV calcium therapy in extreme cases
	Hydration therapy
	Loop diuretics

Derived from Abrams and Tiosano [1]

Clinical Pearls

1. Hypoglycemia is a common cause of jitteriness in a neonate, but it is not the only possible cause.
2. Neonatal hypocalcemia is strongly associated with gestational diabetes, and the degree of hypocalcemia correlates to the severity of gestational diabetes.
3. Intravenous calcium administration, be it bolus doses or continuous infusions, should always be given with caution and while on continuous cardiac monitor.
4. Asymptomatic neonatal hypocalcemia will likely resolve with good enteral nutrition alone.
5. Neonatal hypermagnesemia is always the result of exogenous administration.
6. Hypotonia is the most common symptom of neonatal hypermagnesemia, but hypermagnesemia can also cause respiratory depression which may require support of respiration while awaiting urinary excretion of excess magnesium.
7. Because magnesium levels affect parathyroid function, it can be difficult to correct hypocalcemia in the face of concurrent hypomagnesemia.

Further Reading

1. Abrams SA, Tiosano D. Disorders of Calcium, Phosphorous, and Magnesium Metabolism in the Neonate. In: Martin RJ, Fanaroff AA, Walsh MC, editors. Fanaroff & Martin's Neonatal-Perinatal Medicine: Diseases of the Fetus and Infant. 10th ed. Philadelphia: Elsevier Saunders; 2015. p. 1460–89.
2. Coulter M, Colvin C, Korf B, Messiaen L, Tuanama B, Crowley M, Crossman DK, McCormick K. Hypomagnesemia due to two novel TRPM6 mutations. J Pediatr Endocrinol Metab. 2015;28:1373–8.
3. García Soblechero E, Ferrer Castillo MT, Jiménez Crespo B, Domínguez Quintero ML, González FC. Neonatal hypercalcemia due to a homozygous mutation in the calcium-sensing receptor: failure of cinacalcet. Neonatology. 2013;104(2):104–8.
4. Kubicka Z, Little GA. Transient Metabolic Disturbances in the Newborn. In: Campbell DE, editor. Neonatology for Primary Care. American Academy of Pediatrics; 2015. p. 491–500.
5. Thomas TC, Smith JM, White PC, Adhikari S. Transient neonatal hypocalcemia: presentation and outcomes. Pediatrics. 2012;12:e1461–7.

12 Nutrition in the Newborn

Stephanie Tong-Miller and Henry H. Bernstein

Introduction

It is important that pregnant women be educated on different options for feeding prior to delivery. Breastfeeding is the ideal source of infant nutrition. The American Academy of Pediatrics (AAP) recommends breastfeeding for at least 1 year, including exclusively for 6 months. Breastfeeding reduces the incidence of respiratory tract infections, otitis media, gastrointestinal tract infections, and necrotizing enterocolitis in the infant [1, 2]. Breastfed infants are at reduced risk of SIDS; clinical allergic disease such as clinical asthma, atopic dermatitis, and eczema; celiac disease; and inflammatory bowel disease [3–6]. Rates of obesity are significantly lower in children who were breastfed, and there is also a reduced incidence of both type 1 and type 2 diabetes [3, 7, 8] (Fig. 12.1). Researchers have found a correlation between breastfeeding and a reduction in leukemia [9]. Studies also suggest that breastfeeding has cognitive neurodevelopmental benefits for the baby, although there may be confounding factors, such as socioeconomic status, child-rearing environment, the psychobiology of maternal behavior and mother-infant relationships, and maternal intelligence [10–13].

Breastfeeding also notably benefits mothers by decreasing postpartum blood loss and causing a more rapid involution of the uterus. Additionally, breastfeeding has been associated with decreased rates of postpartum depression, diabetes, hypertension, cardiovascular disease, and breast and ovarian cancer [14–16]. Mothers should be encouraged to pump breast milk when actual breastfeeding is not an option. The target goals of Healthy People 2020, a federal initiative of the US Department of Health and Human Services, are listed in Table 12.1.

Breastfeeding mothers should have a healthy diet that includes calcium, protein, iron, and folic acid and continue prenatal vitamins to ensure adequate essential vitamins and minerals that help stimulate the baby's development. The AAP recommends at least 400 IU of vitamin D daily to prevent vitamin D deficiency and rickets in healthy newborns. All breastfed infants should be supplemented with 400 IU daily of vitamin D until the infant is weaned to 1 L or 1 quart daily of vitamin D-fortified formula or whole milk [17]. Whole milk should be started at 1 year of age. Non-breastfed infants should also be supplemented with 400 IU of vitamin D daily, which can include other vitamin D fortified foods.

Supplemental nutrition, in the form of infant formula, may be necessary or desired by the mother. Basic formulas for full-term infants contain 20 kcal per ounce, cow's milk protein, and lactose. To prevent iron deficiency anemia, infants should receive iron-fortified formula.

S. Tong-Miller · H. H. Bernstein (✉)
General Pediatrics, Cohen Children's Medical Center and Zucker School of Medicine at Hofstra/Northwell, New Hyde Park, NY, USA
e-mail: hbernstein@northwell.edu

G. I. Martin, W. Rosenfeld (eds.), *Common Problems in the Newborn Nursery*,
https://doi.org/10.1007/978-3-319-95672-5_12

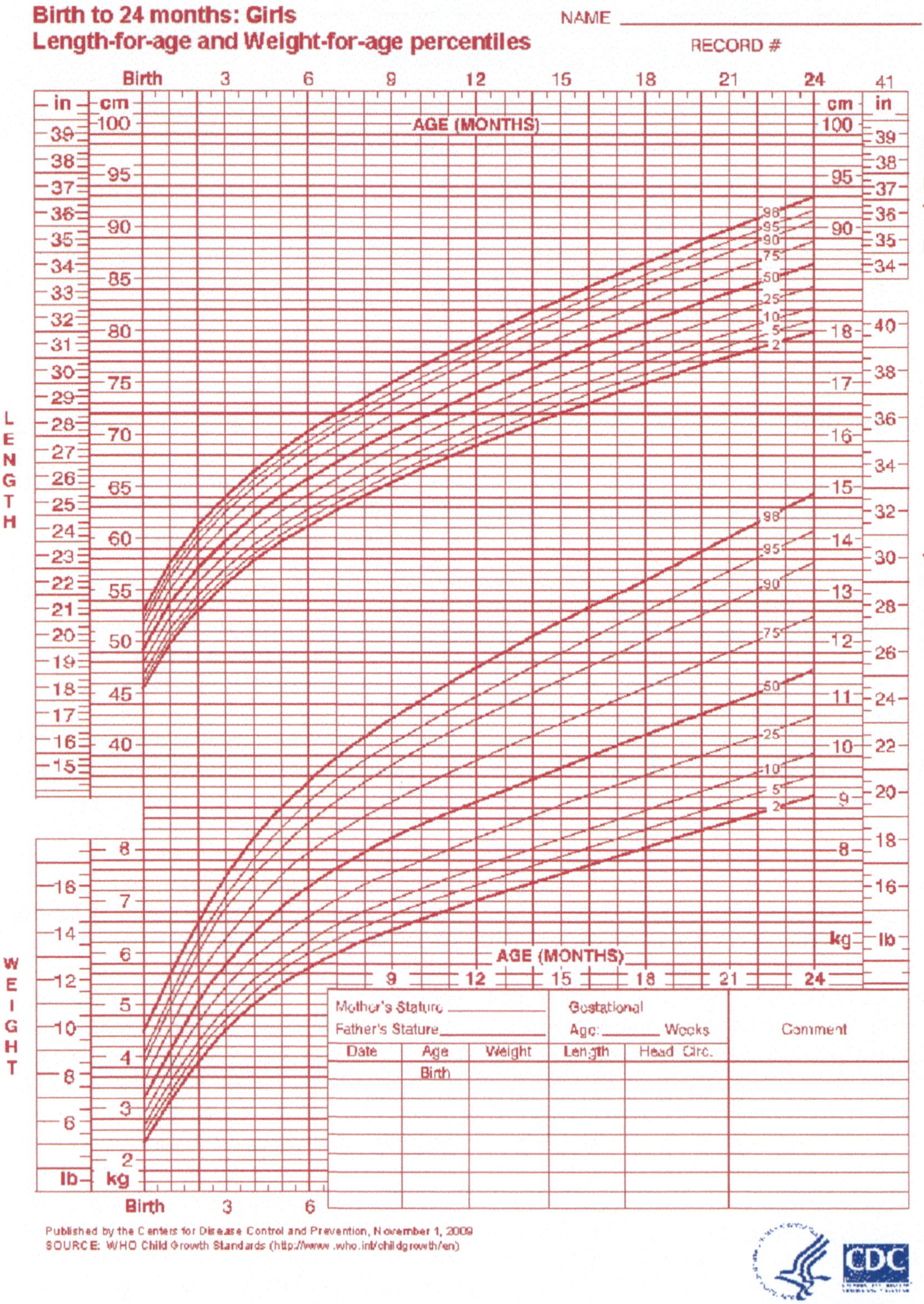

Fig. 12.1 Growth curves for female and male newborns (Source: Centers for Disease Control and Prevention)

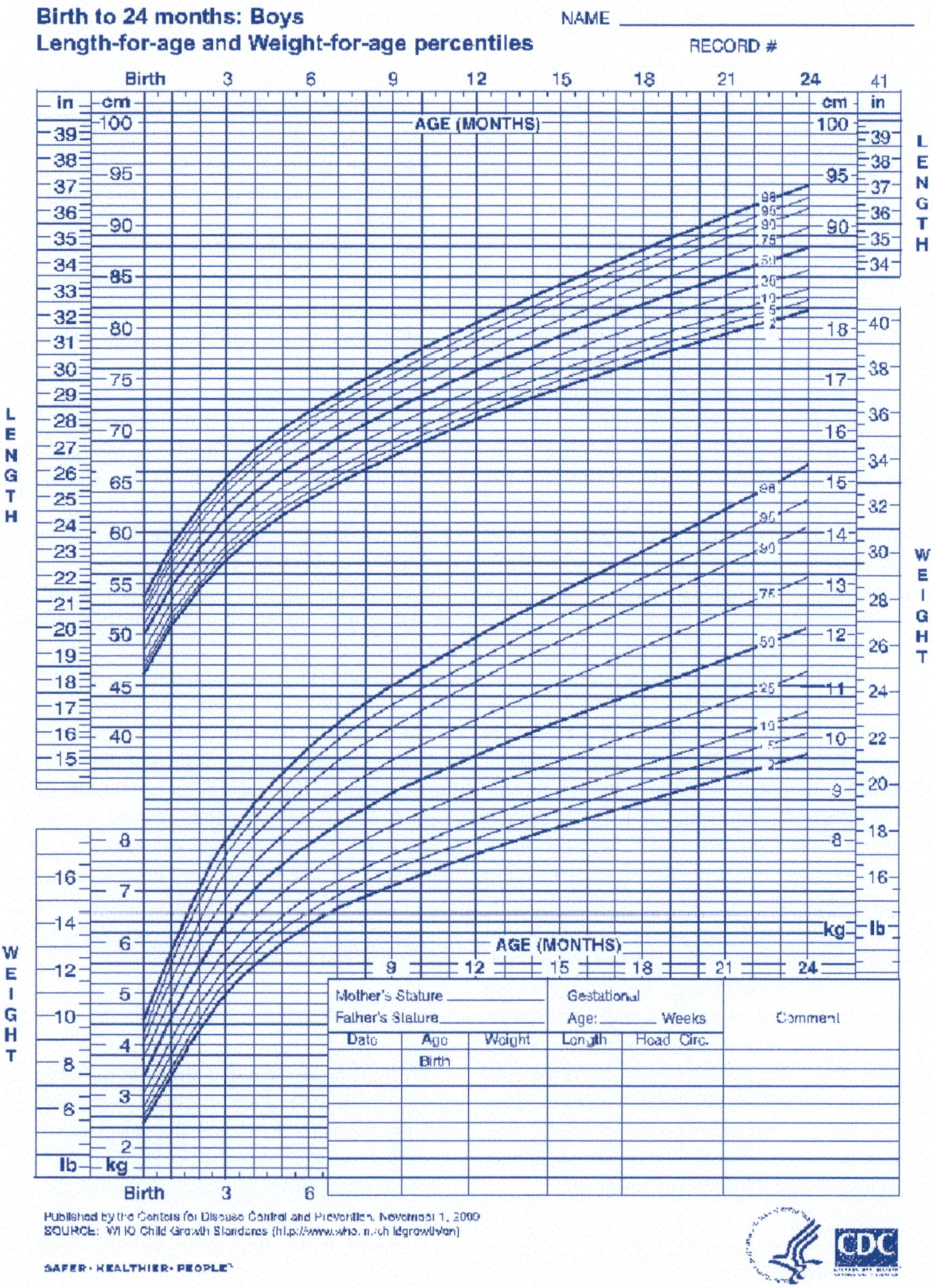

Fig. 12.1 (continued)

Table 12.1 Healthy People 2020 Breastfeeding Goals

Infants who	Target (%)
Ever breastfed	81.9
Breastfed at 6 months	60.6
Breastfed at 1 year	34.1
Exclusively breastfed for 3 months	46.2
Exclusively breastfed for 6 months	25.5

Source: Adapted from Healthypeople.gov

Preterm infants may require enriched formulas that contain more calories per ounce and higher protein concentrations. For infants with feeding intolerance, such as lactose intolerance or milk protein allergy, consider lactose-free formula or elemental formula, respectively [18].

Infant nutrition in the birth hospital is an essential topic in caring for all newborns. What happens in the hospital, even within the first hour of life, can significantly impact how the infant will be fed during the first months of life and have health consequences for families over time. Breastmilk is only produced if milk is first "removed" from the breast, so missed feedings can result in a reduced milk supply.

Mothers may be unable to produce enough milk due to a variety of reasons. If a mother is having difficulty breastfeeding, she should be referred to the birth hospital's lactation consultant – ideally an International Board Certified Lactation Consultant (IBCLC) – who can work with her to ensure that her newborn is establishing a good latch, assess whether she is producing sufficient milk quantities, and address questions and concerns. Mothers should be listened to and supported in their feeding choices. Careful evaluation of the mother-infant dyad is essential, and adaptation of the feeding plan may be necessary. While breastfeeding complications can occur in the hospital, many occur after discharge. Healthcare providers should recognize warning signs and anticipate problems before they negatively impact infant and maternal health and nutrition.

Case Presentation

Maria, a 29-year-old G1P1 mother, just gave birth via cesarean section to a healthy baby boy, John, several hours ago.

Q: What policies can be implemented in the hospital to encourage breastfeeding?

1. Encourage skin-to-skin contact in the delivery room.
2. Establish a liberal policy allowing mothers to have their babies brought from the nursery at any hour.
3. Encourage use of pacifiers.
4. Develop and implement a hospital-wide breastfeeding policy.
5. Offer specialized formulas similar to breast milk.

A: Hospitals are encouraged to strive to meet baby-friendly requirements set forth by the WHO/UNICEF to promote breastfeeding. Under these requirements, a birth hospital can create a written breastfeeding policy and train its staff members to implement it. Pregnant women should be educated on the benefits of breastfeeding and urged to initiate breastfeeding early.

After delivery, mother and baby should be kept together to encourage breastfeeding. Mothers should be offered resources such as access to lactation consultants, "rooming in" with the newborn, and education on newborn feeding cues. Access to formula and pacifiers should be limited until breastfeeding is established. In circumstances where mothers are unable to breastfeed (e.g., baby is premature or mother has a temporary maternal medical contraindication), pumping should be encouraged.

Answer: 1, 4

Maria is concerned that she is not producing enough milk to feed her newborn. You reassure her that her milk will come in, but it can take several days. She wants to know how she can track whether John is getting enough breast milk.

Q: How much milk per feeding should a 3-day-old term newborn take in?

1. 0–5 ml
2. 10–20 ml
3. >30 ml

A: It is important to educate mothers that newborn infants have very small stomachs. The newborn stomach size is appropriately matched to the amount of milk that is produced by mothers who recently gave birth. Newborns can generally digest 0–5 ml (~1 teaspoon) of milk per feeding comfortably on day 1 of life, which then increases to 10–20 ml (~1 tablespoon) by day 3 and more than 30 ml (>1 oz.) by 5 days of age.

As the infant grows, the stomach will expand to accept more liquid per feed. By 1–6 months of age, an exclusively breastfed baby can tolerate between 19 and 30 oz. Breastfed babies on average get 3 ounces per feed; therefore 8 feeds a day will give a total of 24 oz. of breastmilk [20].

Answer: 2

Maria tells the lactation consultant that she feeds John for about 15 min every 2 h. She doesn't remember how many stools or wet diapers John has had, but if she had to guess, it would be 1–2 stools and 3 wet diapers. The stools were dark-colored.

Q: Which of these findings is concerning?

1. Stool color is unusual.
2. Too few stools, so baby may not be getting enough milk.
3. Too few wet diapers, so baby is dehydrated.
4. These findings are normal.

A: A baby who is getting enough milk will have one or two bowel movements per day and an increasing number of them over the next week. Stools are initially black and tarry (meconium) but quickly progress to yellow and seedy by a week of age. When a mother's milk production increases, the baby will often stool with each feeding for the first month of life. During the first week of life, a baby should urinate the same number of times per day as their number of days of life leading up to an average of 6 to 8 times a day by 1 week of age [21]. See Table 12.2 for details on the numbers of stool and wet diapers during the first 5 days of life.

Table 12.2 Breastfed newborn intake/output norms [19]

Day	Age (h)	Milk volume per feeding (mL)	No. of feeds	No. of voids	No. of stools
1	0–24	0–5	>6	≥1	≥1
2	24–48	5–10	≥8	2–3	1–2
3	48–72	10–20	≥8	4–6	≥3
4	72–96	20–30	≥8	4–6	≥4
5	>96	>30	≥8	6–8	≥4

The newborn should void within 24 h and stool within 48 h of birth

Answer: 4

Despite these reassurances, Maria is still concerned about her milk supply.

Q: How would you advise her?

1. Keep a log of feeding and elimination patterns.
2. Supplement with formula.
3. Recommend keeping the baby skin to skin often.
4. Recommend fenugreek herbal supplement.
5. Recommend a galactagogue, like domperidone or metoclopramide.
6. Hand expression.

A: There is no panacea for low breast milk supply, but counseling families about what to expect, working with them individually, and employing evidence-based strategies can help. Keeping a log of feeding and elimination patterns can help the mother and her providers assess breastfeeding progress.

Skin-to-skin contact increases milk supply by promoting frequent feedings. It is best practice for infants to room-in with their mothers to facilitate skin-to-skin contact and feeding on cue. There are no galactagogues or herbal products currently recommended by the Academy of Breastfeeding Medicine (ABM) or AAP because studies of efficacy have been inconclusive or negative [22]. Some may not even be safe [23]. All breastfeeding mothers should be taught how to hand express breast milk effectively. This will increase milk supply by increasing perception of demand, provide milk for the baby if they cannot feed at the breast, relieve mastitis, and alleviate fears of low milk supply.

Expressed human milk and formula can be fed to infants in a variety of ways, and each mother-infant dyad should be assessed individually for the method that is right for them. Factors to consider include cost and availability, ease of use and cleaning, stress to the infant, adequacy of milk intake, anticipated time period for usage, maternal preference, staff expertise, and whether the method supports development of breastfeeding skills [24]. Some studies suggest that the use of teats or artificial nipples (such as those on bottles) may decrease the likelihood of exclusive breastfeeding [24–26]. Step 9 of the WHO's Ten Steps to Successful Breastfeeding indicates that no artificial teats or pacifiers should be given to breastfeeding infants, and cup feeding is preferred [27]. The AAP qualifies this recommendation by indicating that pacifier use should be delayed until breastfeeding is well established, usually about 3 to 4 weeks after birth [28]. Thus, bottle-feeding and use of artificial teats should be delayed for the same amount of time, if possible.

Answer: 1, 3, 6

Maria tries hand expression and is concerned by the thick consistency of her milk. She asks if this is normal.

Q: How should you respond?

1. This is normal.
2. She is dehydrated and should drink more water.
3. She may have a yeast infection, so appropriate testing should be ordered.

A: Human milk has a unique composition that changes over time in response to the infant's needs. Colostrum, the first milk that is produced and released, has a thicker, yellowish consistency, so the mother should not be concerned about this milk. It contains a high concentration of antibodies, immunoglobulins, and proteins to help build her newborn's immune system. It also has laxative properties to help the infants pass early stools.

Answer: 1

Q: You examine John on day 2 of life. John's weight loss is 8.5% down from his birth weight. He is being exclusively breastfed (birth weight, 3.250 kg; current weight, 2.973 kg).

Are you concerned about John's weight loss?

1. Yes, weight loss between 7% and 10% should be evaluated.
2. No, formula supplementation now will help the infant gain weight.

A: Infants should lose no more than 10% of their birth weight and have no further weight loss by day 5 of life. Weight loss of 7% or more should be evaluated and followed up closely [29]. If such weight loss is noted with breastfeeding, supplementation is not immediately necessary. However, a thorough evaluation of the breastfeeding dyad by a physician and lactation consultant should be conducted, including observation of feedings and evaluation of elimination patterns. They may be able to help correct any issues that may be contributing to weight loss.

Answer: 1

Q: What aspects of the dyad's history may be related to this weight loss?

1. Infant was delivered by C-section.
2. Mother is under 30.
3. Infant is male.
4. Infant is exclusively breastfed.
5. Full term.

A: Infants delivered by C-section are more likely to lose more weight, because of possible delayed milk production and lactation difficulty in the mother [30–32]. Older age has been positively associated with increased weight loss in newborns, suggesting that John's weight loss is more likely caused by other factors [33, 34]. Gender of the infant has not been shown to influence newborn weight loss [33]. Exclusive breastfeeding, however, is associated with newborn weight loss in several studies [30, 31, 35], but the association between breastfeeding and neonatal weight loss can be addressed by carefully monitoring infant weight, ensuring that breastfeeding is evaluated and supported effectively, and addressing any excess weight loss promptly [36]. Full-term infants are not as likely to experience more weight loss. Rather, preterm babies tend to display postnatal growth retardation [37]. Additionally, primiparity and long labor (>14 h) have also been associated with suboptimal breastfeeding and weight loss [38]. Presence of any of these risk factors may indicate the need for special care and follow-up.

Answer: 1, 4

Maria has been exclusively breastfeeding, but recently, she has been experiencing some nipple pain and describes being perpetually exhausted. She asks you if she would still experience all the benefits of breastfeeding if she supplements occasionally with formula.

Q: Which of these statements might you include in your response to Maria?

1. Though there are benefits to breastfeeding exclusively, breastfeeding and formula feeding provide similar nutrition, so supplementing occasionally will not make a difference.
2. Nipple pain is normal and she just has to push through until the nipples toughen up.
3. Maria must continue breastfeeding; her baby will not be healthy if she does not.

A: Breastfeeding should not cause nipple pain. A lactation counselor can assist with assessing and correcting latch and positioning to prevent pain. There are demonstrated benefits to breastfeeding exclusively that include development of the infant gut microbiome, protection from future infections, and facilitation of iron absorption and digestion. Unlike formula, breast milk contains living properties such as bioactive proteins, enzymes, immune cells, growth factors, and hormones that help the baby develop and grow [39]. However, formula does contain the necessary nutrients for growth and development. Ultimately, breastfeeding is the mother's choice – though it should be a fully informed one. All mothers should be supported in their breastfeeding and feeding goals, and no one should be shamed for not being able to breastfeed or simply not choosing to do so.

You call in a lactation consultant to help address the weight loss and nipple pain. She sees that the baby's position and latch angle may be causing some of the nipple pain that Jane is experiencing. She shows Jane some different positions to try. She lets her know about the hospital's breastfeeding support group and encourages her to attend.

There is no picture of a "perfect" latch, but there are elements of the latch that are important to focus on. Certain factors may lead to inadequate intake for the infant and subsequent weight loss, as well as pain for the mother.

Elements of a good latch include the following:

- *Body Positioning*: The infant's entire body with head, hips, and shoulders aligned should be turned toward the mother's body. Their arms and hands should be around the breast so that their hand motions can stimulate oxytocin release and milk letdown. The mother's hand should support the infant's head at the base of the neck rather than the back of the head.
- *Latch Observation*: The infant's mouth should open wide to initiate the latch, and the bottom lip and tongue, not the top lip, should touch the breast first. The infant's chin should be firmly touching the breast, the nose should be close to or touching the breast, and more than just the nipple should be in their mouth. The infant's bottom lip should be covering more of the areola than the top lip so that the nipple is not being sucked on directly. The infant's mouth should be open wide with both the top and bottom lips sealed (not turned inwards toward their mouth) on the breast. The infant's cheek should be rounded, not dimpled.

- *Nipple Appearance*: The mother should feel a tugging sensation as the infant feeds but little discomfort. Her nipple should appear similar pre-feeding and post-feeding. If the nipple is shaped differently or discolored after breastfeeding, this may indicate that the latch is not ideal and could cause pain.

All of these "ideal" elements are not necessary for an effective latch, and it may be difficult to evaluate some of these elements with different mother-infant dyads. If breastfeeding is working for the dyad – the baby is swallowing milk and the mother is not experiencing pain – then there is no need to adjust it. Observing and hearing gulping and swallowing during the latch is a good indication that the infant is ingesting milk. Pauses in sucking patterns and a more pronounced and slightly horizontal movement of the jaw indicate swallowing. It may be difficult to tell if swallowing is actually occurring, so keeping track of stooling, urination, and weight gain can help in making a final determination about how to proceed with feeding [40].

A lactation consultant is an expert in breastfeeding and best able to evaluate the latch most effectively. However, everyone who works with newborns should be able to provide basic breastfeeding counsel. Online video resources are helpful in learning to recognize these latch elements and jaw movements – see additional resources at the end of the chapter.

Answer: 1

Q: How would you advise Maria about the exhaustion she reports to be experiencing?

1. Tell her to start pumping so that she can store breast milk and her partner can feed John while she sleeps.
2. Sympathize with her experience and express an understanding that breastfeeding can be difficult, but let her know that many mothers often find it easier to continue by as long as 2 weeks.
3. Tell her to switch to formula if she is having trouble sleeping.

A: Sympathize with and support Maria in her decision to breastfeed, for breastfeeding is often tiring, especially early on. The first few days after delivery are crucial for establishing exclusivity. There is a critical period on the second to third day of life when women are most concerned about not producing enough milk and are often faced with pain and exhaustion.

Every mother-infant dyad's experience is different, but many mothers report that over time breastfeeding becomes easier and less time-consuming than bottle-feeding [41]. After breastfeeding is established, expressing breast milk may be a good way to share feeding responsibilities with other caretakers and can be important for mothers who are returning to work. Mothers should be reminded to continue breastfeeding or expressing milk at regular intervals in order to maintain their milk production even when there is an ample supply of stored milk.

Babies should feed at least 8–12 times a day. Newborns usually nurse on their mothers' breasts every 2–3 h for around 15–20 min each feeding. However, there is no set time for feedings, and they may vary in length, depending on when the baby is satisfied.

Mothers should look for their infants' hunger cues. When a baby is hungry, they will become more alert, put their hands or fingers on their mouth, make sucking motions, stick out their tongue, smack their lips, kick or squirm, or begin rooting (moving the jaw and mouth or head in search of the breast). If they begin crying, this is usually a late signal that they want to eat and are now very hungry.

Cluster feeding occurs in the early days when the baby may take longer at each feed, starting and finishing after 20–30 min and then wanting to feed again shortly thereafter. Babies may engage in cluster feeding in the early weeks or months, if they are sleeping for longer periods, or are experiencing a growth spurt. If moms are not expecting this, they may incorrectly interpret this frequent feeding as an indicator that they are not making enough milk. Instead, these frequent feeds allow the baby to get adequate calories and encourage more milk production to meet its needs during growth spurts. As they become older, the time between feedings will increase as the capacity of their stomachs becomes larger [42].

Answer: 2

Q: After this evaluation, how would you proceed?

1. Keep Maria and her newborn John in the hospital for one more day to observe if there is any further weight loss.
2. Discharge Maria and John, but ensure that they have a follow-up appointment within 24–48 h scheduled and confirmed.

A: All evaluation metrics indicate that John is feeding sufficiently. As long as an appointment to check for weight gain is scheduled and confirmed, discharge at this point is reasonable. Maria should be provided with resources to call if any issues come up while breastfeeding, including the number of a local lactation consultant.

Answer: 2

Case Presentation

Anna is a 31-year-old now G2P2002 mother, with a history of HIV. She formula fed her older child but heard that breastfeeding is more beneficial than formula.

Q: How do you respond?

1. She should breastfeed this child since breastfeeding is more beneficial.
2. HIV is a contraindication to breastfeeding; she should formula feed her baby.

A: In the U.S., HIV is a contraindication to breastfeeding, as the HIV virus can be transmitted from mother to infant through breast milk. Mothers are advised to seek alternatives to breastfeeding given that formula and clean water are readily available.

Other contraindications include active pulmonary tuberculosis and active herpes. When either of these infections are present, mothers are encouraged to formula feed instead of breastfeed. In contrast, maternal hepatitis A, B, and C are generally not passed to the infant through breast milk. However, the infant must receive the first dose of hepatitis B vaccine within 24 h of birth. Of note is that cytomegalovirus is a risk to premature infants, but not full-term infants who are breastfed.

Furthermore, mothers who develop fevers or other signs of non-life-threatening infections may express concern about harm to the infant when breastfeeding. In general, the infants have already been exposed to the infection, so the mother should continue breastfeeding or expressing breast milk. The breast milk will actually provide antibodies and other anti-infective agents to protect the infant. Finally, breastfeeding while the mother has mastitis is safe for the infant and may actually help the mother recover and heal more quickly [43].

Answer: 2

Infants with metabolic disorders that prevent them from breaking down lactose in breast milk, such as galactosemia, should not be breastfed. Other metabolic disorders may not prevent successful breastfeeding; babies with phenylketonuria can breastfeed while being monitored for blood phenylalanine levels because of the low phenylalanine concentrations in breast milk. Taking oral contraceptives is not necessarily a contraindication, but estrogen-containing contraceptives can have a significant effect on milk supply, so they are not recommended for lactating mothers especially before breastfeeding is well established. They may also increase risk of thromboembolism before 3 weeks postpartum. However, progestin-only contraceptives generally have not been associated with reduced milk supply and can be used [44].

Mothers are not advised to breastfeed while taking herbals because they may contain active ingredients that are not controlled or regulated, which can negatively impact the young infant.

When mothers have questions about what medications they can and cannot take, they may consult LactMed (https://toxnet.nlm.nih.gov/newtoxnet/lactmed.htm), a free online database that provides information on the effects of drugs and other chemicals on breastfeeding. LactMed provides further information on whether drugs can be used while breastfeeding and suggests alternatives when appropriate, so that mothers can best make informed decisions about whether to breastfeed or formula feed [45].

Overall, mothers should be supported in making informed decisions about whether to breastfeed or formula feed. While breastfeeding is most often recommended because of its health benefits for the mother and child, some mothers may have various medical or personal reasons for choosing to formula feed. Their decisions should be respected. Additionally, mothers who want to breastfeed and have no contraindications but felt the need to supplement in the hospital for any reason should be given anticipatory guidance in transitioning to breastfeeding to their personal desired extent. They should be reassured that the need for formula may not persist and told how to increase or maintain their milk supply while supplementing.

Anna decides to formula feed her newborn. She is confused about the many brands of formula on the market and wants to choose the best one for her baby. She also wants to know if she can supplement formula feedings with cow's milk, as she says that "real" milk will provide additional benefits beyond what formula can provide.

Q: How should you advise her?

1. Anna can give her baby warmed cow's milk in between feedings of formula.
2. Anna should avoid cow's milk, but giving goat's milk or soy milk to her baby is fine.
3. Besides formula, the only additional liquid that Anna should give her baby is plain water.
4. Anna should only give her baby formula.

A: Iron-fortified infant formula is the acceptable and recommended substitute for breast milk during the first year of life for a full-term infant. As long as formula is iron-fortified, different brands tend to provide similar benefits. Anna should be advised not to give cow's milk to her baby, as infants fed with cow's milk in the first year are at higher risk for iron-deficiency anemia and disruption of intestinal microbial environment. Parents should also avoid other low-iron breast milk substitutes such as goat milk, soy milk, or low-iron formulas, although soy-based and lactose-free formulas may be used in cases such as when the infant has lactose intolerance [46, 47]. Giving plain water alone (i.e., not mixed with formula) is never recommended for young babies as it may dilute out the salt in the body, causing significant medical problems.

In the first few weeks, formula-fed infants generally ingest 2–3 oz. every 3–4 h or about 6–8 times per day. They usually take longer, less frequent feedings than breastfed infants. Anna should feed her infant when he displays signs of hunger, such as putting his hand toward his mouth, sucking, rooting, grimacing, or fussing. Young infants will then turn their heads away, lose interest in eating, or close their mouths when they are full after a feeding. During feeding, the parent can bond with the infant by holding the infant close, in a semi-upright position, and looking into the eyes of the baby. Prepared formula should be used right away and at least within 24 h. At the end of the infant's first month, they should take in about 4 oz. (120 ml) every 4 h, and at the end of 6 months, they should take in 6–8 oz. (180–240 ml) every 5–6 h [48].

Answer: 4

Case Presentation

Anna and her baby are ready for discharge, and she has a few questions about her baby's nutrition at home.

Q: How much weight gain do you expect per day during the early months of life?

1. <0.5 oz.
2. 0.5–1 oz.
3. 1.5 oz.
4. 2 oz.

A: Full-term infants generally should gain about 1 oz. per day in the early months of life.

They are expected to double their birth weight by 4 months of age and triple their birth weight by 1 year. Regardless of how a mother chooses to feed her child, weight gain should be monitored according to the appropriate growth curve. The baby should regain their birth weight no later than 2 weeks. Below are the WHO growth curves for breastfed female and male infants. The CDC and AAP recommend these growth curves as the standards to be used for children under 24 months.

Answer: 2

Q: How would you tell Maria and Anna to heat up pumped breast milk or formula?

1. Microwave.
2. Stove top (be sure to prevent boiling).
3. Run warm water over the bottle.
4. It does not need to be warmed up.

A: Formula or pumped breast milk should be heated by running warm water over the bottle, so that the milk is brought to room temperature. After warming, the caretaker can test the temperature of the milk on his/her arm. In contrast, using a microwave or stovetop might cause uneven heating and create hot pockets that may scald the infant when feeding. Note that prepared formula should be used right away or at least within 24 h.

Mothers should wash their hands and appropriate pumping equipment with soap and water before expressing breast milk. Breast milk should be labeled with the date expressed so that the oldest milk can be used first. Guidelines for storing breast milk are in Table 12.3.

Answer: 3

Besides their patient-centered medical home, it is important to inform patients of all the available resources to assure them that they are not alone if they confront further challenges. Providers should maintain a list of local and national resources that they can share with mothers. Local resources include nearby Women, Infants, and Children (WIC) programs, community support groups (e.g., La Leche League, Baby Café, hospital-based breastfeeding groups, faith-based groups), and private practice lactation consultants. Nationally available resources include online communities such as La Leche League International, mobile applications, and breastfeeding helplines:

- La Leche League Breastfeeding Helpline (available 24/7 in English and Spanish) – 1-877-452-5324
- US Office of Women's Health phone line (Mon-Fri 9 am–6 pm EST in English and Spanish) – 1-800-994-9662

Table 12.3 Storage duration of fresh human milk for use with healthy full-term infants

Location	Temperature	Duration	Comments
Countertop, table	Room temperature (up to 77°F or 25°C)	6–8 h	Containers should be covered and kept as cool as possible; covering the container with a cool towel may keep milk cooler
Insulated cooler bag	5–39°F or −15–4°C	24 h	Keep ice packs in contact with milk containers at all times, limit opening cooler bag
Refrigerator	39 °F or 4 °C	5 days	Store milk in the back of the main body of the refrigerator
Freezer			Store milk toward the back of the freezer, where temperature is most constant. Milk stored for longer durations in the ranges listed is safe, but some of the lipids in the milk undergo degradation resulting in lower quality
Freezer compartment of a refrigerator	5 °F or – 15 °C	2 weeks	
Freezer compartment of refrigerator with separate doors	0°F or −18°C	3–6 months	
Chest or upright deep freezer	−4°F or −20°C	6–12 months	

Source: Centers for Disease Control and Prevention

Clinical Pearls

- Families should be provided with all necessary information and support to make an informed decision about feeding choices for their newborn.
- Breastfeeding is the ideal source of infant nutrition – it offers many benefits to both infant and mother.
- The American Academy of Pediatrics recommends breastfeeding for at least 1 year and exclusively for 6 months.
- Exclusive breastfeeding provides additional benefits beyond mixed feeding strategies.
- Though all maternal-infant healthcare providers should be able to provide basic breastfeeding counsel, the opportunity to meet with a professional lactation expert in the hospital and whenever any issues arise after discharge is valuable for postpartum mothers.
- If infants lose more than 7–10% of their birth weight, careful evaluation of the mother-infant dyad should be conducted, but such weight loss does not necessarily require formula supplementation for an infant that is being breastfed.
- All mothers should be supported in their breastfeeding and feeding goals. No one should be shamed for not being able to breastfeed or simply not choosing to do so.
- Providers should be knowledgeable about breastfeeding and formula feeding and maintain a list of local and national resources that they can share with mothers.

Acknowledgments The comprehensive literature reviews and detailed editorial assistance of research assistants Victoria Chi, Shannon Cleary, Angie Lee, Irene Song, Yingna Wang, Yun Chao Chen and Maggie Sherin at Cohen Children's Medical Center are greatly appreciated.

References

1. Chantry CJ, Howard CR, Auinger P. Full breastfeeding duration and associated decrease in respiratory tract infection in US children. Pediatrics. 2006;117(2):425–32.
2. Quigley MA, Kelly YJ, Sacker A. Breastfeeding and hospitalization for diarrheal and respiratory infection in the United Kingdom millennium cohort study. Pediatrics. 2007;119(4)
3. Ip S, Chung M, Raman G, et al. Tufts-New England Medical Center Evidence-based Practice Center. Breastfeeding and maternal and infant health outcomes in developed countries. Evid Rep Technol Assess (Full Rep). 2007;153(153):1–186.
4. Greer FR, Sicherer SH, Burks AW. American Academy of Pediatrics Committee on nutrition, American Academy of Pediatrics section on allergy and immunology. Effects of early nutritional interventions on the development of atopic disease in infants and children: the role of maternal dietary restriction, breastfeeding, timing of introduction of complementary foods, and hydrolyzed formulas. Pediatrics. 2008;121(1):183–91.
5. Akobeng AK, Ramanan AV, Buchan I, Heller RF. Effect of breast feeding on risk of coeliac disease: a systematic review and meta-analysis of observational studies. Arch Dis Child. 2006;91(1):39–43.
6. Barclay AR, Russell RK, Wilson ML, Gilmour WH, Satsangi J, Wilson DC. Systematic review: the role of breastfeeding in the development of pediatric inflammatory bowel disease. J Pediatr. 2009;155(3):421–6.
7. Perrine CG, Shealy KM, Scanlon KS, et al. Centers for Disease Control and Prevention (CDC). Vital signs: hospital practices to support breastfeeding—United States, 2007 and 2009. MMWR Morb Mortal Wkly Rep. 2011;60(30):1020–5.
8. Das UN. Breastfeeding prevents type 2 diabetes mellitus: but, how and why? Am J Clin Nutr. 2007;85(5):1436–7.
9. Bener A, Hoffmann GF, Afify Z, Rasul K, Tewfik I. Does prolonged breastfeeding reduce the risk for childhood leukemia and lymphomas? Minerva Pediatr. 2008;60(2):155–61.
10. Der G, Batty GD, Deary IJ. Effects of breast feeding on intelligence in children: prospective study, sibling pairs analysis, and meta-analysis. BMJ. 2006;333(7575):945.
11. Lucas A, Cole TJ, Morley R, Lucas PJ, Davis JA, Bamford MF, Crowle P, Dossetor JF, Pearse R, Boon A. Factors associated with maternal choice to provide breast milk for low birthweight infants. Arch Dis Child. 1988;63(1):48–52.
12. Long term effects of breastfeeding: a systematic review. World Health Organization. 2013:57–67. http://apps.who.int/iris/bitstream/10665/79198/1/9789241505307_eng.pdf?ua=1. Accessed Aug 11, 2017.

13. Koo W, Tank S, Martin S, Shi R. Human milk and neurodevelopment in children with very low birth weight: a systematic review. Nutr J. 2014;13:94.
14. Henderson JJ, Evans SF, Straton JA, Priest SR, Hagan R. Impact of postnatal depression on breastfeeding duration. Birth. 2003;30(3):175–80.
15. Stuebe AM, Rich-Edwards JW, Willett WC, Manson JE, Michels KB. Duration of lactation and incidence of type 2 diabetes. JAMA. 2005;294(20):2601–10.
16. Collaborative Group on Hormonal Factors in Breast Cancer. Breast cancer and breastfeeding: collaborative reanalysis of individual data from 47 epidemiological studies in 30 countries, including 50302 women with breast cancer and 96973 women without the disease. Lancet. 2002;360(9328):187–19.
17. Wagner C, Greer F. Prevention of rickets and vitamin D deficiency in infants, children, and adolescents. Pediatrics. 2008;111(4):908.
18. O'Connor M. Infant Formula. Am Fam Physician. 2009;79(7):565–70.
19. Schanler RJ. Breastfeeding handbook for physicians. 2nd ed. Elk Grove Village: American Academy of Pediatrics and the American College of Obstetricians and Gynecologists; 2014. p. 93. Table 7–4.
20. Making Breastmilk. Office on Women's Health, U.S. Department of Health and Human Services. Womenshealth.gov https://www.womenshealth.gov/breastfeeding/learning-breastfeed/making-breastmilk#10 Updated August 1, 2017. Accessed September 29, 2017.
21. How to Tell if a Baby is Getting Enough Milk. Healthychildren.org https://www.healthychildren.org/English/ages-stages/baby/breastfeeding/pages/How-to-Tell-if-Baby-is-Getting-Enough-Milk.aspx Updated November 11, 2015. Accessed September 29, 2017.
22. The Academy of Breastfeeding Medicine Protocol Committee. ABM clinical protocol #9: use of Galactogogues in initiating or augmenting the rate of maternal milk secretion (first revision January 2011). Breastfeed Med. 2011;6(1):41–9.
23. Sachs HC. Committee on drugs. The transfer of drugs and therapeutics into human breast milk: an update on selected topics. Pediatrics. 2013;132(3):796–809.
24. Kellams A, Harrel C, Omage S, Gregory C, Rosen-Carole C. The academy of breastfeeding medicine. ABM clinical protocol #3: supplementary feedings in the healthy term breastfed neonate, revised 2017. Breastfeed Med. 2017;12(3):1–11.
25. Howard CR, Howard FM, Lanphear B, Eberly S, deBlieck EA, Oakes D, Lawrence RA. Randomized clinical trial of pacifier use and bottle-feeding or cupfeeding and their effect on breastfeeding. Pediatrics. 2003;111(3):511–8.
26. Flint A, New K, Davies MW. Cup feeding versus other forms of supplemental enteral feeding for newborn infants unable to fully breastfeed. Cochrane Database Syst Rev. 2016;8:1–41.
27. World Health Organization: Division of Child Health and Development. Evidence for the ten steps to successful breastfeeding. 1998;98:9.
28. Section on Breastfeeding. Breastfeeding and the use of human milk. Pediatrics. 2012;129(3):827–41.
29. Riordan J, Wambach K. Breastfeeding and human lactation. Burlington: Jones & Bartlett Learning; 2009.
30. Flaherman V, Schaefer E, Kuzniewicz M, Li S, Walsh E, Paul I. Early weight loss nomograms for exclusively breastfed newborns. Pediatrics. 2015;135(1)
31. Manganaro R, Mamí C, Marrone T, Marseglia L, Gemelli M. Incidence of dehydration and hypernatremia in exclusively breast-fed infants. J Pediatr. 2001;139(5):673–5.
32. Preer GL, Newby PK, Philipp BL. Weight loss in exclusively breastfed infants delivered by cesarean birth. J Hum Lact. 2012;28(2):153–8.
33. Mezzacappa M, Ferreira B. Excessive weight loss in exclusively breastfed full-term newborns in a baby-friendly hospital. Rev Paul Pediatr. 2016;34(3):281–6.
34. Fonseca MJ, Severo M, Barros H, Santos AC. Determinants of weight changes during the first 96 hours of life in full-term newborns. Birth. 2014;41(2):160–8.
35. Macdonald PD, Ross SR, Grant L, Young D. Neonatal weight loss in breast and formula fed infants. Arch Dis Child Fetal Nenotal Ed. 2003;88(6):F472–6.
36. Davanzo R, Cannioto Z, Ronfani L, Monasta L, Demarini S. Breastfeeding and neonatal weight loss in healthy term infants. J Hum Lact. 2013;29(1):45–53.
37. Fenton T. A new growth chart for preterm babies: Babson and Benda's chart updated with recent data and a new format. BMC Pediatr. 2003;3(13)
38. Dewey KG, Nommsen-Rivers LA, Heinig MJ, Cohen RJ. Risk factors for suboptimal infant breastfeeding behavior, delayed onset of lactation, and excess neonatal weight loss. Pediatrics. 2003;112:607–19.
39. O'Sullivan A, Farver M, Smilowitz J. The influence of early infant-feeding practices on the intestinal microbiome and body composition in infants. Nutr Metab Insights. 2015;8(Suppl 1):1–9.
40. Cadwell K, Turner-Maffei C. Pocket guide for lactation management. 2nd ed. Burlington: Jones & Bartlett Learning; 2014. Appendix G.
41. Mohrbacher N, Kendall-Tackett K, Newman J. Breastfeeding made simple: seven natural laws for nursing mothers. 2nd ed: New Harbringer Publications, Inc; 2010.
42. Breastfeeding Program. Arizona Department of Health Services. http://www.azdhs.gov/prevention/nutrition-physical-activity/breastfeeding/index.php#providers-normal. Accessed September 29, 2017.
43. American Academy of Pediatrics. Bright futures: nutrition issues and concerns. Elk Grove Village: Bright Futures; 2011. p. 113–219. https://brightfutures.aap.org/Bright%20Futures%20Documents/BFNutrition3rdEdition_issuesConcerns.pdf. Accessed October 2, 2017.

44. Berens P, Labbok M. The academy of breastfeeding medicine. ABM clinical protocol #13: contraception during breastfeeding, revised 2015. Breastfeed Med. 2015;10(1):3–12.
45. DiMaggio DM, Cox A, Porto AF. Updates in infant nutrition. Pediatr Rev. 2017;38:449–62.
46. American Academy of Pediatrics. Bright futures: nutrition supervision. Elk Grove Village: Bright Futures; 2011. p. 17–111. https://brightfutures.aap.org/Bright%20Futures%20Documents/BFNutrition3rdEditionSupervision.pdf. Accessed October 2, 2017.
47. Bunik M. The Pediatrician's role in encouraging exclusive breastfeeding. Pediatr Rev. 2017;38(8):353–68.
48. Amount and Schedule of Formula Feedings. Healthychildren.org https://www.healthychildren.org/English/ages-stages/baby/feeding-nutrition/Pages/Amount-and-Schedule-of-Formula-Feedings.aspx. Updated November 21, 2015. Accessed November 9, 2017.

Additional Resources for Provider Education

Centers for Disease Control and Prevention: https://www.cdc.gov/breastfeeding/index.htm.

HealthyChildren.org (American Academy of Pediatrics: https://www.healthychildren.org/English/ages-stages/baby/breastfeeding/Pages/default.aspx.

Academy of Breastfeeding Medicine Clinical Protocols: http://www.bfmed.org/Resources/Protocols.aspx.

Videos from the International Breastfeeding Centre: https://ibconline.ca/breastfeeding-videos-english/.

Cardiology in the Newborn Nursery

13

Bruce D. Sindel and Joseph Ahdoot

Introduction

Incidence of Congenital Heart Disease

The incidence of congenital heart disease has been reported to range from as low as 4/1000 live births [1] to as high as 12.3/1000 live births [2]. The low numbers probably relate to the era prior to 2D echocardiography and ready availability of pediatric cardiology. The higher number appears to depend on how many less significant lesions are included (if tiny VSDs and other trivial lesions are included, the number may be as high as 75/1000 live births). It is likely that the incidence of significant congenital heart disease is approximately 6–9/1000 live births [3, 4] with approximately one quarter of these being critical congenital heart disease [5]. Either way congenital heart disease presents a significant problem for the healthcare provider.

B. D. Sindel, MD (✉)
Neonatal Intensive Care Unit, Pediatrix Medical Group, a MEDNAX Company, Citrus Valley Medical Center—Queen of the Valley Campus, West Covina, CA, USA

Western University of Health Sciences, Pomona, CA, USA

J. Ahdoot, MD
Pacific Pediatric Cardiology Medical Group, Keck School of Medicine, Children's Hospital of Los Angeles, Los Angeles, CA, USA

David Geffen School of Medicine at UCLA, Mattel Children's Hospital, Los Angeles, CA, USA

Embryology

The heart is the first organ to function in the embryo, beginning to beat at approximately 22–23 days and blood flow beginning in the fourth week when the nutritional and oxygen needs of the growing embryo can no longer be met by diffusion from the placenta. The heart initially forms from the mesoderm with two tubes located on either side of the trilaminar embryo in the cranial region. Looking down on a cross section of the early embryo (approximately Day 18), you can see multiple blood islands dispersed throughout the embryo (Fig. 13.1). At the cranial end, these blood islands are actually the primitive heart tubes.

The disclike embryo then undergoes the process of folding, in which both the cranial and lateral ends fold vertically. This brings the heart-forming region to the ventral (frontal) position. As the lateral folds develop, the heart tubes gradually approach each other (Day 21) and fuse to form a single heart tube (Fig. 13.2). This fusion begins at the cranial end of the tubes and extends caudally until a single tube is formed.

The tubular heart then elongates and develops alternating dilatations and constrictions. The bulbus cordis, ventricle, and atrium appear first, but

G. I. Martin, W. Rosenfeld (eds.), *Common Problems in the Newborn Nursery*,
https://doi.org/10.1007/978-3-319-95672-5_13

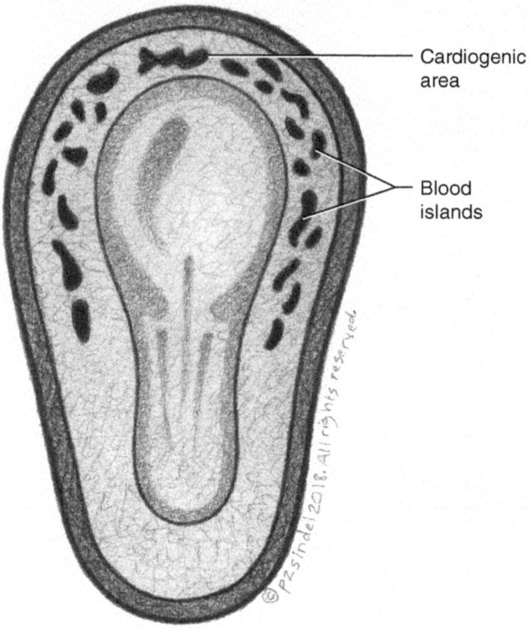

Fig. 13.1 Looking down on a cross section of the trilaminar embryo on Day 18, you see blood islands scattered in the mesodermal portion. These develop into the cardiovascular system. The blood island in the cranial (top) region fuses to become the primitive heart tubes

the truncus arteriosus and sinus venosus soon appear (Day 22 – Fig. 13.3).

The truncus arteriosus is continuous caudally with the bulbus cordis, and cranially it enlarges slightly to form the aortic sac, from which the aortic arches arise. Caudally to the atrium is the sinus venous, which is a large venous sinus that receives the umbilical, vitelline, and common cardinal veins from the chorion (primitive placenta), yolk sac, and embryo, respectively.

The arterial and venous ends of the heart tube are fixed by the branchial arches and the septum transversum, respectively. Since the bulbus cordis and the ventricle grow faster than the other regions (Day 23 – Fig. 13.4), the heart tube bends upon itself, forming a U-shaped bulboventricular loop (Day 24 – Fig. 13.5). Later the S-shaped heart forms (Day 35 – Fig. 13.6).

As the primitive heart bends, the atrium and the sinus venosus come to lie dorsal to the bulbus cordis, truncus arteriosus, and ventricle. By this stage the sinus venosus has developed lateral expansions called the right and left horns.

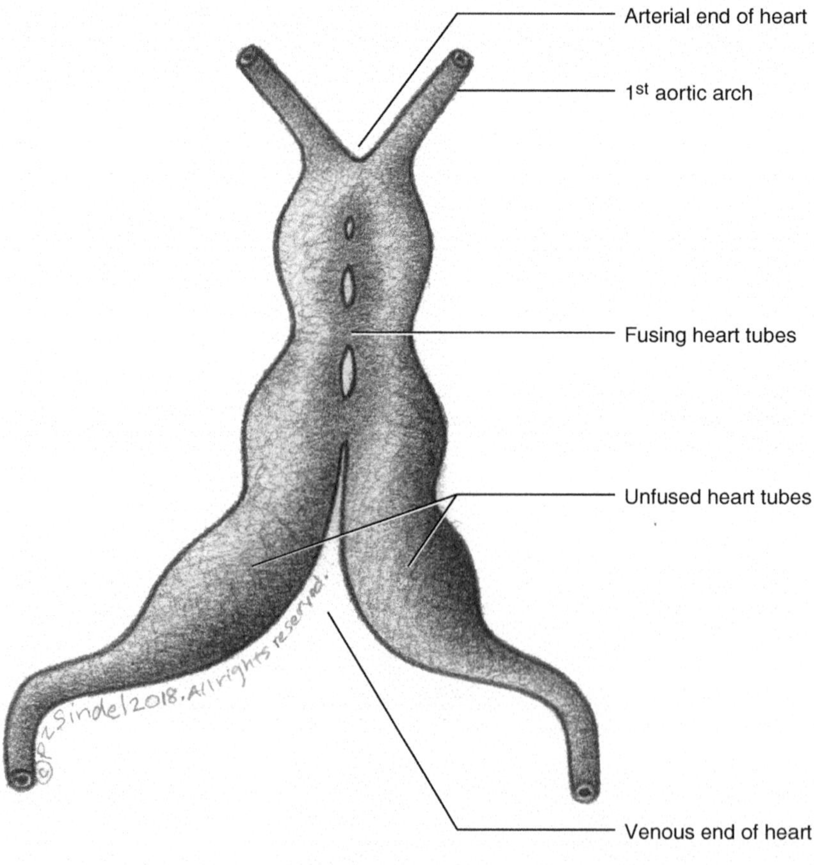

Fig. 13.2 The primitive heart tubes starting to fuse on Day 21, starting from the cranial (top) region

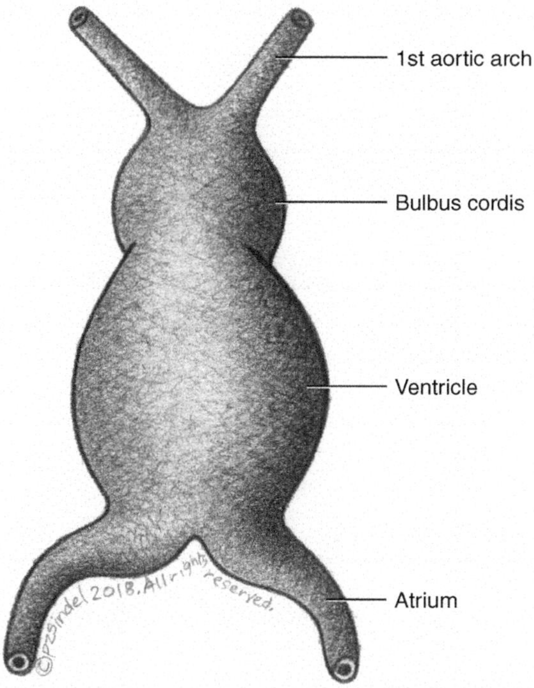

Fig. 13.3 Day 22 – Moving from the cranial to the caudal area (top to bottom) – truncus arteriosus (right where the vessels bifurcate), followed by the bulbus cordis and the primitive ventricle. Just caudal (below) the ventricle is the primitive atrium and most caudal is the sinus venosus

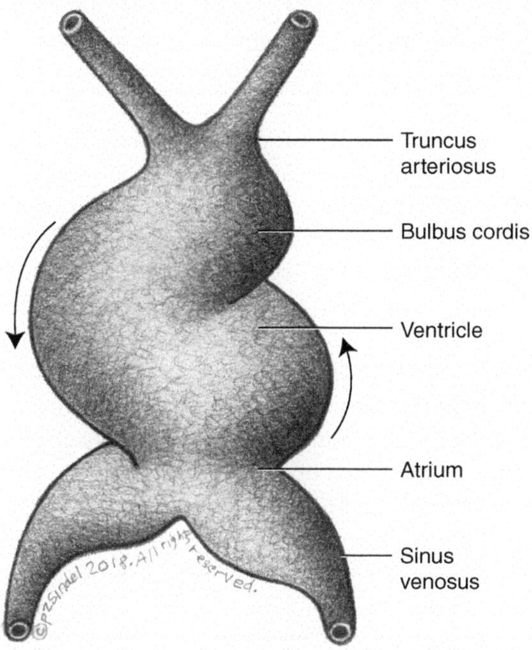

Fig. 13.4 Day 23 – The entire structure continues to grow with the bulbus cordis and the primitive ventricle growing more rapidly causing the primitive heart to bend (rotate) upon itself

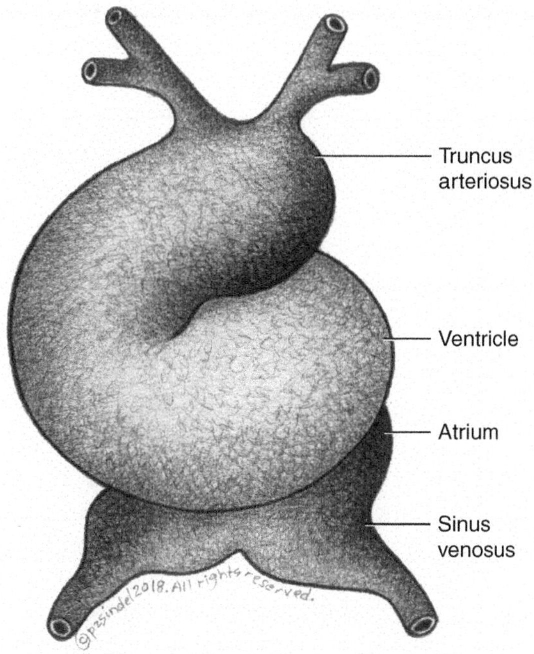

Fig. 13.5 Day 24 – The process continues forming the "U-shaped" bulboventricular loop

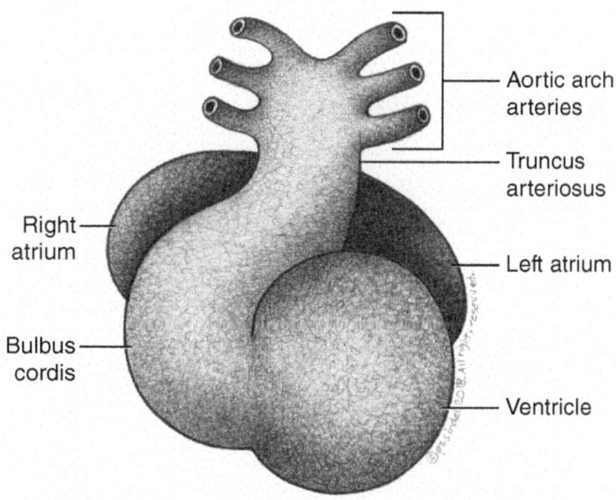

Fig. 13.6 Day 35 – The "S-shaped" heart is formed and the atria have rotated cranially and are now superior to the ventricle

Circulation Through the Primitive Heart

The contractions of the primitive heart begin by Days 22–23; these are myogenic in origin. The muscle layers of the atrium and ventricle are continuous and contractions occur in peristalsis-like waves that begin in the sinus venosus.

During the first week, the circulation through the heart and the embryo is of the ebb-and-flow type. By the end of the fourth week, coordinated contractions of the heart result in a unidirectional flow.

Blood returns to the sinus venosus from (1) the embryo, via the common cardinal veins; (2) the developing placenta, via the umbilical veins; and (3) the yolk sac, via the vitelline veins. Blood from the sinus venosus enters the atrium via the sinoatrial orifice. Its flow is controlled by the sinoatrial valves, which fuse cranially to form a marked projection, the septum spurium in the roof of the right side of the atrium. The blood then passes through the atrioventricular canal into the ventricle. When the ventricle contracts, the blood is pumped through the bulbus cordis and truncus arteriosus into the aortic sac, from which it passes to the aortic arches of the branchial arches. The blood then passes to the dorsal aortae for distribution to the embryo, yolk sac, and placenta.

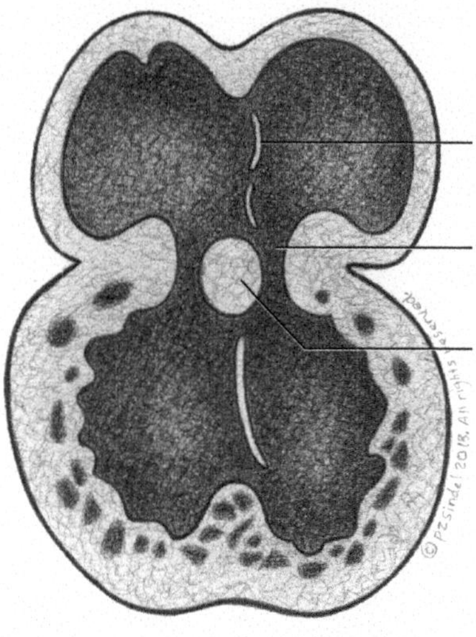

Fig. 13.7 Fourth week – there is a single atrium with the beginnings of the septum primum, the atrioventricular canals divided by the dorsal endocardial cushion and a single ventricle with the beginning of the intraventricular septum forming

Partitioning of the Atrioventricular Canal, the Atria, the Ventricles, and the Great Vessels

Partitioning of the atrioventricular canal, the atria, and the ventricles begins around the middle of the fourth week and is essentially complete by the end of the fifth week. These processes occur concurrently. During the fourth week, bulges form on the dorsal and ventral walls of the atrioventricular canal which are called the endocardial cushions (Fig. 13.7).

During the fifth week, the endocardial cushions fuse, forming the septum of the atrioventricular canal, which divides it into the right and left atrioventricular canals.

The primitive atrium is divided into right and left atrium by the formation and fusion of the septum primum and septum secundum. The septum primum also fuses with the fused endocardial cushions. Initially there is a large opening in the septum primum between its caudal free edge and the endocardial cushion called the foramen primum, which is obliterated when the septum fuses with the endocardial cushion. Before this occurs, perforations appear in the dorsal part which coalesce to form the foramen secundum.

Toward the end of the fifth week, another crescent membrane, the septum secundum, grows from the ventrocranial wall of the atrium, immediately to the right of the septum primum. As it grows, it gradually covers the foramen secundum. This forms an incomplete partition and leaves an oval opening, the foramen ovale. The cranial portion of the septum primum gradually disappears; the remaining part that attaches to the endocardial cushion forms the valve for the foramen ovale. Before birth, the foramen ovale allows almost all the blood from the inferior vena cava to pass through into the left atrium. After birth. The foramen ovale closes, and the interatrial septum becomes a complete partition when the septum primum fuses with the septum secundum.

Initially the sinus venosus is a separate chamber of the heart and opens into the caudal wall of the right atrium. The left horn of the sinus venosus becomes the coronary sinus and the right horn becomes incorporated into the wall of the right atrium.

Most of the left atrium is derived from the primitive pulmonary vein, which develops as an outgrowth of the dorsal atrial wall just to the left of the septum primum. As the atrium expands, the primitive pulmonary vein and its main branches are gradually incorporated into the wall of the left atrium, which results in four pulmonary veins with separate openings into the atrium.

Division of the primitive ventricle into right and left ventricles begins with a muscular ridge or fold, the interventricular septum, in the floor of the ventricle near the apex, which grows actively into the muscular portion of the interventricular septum. This results in a crescentic interventricular foramen between the free edge of the interventricular septum and the fused endocardial cushions, which permits communication between the right and left ventricle until the end of the seventh week. Closure results from the fusion of the subendocardial tissue from three sources: (1) the right bulbar ridge, (2) the left bulbar ridge, and (3) the fused atrioventricular endocardial cushion.

During the fifth week, bulges form on the walls of the bulbus cordis. Similar truncal ridges form in the truncus arteriosus and are continuous with the bulbar ridges. This results in a spiral aorticopulmonary septum when these ridges fuse and divide the bulbus cordis and the truncus arteriosus into the aorta and pulmonary trunk. The spiral nature of the ridges causes the pulmonary trunk to twist around the ascending aorta. The bulbus cordis is gradually incorporated into the walls of the ventricles becoming the conus arteriosus which gives rise to the pulmonary trunk in the right ventricle and the aortic vestibule which is the part of the ventricular cavity just inferior to the aortic valve of the left ventricle.

Case Presentation

You arrive at the hospital for your morning rounds and proceed to the mother-baby unit to see your newborns when Charge Nurse Helen spots you. "Great, doctor, you're here. The nurse for baby girl Grace in room 2120 wanted me to inform you that she heard a murmur while doing her assessment."

What should you do next?

(A) Order a chest X-ray.
(B) Order an echocardiogram.
(C) Obtain further history and perform a complete physical exam.
(D) Order a pediatric cardiology consultation.
(E) A and B.

You thank Helen and ask her to send the bedside nurse, Kasey, over to see you. You review the chart and discover the baby is 39 weeks and 5 days, birth weight 3565 grams born to a 24-year-old gravida 1 para 0, blood type O positive, rubella immune, VDRL nonreactive, hepatitis B surface antigen negative, and group B strep negative. Pregnancy was uncomplicated. There was no history of maternal diabetes, hypertension, or systemic lupus erythematosus (SLE). There was no history of maternal drugs (legal and illicit) or alcohol use during pregnancy. Fetal ultrasound was reported as normal. Mother presented to the hospital early in the AM on the day of delivery in early labor and was admitted to an LDR room. She delivered the baby vaginally at 14:05 after 12 h of labor. Membranes were ruptured 2 h prior to delivery. Mother was afebrile prior to delivery. APGAR scores were 9 and 9 at 1 and 5 min, respectively.

Nurse Kasey arrives and informs you that the baby has acted normally since delivery. She was placed skin-to-skin with mother after delivery and immediately began to nuzzle and breastfeed. The baby has continued to nurse well since delivery and has had several wet diapers and stools. There were no problems at all until she heard a systolic murmur during her early morning assessment. She didn't notify you earlier as she knew you would be there shortly to make morning rounds. You thank her for the information and proceed to the mother's room where you introduce yourself and examine the baby.

Answer: C

You find she is a well-appearing full-term female infant in no distress. Vital signs (heart rate, respiratory rate, and temperature) are normal. She is alert and active and cries appropriately. Head has 2+ molding without a cephalohematoma or caput succedaneum. Anterior fontanel is open and flat. Eyes and ears are normal; nose and throat are clear. Palate is intact. Neck is supple.

Chest shows clear breath sounds with good air entry. Heart shows normal S1 and S2 with a 3/6 crescendo murmur best heard along the upper left sternal border. Femoral pulses are 2+ and symmetrical. Abdomen is soft, non-distended, and non-tender without organomegaly. Genitals reveal a normal female. Anus is patent. Spine is intact. Extremities are normal. Skin is pink, clear, and well perfused without rashes. Baby appears neurologically intact with normal Moro, grasp, and suck reflexes.

What should you do next?

(A) Order an ECG.
(B) Order a chest X-ray.
(C) Order an echocardiogram.
(D) Check oxygen saturations and four-extremity blood pressures.
(E) Order a pediatric cardiology consultation.

Oxygen saturation testing will provide the most useful information at this point [6]. It will help you differentiate whether the murmur represents a cyanotic versus an acyanotic lesion. Pulse oximetry is inexpensive, readily available, and easy to perform. Oxygen saturations should be performed using two different sites, the right hand and either lower extremity (please see next case). Four-extremity blood pressures (BPs) are also easy to perform and may help differentiate the type of non-cyanotic CHD the baby may have and the need for emergent therapy.

Answer: D

You explain your findings to the parents and explain that you need to perform some further testing to determine if the baby's heart is normal or abnormal. You find Nurse Kasey and tell her you agree that the baby has a murmur and ask her to obtain oxygen saturation readings, from the right hand and foot. She brings the pulse oximeter and two sensors. The saturations were noted to 99–100% on both upper and lower extremities. The four-extremity BPs are right arm 65/42 mean 56, left arm 64/44 mean 55, right leg 62/45 mean 50, and left leg 60/43 mean 48.

The next appropriate step is:

(A) Order an echocardiogram.
(B) Order an electrocardiogram.
(C) Order a chest X-ray.
(D) Order a pediatric cardiology consult.
(E) B and C.

Either an echocardiogram or consult by a pediatric cardiologist has been shown to be most cost-effective at this point [7]. Unless you have detected an abnormal rhythm, an electrocardiogram is not likely to provide any helpful information at this point. The chest X-ray can provide some useful information such as the size and shape of the cardiac shadow and whether the pulmonary blood flow is normal, increased, or decreased. This information can be useful if the baby is unstable. One study showed that the chest X-ray did not contribute to the overall management of the patient at this point [8] . With the ready availability of pediatric cardiology or the use of telemedicine to obtain a timely reading, echocardiograms should be readily available and will provide a specific diagnosis. The pediatric cardiologist can decide if and when a chest X-ray and/or ECG need to be done.

You order an echocardiogram, which is done within an hour. About an hour after it was completed, you receive a phone call from the pediatric cardiologist who was able to access the study over the Internet. She tells you that the baby has a moderately stenotic aortic valve. She tells you to transfer the baby to the NICU for monitoring, and she will be in to evaluate the infant and check for the need of further testing/therapy (cardiac catheterization and/or surgical valve replacement).

Answer: A and D

Newborn with Murmur

The approach to the newborn with a murmur must include a thorough history, physical examination, and appropriate testing.

The evaluation begins with a primary survey to better understand the acuity and to be able to respond appropriately. Patients in respiratory distress and impending failure or shock must be transferred to the NICU for immediate stabilization of respiratory and hemodynamic status. Once under intensive care, the clinician will likely choose to perform a chest X-ray and ECG as initial evaluation and thereafter perform an echocardiogram to delineate the details of the cardiac anatomy. When evaluating a stable newborn, the echocardiogram is likely the first test ordered and may be all the patient requires before discharge home. In all cases, a pediatric cardiologist should review the data and formally consult or guide the neonatal team.

Some of the most frequent signs of heart failure are tachypnea, inability to nipple feeds, lethargy, and irritability.

Some of the most frequent symptoms of heart failure are tachypnea, tachycardia, hypotension, temperature instability, poor pulses, poor perfusion, and hepatomegaly.

The clinician must have a full understanding of the maternal prenatal history, perinatal events, as well as postnatal newborn adaptation to his/her new environment.

Which of the following maternal clinical findings are associated with congenital heart disease in the newborn?

1. Diabetes
2. Hypertension
3. Maternal systemic lupus erythematosus (SLE)
4. Previous infant with congenital heart disease
5. 1,3, and 4

Infants of diabetic mothers and mothers with previous history of children with congenital heart disease are at higher risk for having children with cardiac defects. Maternal lupus is associated with complete heart block in the newborn.

After a thorough history is obtained, a complete physical examination must be performed. The salient features in a newborn cardiac physical exam are vital signs including pulse oximetry and four-extremity blood pressures, auscultation for abnormal cardiac sounds, evaluation for respiratory distress, hepatosplenomegaly, poor pulses, and perfusion.

If the newborn fails the newborn screening exam or shows clear signs of cyanosis, he or she must be transferred to the NICU for further evaluation.

If the newborn shows signs of respiratory distress or congestive heart failure, he/she must be transferred to the NICU for management regardless of oxygen saturations.

There are potentially hundreds of combinations of different cardiac malformations. It is extremely challenging to describe each defect and the appropriate clinical management. Dividing the defects into two categories, cyanotic and non-cyanotic defects. These categories can be further divided to better manage the long differential diagnosis for cardiac defects.

Non-cyanotic lesions can be further divided into ductal-dependent and non-ductal-dependent lesions. Ductal-dependent lesions are usually associated with obstructive defects such as coarctation of the aorta, critical aortic stenosis, or critical pulmonic stenosis. In these patients every effort must be made to maintain patency of the ductus arteriosus to ensure hemodynamic stability. Non-ductal-dependent lesions can be further divided into left to right shunts and valvular abnormalities. Left to right shunts include atrial septal defects, ventricular septal defects, complete atrioventricular canal defects, patent ductus arteriosus, and aortopulmonary window. Valvular abnormalities range in location and severity and are best quantified by further imaging, such as echocardiography.

Answer: 5

What is the most likely diagnosis in a preterm, ventilator-dependent infant in the NICU with continuous murmur heard throughout the precordium and bounding pulses?

(A) ASD
(B) VSD
(C) PDA
(D) Atrioventricular canal defect

Answer: C

What is the most likely diagnosis in a 3-day-old infant with a holosystolic murmur heard best along the left lower sternal border?

(A) ASD
(B) VSD
(C) PDA
(D) Atrioventricular canal defect

Answer: B

What is the most likely diagnosis in a 1-day-old infant with 3/6 crescendo systolic murmur best heard along the upper sternal border?

(A) Pulmonic stenosis
(B) Tricuspid stenosis
(C) Aortic stenosis
(D) Mitral stenosis
(E) A and C
(F) B and D

Answer: E

What is the most likely diagnosis in a 2-day-old infant with diastolic murmur heard throughout the precordium?

(A) Mitral stenosis
(B) Tricuspid stenosis
(C) Aortic insufficiency
(D) Pulmonic insufficiency
(E) All of the above

Answer: E

Case Presentation

You are asked to evaluate a 3-day-old infant, shortly before discharge home, who was product of a cesarean section at term with APGAR score of 9 at 1 and 5 min, respectively. Mother is concerned because the baby has been crying, irritable, and suddenly unable to feed. The perinatal history was unremarkable and patient passed the newborn screen for cyanotic congenital heart disease. Upon exam he is found to have a long systolic murmur best heard over his back. He has poor perfusion throughout with diminished pulses in the lower extremities.

What should be the next step in evaluating the patient?

(A) CXR
(B) ECG
(C) Four-extremity blood pressure and pulse oximetry
(D) CBC

The differential diagnosis for a newborn with this presentation always includes possible sepsis. A long systolic murmur and poor pulses in the lower in extremities lead us to believe a cardiac defect is likely in this case. The patient was initially well and very rapidly went on to appear in shock. Checking four-extremity blood pressures is indicated when differential pulses are suspected in the initial evaluation. Documenting a significant gradient between the right upper and lower extremities helps navigate through your differential diagnosis for non-cyanotic congenital heart disease. The most likely diagnosis in this patient is coarctation of the aorta. This case illustrates the effects of one of the most important anatomic changes in cardiac structure in the newborn period, closure of the ductus arteriosus. The ductus arteriosus normally closes within the first few minutes after birth; however, this transition may be delayed for hours, days, and even weeks. In this case, as the ductus arteriosus closed, the patient manifested the hallmark symptoms of poor perfusion to the lower extremities, pressure gradient between the extremities, and compensated shock. The diagnosis is confirmed by echocardiography and patients commonly respond well to starting prostaglandin E1 (PGE).

Answer: C

Case Presentation

A 3-week-old infant presents to the emergency department with temp of 100.6. Although the patient was very vigorous at birth, the mother has noticed a significant difference in his behavior in the past week. He appears hungry but is unable to finish his feeds. He is very sweaty and breathes rapidly after taking only one ounce of formula. In the emergency department, his respiratory rate is 60 breaths per minute, heart rate is 160 beats per minute, and his oxygen saturation is 98%. On examination he has a 3/6 holosystolic murmur along the left sternal border. The liver is palpated 4 cm below the right costal margin and the capillary refill is 5 sec.

What is the most likely diagnosis?

(A) Small muscular VSD
(B) Small PDA
(C) Large VSD
(D) Small ASD

One of the most important changes in newborn physiology is the transition from fetal circulation. The pulmonary vascular resistance (PVR) and pulmonary artery pressures are normally elevated in the newborn. Elevated PVR translates to high pulmonary artery and ultimately high right ventricular pressures. Right-sided pressures can be as high as the pressures in the aorta and the left ventricle. If the pressures in the right and left ventricle are nearly equal, the degree of left to right shunting is minimal and the patient appears healthy. Sometime in the first 60 days of life, the pulmonary vascular resistance drops to levels commonly seen in adults. As the pulmonary vascular resistance decreases, the pressures on the right side become substantially lower than the pressures on the left side. This increases the pressure gradient between the chambers and increases the degree of left to right shunting. For this reason, a patient with a large PDA or VSD may appear very healthy at birth but progresses to congestive heart failure sometime in the first 2 months of age. This is a common presentation for infants with large left to right shunts.

Answer: C

When encountering a non-cyanotic patient with signs of congestive heart failure, a chest X-ray and ECG may be extremely helpful in the evaluation and management. An ECG can be used to rule out arrhythmias as a cause of congestive heart failure. A chest X-ray can help assess the degree of left to right shunting, pulmonary perfusion, and superimposed compounding abnormalities such as infectious or pulmonary disease. We believe that routine chest X-rays and ECGs are extremely helpful in the initial management of these patients.

The next step in evaluating the patient is to perform an echocardiogram. These studies can illustrate anatomic abnormalities and tailor specific management protocols for each cardiac defect. The patient with a small left to right shunt who is hemodynamically stable will be scheduled for outpatient follow-up. The patient with large left to right shunt will require anti-congestive therapy, maximum nutritional intake, and ultimately transcatheter and/or surgical intervention. The patients with obstructive lesions such as coarctation of the aorta, critical aortic stenosis, and critical pulmonic stenosis must be treated with PGE until palliated by surgical or transcatheter interventions. Valvular disease has a wide range of clinical presentations. Mild valvular disease is followed in an outpatient basis. Moderate valvular disease may respond to anti-congestive therapy. Severe valvular disease often requires surgical or transcatheter intervention.

The most important approach to anti-congestive therapy is to increase inotropic support, decrease systemic afterload, and decrease preload. Examples of inotropic agents include digoxin, dopamine, epinephrine, and milrinone (milrinone also decreases afterload). Diuretics such as lasix, diuril, and aldactone help to decrease preload. Afterload reducing agents include ACE inhibitors (enalapril), beta-blockers (carvedilol), sildenafil, and milrinone. These medications can be used in different combinations in the inpatient or outpatient setting to help stabilize the patients as a bridge to palliation (Tables 13.1 and 13.2).

Table 13.1 Workup of newborn with murmur

1. Hemodynamically stable newborn
(a) Echocardiogram
(b) ECG if suspected arrhythmia
(c) Pediatric cardiology consult
2. Hemodynamically unstable newborn
(a) Transfer to NICU
(b) Stabilize cardiac and respiratory status
(c) Four-extremity blood pressures and pulse oximetry
(d) CXR and ECG
(e) Echocardiogram
(f) Pediatric cardiology consult

Table 13.2 Differential diagnosis for non-cyanotic newborn with murmur

(a) Left to right shunts
(i) ASD
(ii) VSD
(iii) PDA
(b) Obstructive lesions
(i) LVOT obstruction, coarctation of the aorta
(ii) RVOT obstruction
(iii) Brach PS
(c) Valvular insufficiency
(i) Aortic
(ii) Pulmonic
(iii) Mitral
(iv) Tricuspid

Case Presentation

You are called by Nurse Rachel who informs you that she is taking care of baby boy Clark. She performed CCHD testing at approximately 24 h of age per protocol and the baby failed. The saturations were 92% in the right hand and foot. You ask if she repeated the test.

Should the nurse have repeated the test?

(A) Yes, twice 15 min apart
(B) Yes, 3 times 1 h apart
(C) Yes, 3 times half our apart
(D) No need to repeat the test

A screen is considered failed, if any oxygen saturation measures <90% (in the initial or repeat screen), oxygen saturation of <95% in the right hand and foot on three measures, each separated by 1 h, or if a >3% absolute difference exists in oxygen saturations between the right hand and foot on three different measures, each separated by 1 h [9].

Any screening with an oxygen saturation measure > = 95% in the right hand or foot with a = <3% absolute difference between the right hand and foot is considered a passed screen, and no repeat is necessary.

Answer: B

The nurse informs you that she followed the protocol and repeated the screen 3 times each separated by 1 h. You remembered that you examine the baby earlier in the day when you made rounds. The baby was born by repeat C-section at 39 weeks and 3 days, the day before at 17:13 to a 26-year-old gravida 2 para 1 mother who was blood type O+, rubella immune, VDRL nonreactive, hepatitis B surface antigen negative, and group B strep negative. The baby required no resuscitation and APGAR scores were 9 and 9 at 1 and 5 m, respectively.

What should you do next?

(A) Evaluate the baby.
(B) Observe the baby for a period of time to see if the saturations improve.
(C) Order a chest X-ray.
(D) Order an echocardiogram.
(E) Obtain a pediatric cardiology consult.

Perform a careful physical examination to assess possible non-cardiac causes of low saturations, such as a pneumothorax, pneumonia, transient tachypnea of the newborn, etc.

Answer C is partially correct as a chest X-ray may be helpful in diagnosing respiratory conditions that might cause decreased saturations. It will also give you cardiac shadow size and shape along with pulmonary blood flow.

You are too far away to be able to go to the hospital in a timely manner, so you page the pediatric hospitalist on-call to ask him to please evaluate the baby for you. He calls you back in

15 min after completing his evaluation and informs you that the baby is stable, with no signs of respiratory distress or respiratory disease.

Answer: A

What should you do next?

(A) Observe the baby for a period of time to see if the saturations improve.
(B) Order an echocardiogram.
(C) Obtain a pediatric cardiology consult.
(D) Transfer the baby to the NICU.

At this point we need to know if the baby has a cardiac lesion, especially if it is ductal dependent. Answer C could also be correct if there is a pediatric cardiologist immediately available to evaluate the infant. This can be done prior to the echocardiography.

You order an echocardiogram, but the nursing supervisor informs you that they will need to call in the on-call echocardiogram technologist to perform the study and it will take several hours.

Answer: B

What should you do until the echocardiogram can be done?

(A) Transfer the baby to NICU for close monitoring with ready availability of prostaglandin E1.
(B) Observe the baby in the newborn nursery since he is very stable.
(C) Observe the baby in the newborn nursery, but continue oxygen saturation monitoring.
(D) Throw a temper tantrum until the nursing supervisor agrees to have the echocardiogram performed sooner.

Since you do not know if the baby has a ductal-dependent lesion which could turn critical quickly if the PDA closes, the baby needs to be monitored closely where there are personnel that can recognize the baby's condition and respond quickly by starting PGE1.

You call the neonatologist on-call, explain the situation, and ask for the baby to be transferred to the NICU. The neonatologist agrees and transfers the baby. The baby remained stable while monitored in the NICU. Chest X-ray revealed increased size of the cardiothymic shadow and increased pulmonary flow. A hyperoxia test was performed, and saturations and arterial PO2 did not improve significantly, suggesting likely cyanotic congenital heart disease. The echocardiogram was completed and confirms a diagnoses of transposition of the great vessels (ductal dependent). The pediatric cardiologist suggests that the baby be started on low-dose PGE1 (0.03 mcg/kg/min) while the transfer to the local pediatric cardiac center is arranged. The baby is transferred early the next morning and had an arterial switch performed. The baby did well post-op.

Answer: A

Case Presentation

You are asked to evaluate a newborn with respiratory distress and persistent cyanosis in the delivery room. The perinatal history was unremarkable and the patient was delivered vaginally without any complications. Pulse oximetry documents saturations of 78% on room air and the patient appears to have mild tachypnea and subcostal retraction. After transfer to the neonatal ICU, the patient is stabilized and placed on 100% oxygen for 10 min. Blood gas and Pulse oximetry are obtained to evaluate the patient's response to Oxygen therapy.

Match the clinical findings (Saturations and pO2) with the most likely etiology for cyanosis.

Clinical findings

1. Systemic saturations of 100% and pO2 of 390 ppm
2. Systemic saturations of 85% and pO2 of 90 ppm
3. Systemic saturations of 92% and pO2 of 130%

Etiology for cyanosis

(a) Cardiac
(b) Pulmonary
(c) Mixed etiologies possible persistent fetal circulation

Answer: 1 matches with "b", 2 matches with "a", and 3 matches with "c"

Patients with significant improvement in oxygen saturation and arterial pO2 are likely to have pulmonary disease. In cyanotic congenital heart disease, applying 100% oxygen does not improve systemic saturations. This is primarily due to right to left shunting or complete mixing of systemic and pulmonary venous flows. Patients with modest improvement are likely to have pulmonary disease in conjunction with persistent fetal circulation causing right to left shunting at the atrial (patent foramen ovale) or great arterial (patent ductus arteriosus) levels.

Understanding the differential diagnosis for cyanotic congenital heart disease is extremely helpful in the next step for evaluation and management of the patient. A chest X-ray which evaluates pulmonary blood flow can assist with the differential diagnosis.

When faced with a cyanotic newborn, the clinician should immediately assess the acuity and hemodynamic stability. Although all patients should be transferred to the NICU for further evaluation, those with impending cardiac or respiratory failure will require much more intensive and timely care. The clinician must first stabilize the airway, breathing, and circulation. After the patient is stabilized, more detailed historical information is necessary, and a physical examination is completed. Blood pressures (four extremities), pulse oximetry, chest X-rays, and an electrocardiogram will rule out arrhythmias and possible anatomic cardiac abnormities.

Although most likely causes of cyanosis in the newborn are of respiratory origin, sepsis is always a possible cause for low oxygen saturations after birth. It is often difficult to differentiate between cardiac and respiratory etiologies for cyanosis. The hyperoxia test is very useful and will often help differentiate between pulmonary and cardiac etiologies for cyanosis. To perform the hyperoxia test, first check pulse oximetry and an arterial blood gas including pO2 (partial pressure of dissolved oxygen) at baseline. Then apply 100% oxygen for approximately 10 minutes. Check pulse oximetry and the arterial blood gas again under these conditions.

Case Presentation

While analyzing the CXR on a newborn with cyanotic heart disease, you notice significantly diminished vascular markings in the peripheral lung fields.

What are the most likely diagnoses for this presentation?

1. Tetralogy of Fallot (TOF)
2. Tricuspid atresia
3. Transposition of the great arteries (TGA)
4. Truncus arteriosus
5. Total anomalous pulmonary venous return
6. 1 and 2
7. 3, 4, and 5

Most often there are two possible cardiac diagnoses for any patient with cyanosis and decreased pulmonary vascular markings on CXR: tetralogy of Fallot and tricuspid atresia. Patients with TOF have a long harsh systolic murmurs noted on the physical exam, right axis deviation, and right ventricular hypertrophy on ECG as well as boot-shaped cardiac silhouette on CXR. TOF is the most common cardiac cause for cyanosis in the newborn. Tricuspid atresia presents with continuous murmur (patent ductus arteriosus), small cardiac silhouette on CXR, and diminished right ventricular forces on ECG (Figs. 13.8, 13.9, and 13.10).

Answer: 6

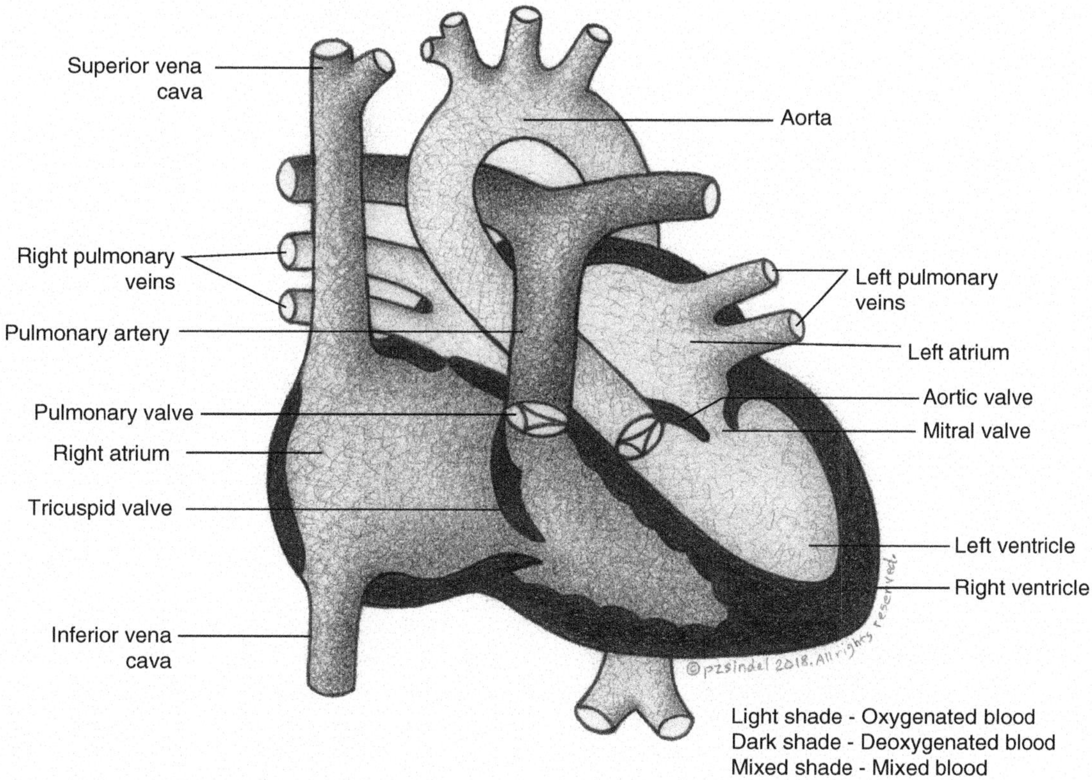

Fig. 13.8 Normal heart

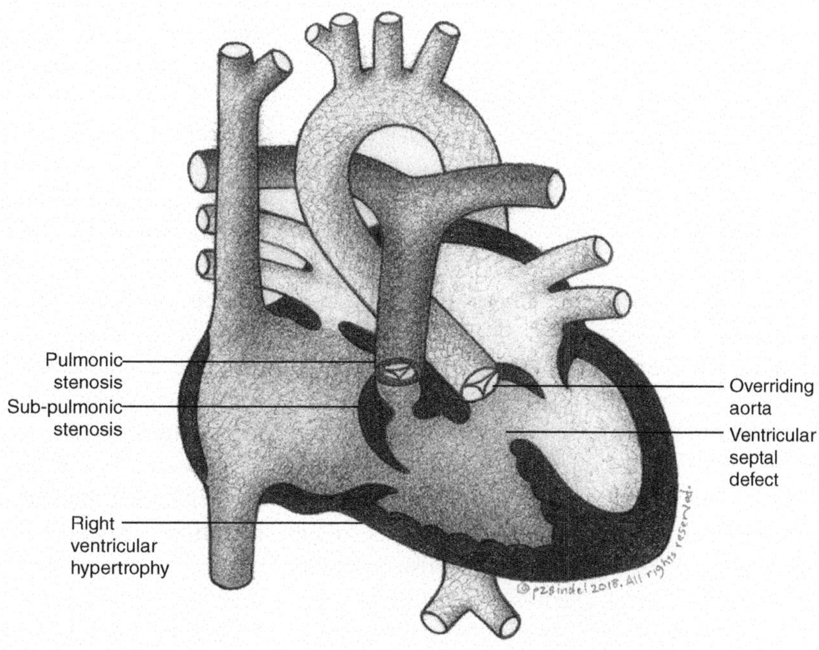

Fig. 13.9 Tetralogy of Fallot

Fig. 13.10 Tricuspid atresia

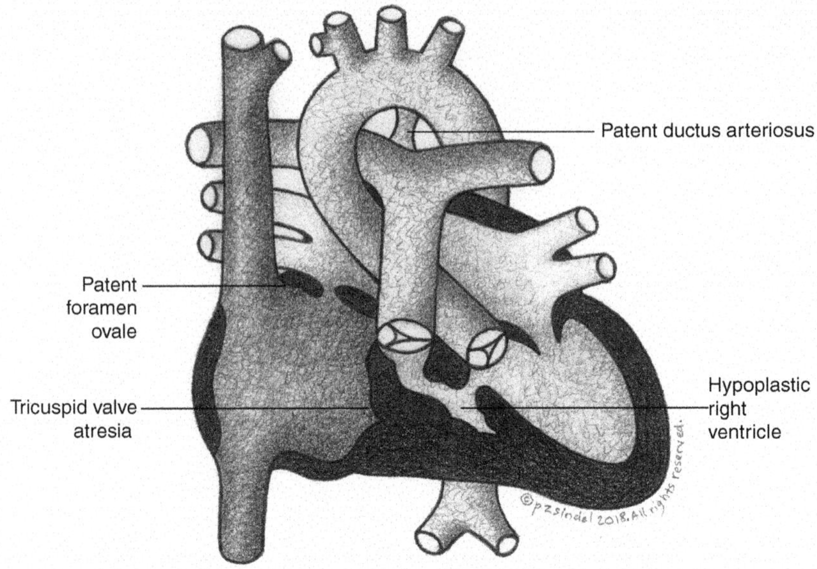

Case Presentation

While analyzing the CXR on a newborn with cyanotic heart disease, you notice significantly increased vascular markings in the peripheral lung fields. What are the most likely diagnoses for this presentation?

1. Tetralogy of Fallot (TOF)
2. Tricuspid atresia
3. Transposition of the great arteries (TGA)
4. Truncus arteriosus
5. Total anomalous pulmonary venous return
6. 1 and 2
7. 3, 4, and 5

Most often there are three possible cardiac diagnoses for any patient with cyanosis and increased pulmonary vascular markings on CXR. Transposition of the great arteries (TGA) is the most common form of cyanotic heart disease noted in the first few minutes after birth. Patients with TGA have a loud, single second heart sound, and the cardiac silhouette on CXR is often described as an egg on a string. Malposition of the great arteries creates a narrow mediastinal shadow on CXR and hence the appearance of a string holding the remainder of the egg-shaped heart. Patients with truncus arteriosus often have a very abnormal truncal (aortic valve) with possible stenosis or insufficiency. These patients have a single second heart sound with systolic and diastolic murmurs of truncal valve disease. Patients with total anomalous pulmonary venous return (TAPVR) have very classic and unique CXR findings including increased pulmonary venous markings (curly B lines) and cardiac silhouette resembling a snowman (Figs. 13.11, 13.12, 13.13, and 13.14).

Answer: 7

There are other forms of very complex cardiac malformations that cause cyanosis. These include single ventricle with aortic obstruction (hypoplastic left heart syndrome) and single ventricle with pulmonary obstruction (hypoplastic right heart syndrome). Epstein's anomaly of the tricuspid valve may also present with cyanosis in the newborn period.

The echocardiogram is the most widely used and effective tool in the initial evaluation of infants and newborns with congenital heart disease. Frequently the clinician does not have immediate access to echocardiography and must depend on his/her clinical skills to stabilize the patient and optimize care until the echocardio-

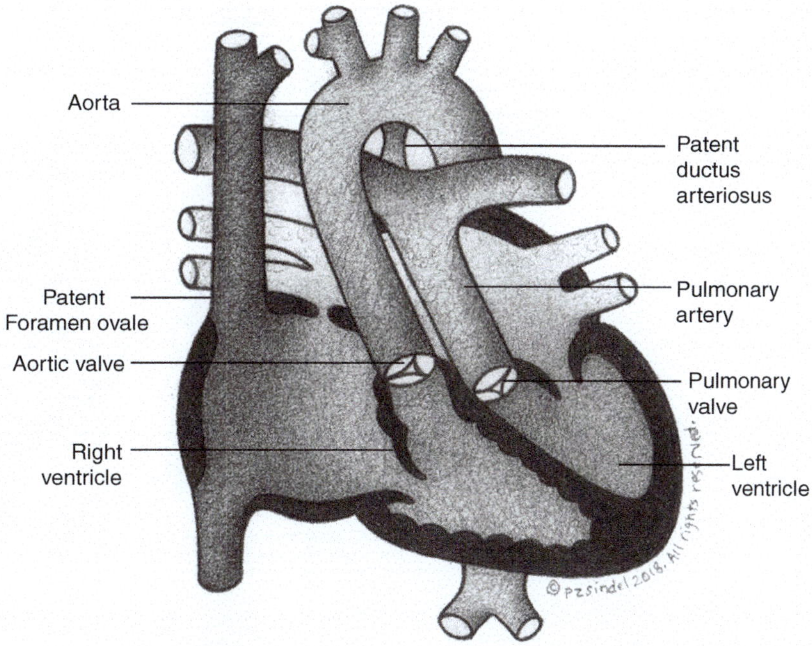

Fig. 13.11 Transposition of great arteries

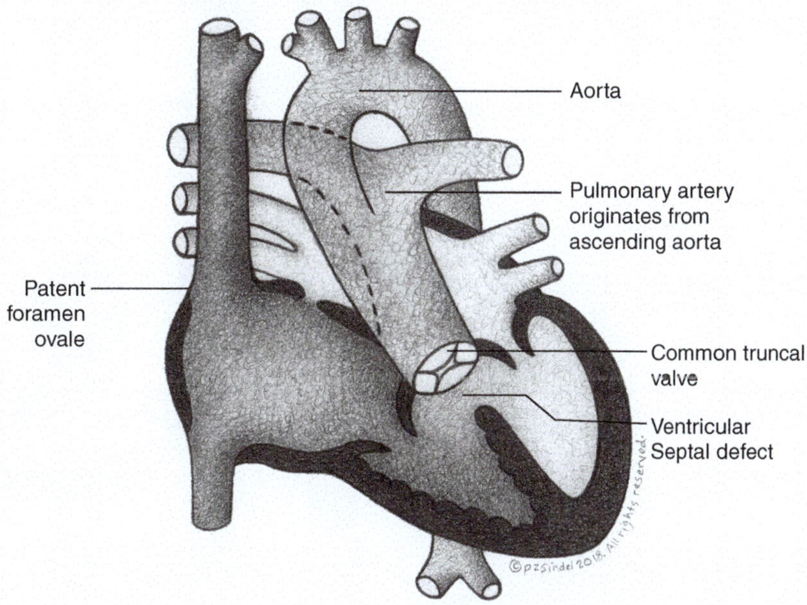

Fig. 13.12 Truncus arteriosus

gram can be performed. A thorough history, physical examination, hyperoxia test, CXR, and ECG will provide sufficient information to commence the appropriate therapeutic modalities.

Eventually the echocardiogram and consultation with a pediatric cardiologist will solidify the details of the cardiac anatomy and guide the clinician in implementing appropriate care. One of the most commonly used therapeutic agents for stabilizing patients with cyanotic congenital heart disease is prostaglandin E1 (PGE). PGE is used to maintain patency of the ductus arteriosus, promoting mixing of oxygenated and deoxygenated blood in TGA, pulmonary blood flow in pul-

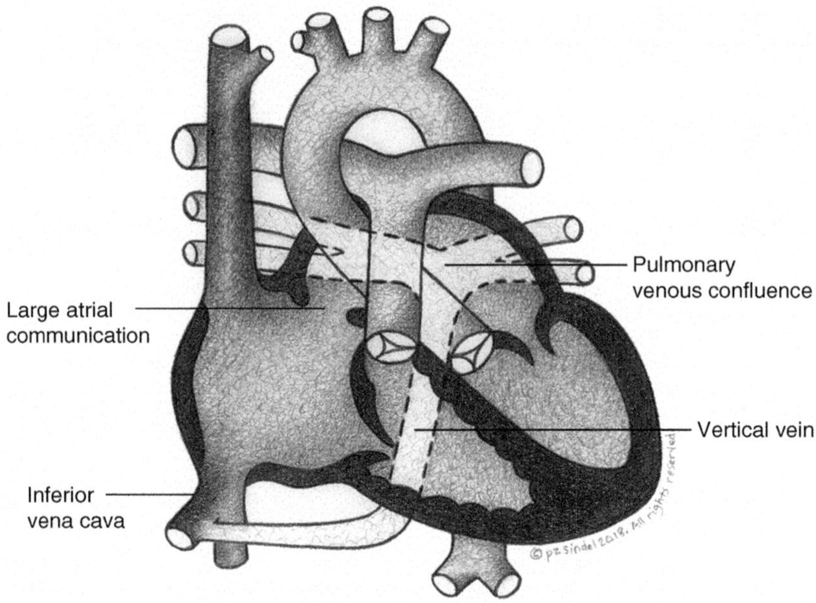

Fig. 13.13 Infracardiac TAPVR

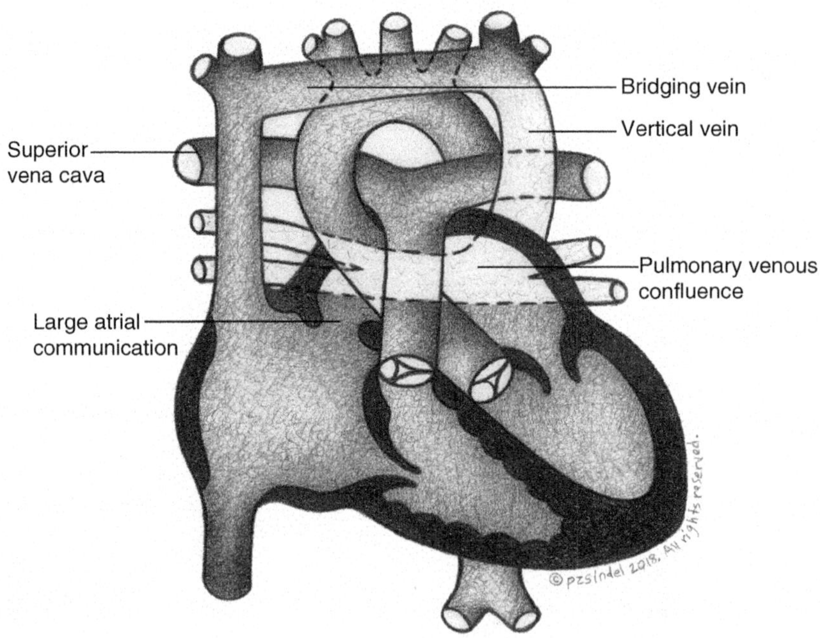

Fig. 13.14 Supracardiac TAPVR

monary obstructive lesions such as TOF and tricuspid atresia, and systemic blood flow in systemic obstructive lesions such as aortic atresia or hypoplastic left heart syndrome.

Other therapeutic modalities include oxygen supplementation, inotropic support, nitric oxide, and extracorporeal membrane oxygenation (ECMO) (Tables 13.3 and 13.4).

Table 13.3 Workup of newborn with documented cyanosis

1. Transfer to neonatal ICU
2. Stabilize cardiac and respiratory status
3. Four-extremity blood pressures and pulse oximetry
4. Hyperoxia test
5. CXR and ECG
6. Echocardiogram
7. Pediatric cardiology consult

Table 13.4 Differential diagnosis for the newborn with cyanotic congenital heart disease

1. Lesions with decreased pulmonary blood flow
(a) Tetralogy of Fallot (b) Tricuspid atresia
2. Lesions with increased pulmonary blood flow
(a) Truncus arteriosus (b) Transposition of great arteries (c) Total anomalous pulmonary venous return (pulmonary venous congestion)
3. Lesions with variable pulmonary blood flow
(a) Single ventricle (hypoplastic left or right ventricle)

Clinical Pearls

- Deviation from normal embryologic development usually results in congenital heart disease.
- Treat congestive heart failure (CHF) appropriately with diuresis and inotropic support.
- Cyanotic newborns without any respiratory symptoms are very likely to have cyanotic congenital heart disease.
- The hyperoxia test can help to differentiate pulmonary and cardiac causes of cyanosis.
- Patients with cardiac cyanosis usually respond well to PGE.
- Cyanosis and CHF are very separate processes that may present simultaneously. However, the mechanisms are distinct and the processes are often mutually exclusive.
- Newborns with cyanosis who fail the hyperoxia test and show decreased pulmonary vascular markings on CXR are likely to have either tricuspid atresia or tetralogy of Fallot.
- Newborns with cyanosis who fail the hyperoxia test and show increased pulmonary vascular markings on CXR are likely to have either transposition of the great arteries, truncus arteriosus, or total anomalous pulmonary venous return.
- Tetralogy of Fallot. Cyanosis, long harsh systolic murmur, decreased pulmonary vascular markings, boot-shaped heart.
- Tricuspid atresia. Cyanosis, decreased pulmonary vascular markings, significantly decreased RV forces on ECG.
- Transposition of great arteries. Cyanosis, increased pulmonary vascular markings, egg on a string (no thymic shadow)
- Truncus arteriosus. Cyanosis, single S2, increased pulmonary vascular markings.
- Total anomalous pulmonary venous return. Cyanosis, increased pulmonary vascular markings, snow man.

Acknowledgments The authors would like to acknowledge and express their deepest gratitude to Phyllis Z Sindel BFA for the wonderful medical illustrations included in this chapter. We could not have completed this work without her participation.

References

1. Ferencz C, Rubin JD, McCarter RJ, et al. Congenital heart disease: prevalence at live birth. Am J Epidemiol. 1985;121:31–6.
2. Hoffman JIE. Incidence of congenital heart disease. I. Postnatal incidence. Pediatr Cardiol. 1995;16:103–13.
3. Hoffman JIE, Kaplan S. The incidence of congenital heart disease. J Am Coll Cardiol. 2002;39:1890–900.
4. Botto LD, Correa A, Erickson JD. Racial and temporal variations in the prevalence of heart defects. Pediatrics. 2001;107:E32.
5. Mahle WT, Newburger JW, Matherne GP, Smith FC, Hoke TR, Kopple R, Gidding SS, Beekman RH 3rd,

Grosse SD, on behalf of the American Heart Association Congenital Heart Defects Committee of the Council on Cardiovascular Disease in the Young, Council on Cardiovascular Nursing, and Interdisciplinary Council on Quality of Care and Outcomes Research; and the American Academy of Pediatrics Section on Cardiology and Cardiovascular Surgery, and the Committee on the Fetus and Newborn. Role of Pulse Oximetry in examining newborns for congenital heart disease: a scientific statement from the American Heart Association and the American Academy of Pediatrics. Circulation. 2009;120:447–58.

6. Turly Y, Yetman RJ, Cromwell PF. Evaluation of a newborn with a Murmur. J Pediatr Health Care. 2013;27(3):226–9.
7. Yi MS, Kimball TR, Tsevat J, Mrus JM, Kotagal UR. Evaluation of heart murmurs in children: cost-effectiveness and practical implications. J Pediatr. 2002;141(4):504–10.
8. Oeppen RS, Fairhurst JJ, Argent JD. Diagnostic value of the chest radiograph in asymptomatic neonates with a cardiac murmur. Clin Radiol. 2002;57:736–40.
9. Kemper AR, Mahle WT, Martin GR, Coolie WC, Kumar P, Morrow WR, Kelm K, Pearson GD, Glidewell J, Grosse SD, Howell RR. Strategies for implementing screening for critical congenital heart disease. Pediatrics. 2011;128(5):e1259–67.

Diagnosis and Management of Nursery Arrhythmia

14

Robert Loitz

Introduction

Cardiac arrhythmias presenting at birth are rare and, in the majority of cases, are asymptomatic and self-limiting. Approximately 1% of newborns are recognized with rhythm abnormalities. The majority display asymptomatic atrial ectopy or benign sinus bradycardia. The challenge is to discern between these benign rhythms and the less frequent hemodynamically significant rhythm disturbances requiring intervention.

Many hemodynamically significant arrhythmias are first noted during prenatal evaluation and perinatal monitoring. Irregular contractions are often evident on fetal ultrasound. Discontinuity on ultrasound of the frequency of atrial and ventricular contractions along with slow fetal pulse rate is a typical presentation of congenital forms of heart block.

Sustained fetal tachyarrhythmias are associated with risk of fetal myocardial dysfunction, intrauterine growth retardation, and possible development of fetal hydrops requiring initiation of antiarrhythmic maternal drug therapy. Neonatal intensive care management is typically prearranged in cases of a symptomatic fetal arrhythmia. Initial recognition or stabilization of these newborns is typically not performed in the well-baby nursery.

Benign asymptomatic rhythm abnormalities and destabilizing symptomatic rhythm disturbances can however first present without prior suspicion in the nursery and must be promptly recognized. Every well-baby nursery needs to be equipped with personnel and equipment allowing the prompt awareness of rhythm abnormalities. Benign arrhythmias require continued monitoring without other intervention. Potentially hemodynamically destabilizing arrhythmias need to be recognized, documented, and monitored with stabilization and therapy initiated prior to transfer to a higher acuity neonatal care unit.

Every well-baby nursery should have trained clinical personnel to recognize the presentation of both benign and symptomatic arrhythmias. On-site and immediately available equipment for diagnosis and monitoring of newborn heart rate and rhythm is mandatory along with the ability to administer first-line drug therapy and other treatments. In the event of acutely destabilizing arrhythmias, personnel trained in emergency life support must be available along with resuscitative equipment, means of delivery of life support medications, and cardioversion capability.

After initial stabilization, hemodynamically significant arrhythmias will require subsequent monitoring and intervention in an NICU setting.

R. Loitz, MD
Pacific Pediatric Cardiology Medical Group, Pasadena, CA, USA

Keck School of Medicine, University of Southern California, Los Angeles, CA, USA

G. I. Martin, W. Rosenfeld (eds.), *Common Problems in the Newborn Nursery*,
https://doi.org/10.1007/978-3-319-95672-5_14

Newborns with benign rhythms will require ongoing routine clinical monitoring prior to discharge home. Arrhythmias persisting at discharge need scheduled cardiology evaluation as outpatients with immediate reassessment if any post-discharge symptoms are suspected.

The Equipped Nursery

The prerequisite for prompt recognition and timely management of nursery arrhythmias is diligent and ongoing clinical observation by on-site medical and nursing personnel including routine serial measurement of heart rate and pulse regularity along with blood pressure, oximetry, respiratory, and perfusion status.

Required equipment includes 12-lead EKG recorder with rhythm strip printout for use in diagnosis and real-time management.

First-line antiarrhythmic drugs need to be on-site or promptly available from the hospital pharmacy. Required drugs (Table 14.1) include propranolol IV/PO, digoxin IV/PO, lidocaine IV, adenosine IV, and prostaglandin E1.

In nursery availability of additional neonatal resuscitation medications including atropine, epinephrine, sodium bicarbonate, and calcium gluconate.

On-site or on-call echocardiography to assess for structural and functional heart abnormality.

Neonatal cardioversion/defibrillator with low-wattage capability and infant-sized electrode pads (Table 14.2).

The cardioversion procedure should be well organized with a protocol which is consistent and includes a step-by-step approach (Table 14.3).

Table 14.2 Neonatal cardioversion required equipment

External pediatric defibrillator
(Typically minimum charge level 2 joules, alternatively may use pediatric-capable adult defibrillator with energy-reducing pads)
Neonatal-sized electrode pads maximum 4.5 cm diameter
Cardiac monitor with strip recorder
Airway management equipment
Antiarrhythmic and resuscitation medications

Table 14.3 Cardioversion procedure (step by step)

Neonatal cardioversion/defibrillation		
Pre-sedation		
Pad placement		
	Anterior/ posterior	Front at left of mid sternum
		Back at left mid-chest (alternatively at subxiphoid apex)
Defibrillator charging		
	Power	*ON*
	Mode	*MANUAL*
	Energy	0.5–1.0 joule/kg to max 2 joule/kg
	Sync mode	Cardioversion *ON*
		Defibrillation *OFF*
	Charge	*CHARGE* button *PRESS*
Clear personnel from bedside		
Administer shock		*SHOCK* button *PRESS*

Table 14.1 Antiarrhythmic medications

Drug dosages			
Propranolol	0.1 mg/kg/dose	Po	Every 6–8 h
	1 mg/kg/dose	IV	Every 6–8 h
Digoxin	Digitalization		
	Preterm		30 mcg/kg/ total dose divided in 3 doses every 12 h
	Full-term		40 mcg/kg/ total dose divided in 3 doses every 12 h
	Maintenance		
	Preterm		5–10 mcg/kg/day divided every 12 h
	Full-term		10 mcg/kg/day divided every 12 h
Lidocaine	1 mg/kg		IV bolus
	50 mcg/kg/min		IV continuous drip
Adenosine	50 mcg/kg		IV bolus increasing to effect every 5 min by
			50 mcg increments to 200 mcg/kg maximum dose
Prostaglandin E1	0.05–0.1 mcg/kg/min		IV infusion with maintenance 0.01–0.05 mcg/kg/min

Bradyarrhythmia

Case Presentation

Full-term female neonate arrives in the well-baby nursery after vaginal delivery appearing well but with an irregular pulse and good perfusion and in no respiratory distress. By palpation heart rate averages 70–90 beats/minute (Fig. 14.1)

1. What immediate management is indicated?
   (A) Transfer to NICU for cardiac monitoring
   (B) 12-lead EKG and 2D echocardiogram
   (C) 12-lead EKG/rhythm strip
   (D) Septic workup
2. What rhythm is displayed on the EKG initially obtained?
   (A) PACs with aberration and nonconduction
   (B) Junctional rhythm with aberrant conduction
   (C) Second-degree AV block
   (D) Ectopic ventricular contractions
3. What initial therapy is indicated?
   (A) Transfer to NICU for cardiac monitoring and possible chronotropic drug support
   (B) Ongoing nursery vital sign monitoring with repeat EKG prior to discharge
   (C) Start low dose oral beta-blocker
   (D) Cardiac consultation including 2D echo evaluation

Answers: 1B 2A 3B

An abnormally slow heart rate, whether regular or irregular, when detected by auscultation or EKG monitoring is indicative of a bradyarrhythmia. The majority of slow heart rate rhythms such as sinus bradycardia or sinus arrhythmia are asymptomatic and self-limiting. Alternatively, severe dysfunction or the sinus node, AV node, or the conduction pathways may present with profoundly low heart rates and impaired cardiac output.

Sinus Bradycardia

Sinus bradycardia presents with slow regular rate less than 90 beats/minute with normal P wave access and PR interval. Lower heart rates are often promoted by increased vagal tone induced by drugs, hypothyroidism, CNS abnormality, and hypoxemia or as a reflex to airway maneuvers or suctioning inducing a vagal reflex. Low rate may also be a presenting feature of prolongation of the QT interval. A 12-lead EKG should be obtained whenever bradycardia is suspected to confirm the absence of heart block or QT prolongation. Assessment should be made for the presence of contributing systemic factors provoking increased vagal tone. Isolated sinus bradycardia is asymptomatic, self-resolving, and does not require antiarrhythmic therapy.

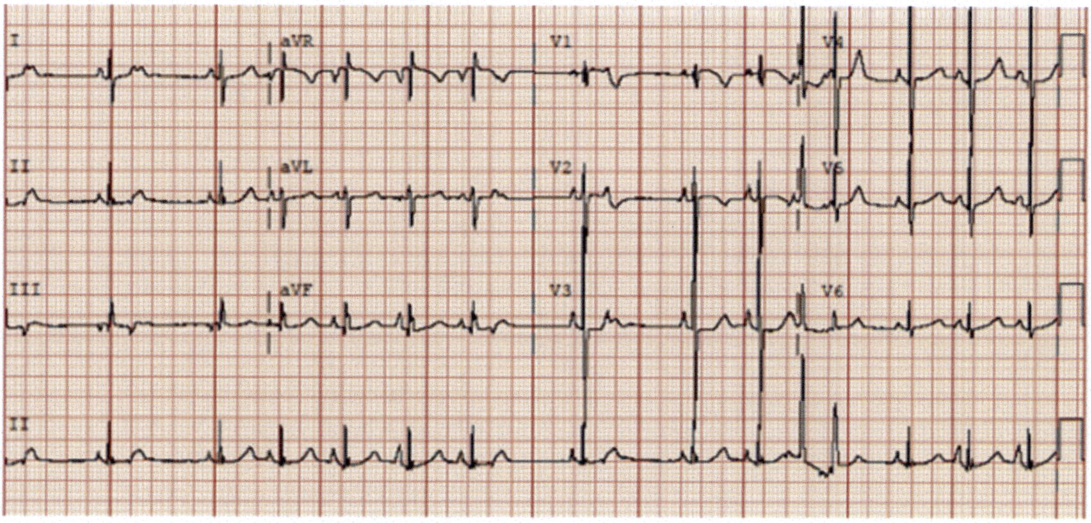

Fig. 14.1 Premature atrial contractions with aberrant conduction

Sinus Arrest

In rare cases the sinus node or, alternatively, the atrial muscle fail to induce a pacemaker impulse resulting in potentially irregular AV node or ventricular escape rhythm. Absence of atrial activity is seen on EKG for multiple cycle lengths potentially inducing severe bradycardia with occasionally irregular escape rhythm response. Atrial pauses greater than 3 sec can result in impaired cardiac output requiring cardiotropic drug therapy. Emergency use of IV atropine or epinephrine is indicated to increase escape rhythm rates prior to transfer to intensive care for assessment of need of pacemaker support.

Atrioventricular Block

An irregular or slow heart rate showing appropriately frequent and normally appearing P waves with intermittent or absent QRS ventricular conduction is the indication of impaired AV node conduction. Slowed but consistent AV node conduction is demonstrated by an increased EKG PR interval greater than 0.16 sec at birth. Intermittent nonconduction will show P waves with occasionally absent succeeding QRS complexes. In approximately 1:20,000 births, complete heart block presents with independent generation of ventricular QRS complexes at a rate not associated with P wave frequency (Fig. 14.2).

In 25–50% of cases, higher level AV node conduction abnormalities are associated with congenital heart deformities and are an indication for 2D echo screening. The most common heart abnormalities seen include congenitally corrected transposition of the great arteries, heterotaxy, seen in AV canal defects especially "polyspenia" or left atrial isomerism.

Profoundly increased vagal tone promoted by abdominal pain, airway manipulation, or CNS abnormality may temporarily impair AV node conduction. Abnormalities in electrolytes such as potassium, magnesium, and calcium need to be eliminated. Pericardial inflammation due to isolated pericarditis or pulmonary disease can induce AV node inflammation resulting in often transient AV node block.

Maternal autoimmune disorders, most prominently systemic lupus erythematosus and Sjogren's syndrome, lead to production of anti-Ro and anti-La maternal antibodies that cross the placenta and result in immune complex damage of the fetal AV node. Most cases of maternal autoimmune-induced fetal AV node injury present with second trimester fetal bradycardia and are an indication for high-risk delivery and immediate neonatal intensive care intervention.

Isolated congenital dysfunction of the AV node or distal conduction pathways can occur in

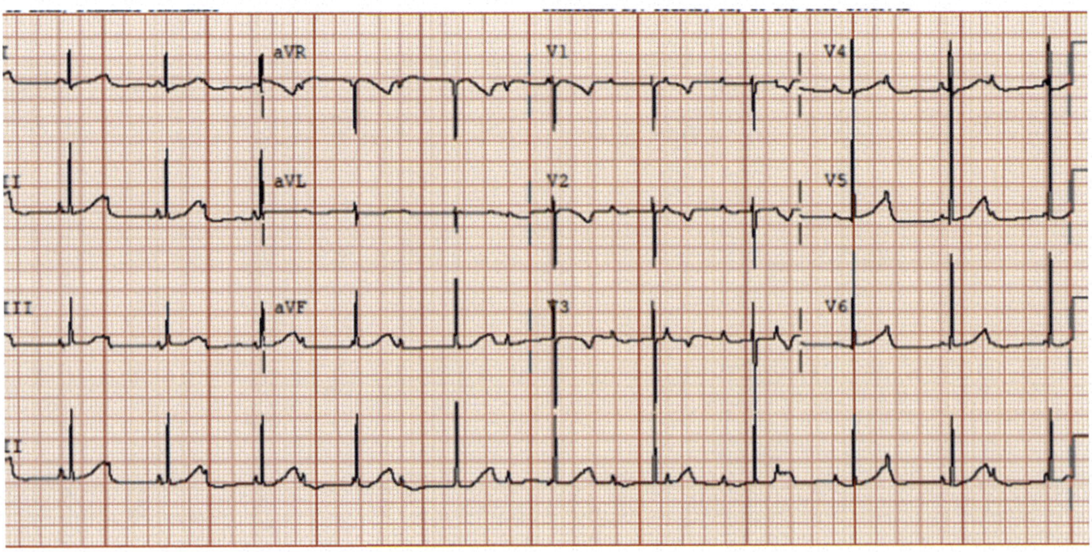

Fig. 14.2 Atrial-ventricular heart block

the absence of other structural heart abnormalities and present with fetal and subsequent neonatal bradycardia.

All cases of higher level AV node dysfunction should be transferred to an intensive care unit. Acute management with chronotropic agents is indicated if impaired cardiac output is suspected. The receiving intensive care unit should have the capability to initiate temporary pacing if an impaired cardiac output state is not stabilized on drug therapy. Permanent pacemaker placement is typically required eventually in neonates with native heart rates less than 55 beats/minute.

Premature Atrial Contraction (PAC)-Induced Bradycardia

A common cause of bradycardia seen almost exclusively in newborns is a reduced ventricular rate resulting from the nonconduction of early and frequent premature atrial contractions. Due to the generally prolonged AV node refractory period seen at birth, rapid atrial impulses occurring during the refractory period are not conducted to the ventricles. Nonconducted P waves will be seen along with abnormal-appearing conducted premature atrial beats. The resultant EKG pattern may mimic a primary AV block but typically differs upon analysis of P wave morphology and coexistence of conducted premature atrial beats. Unlike AV block where P wave axis and appearance are typically normal, the nonconducted P waves will appear similar to those seen in conducted premature atrial beats.

The bradycardia induced by nonconducted premature atrial contractions is rarely symptomatic resolving over the first month of life as atrial automaticity resolves and AV node refractory period shortens. If symptomatic bradycardia occurs, therapy with b-blockers or digoxin may be temporarily used.

Tachyarrhythmias

Case Presentation

A full-term 3.8 kg male with unremarkable prenatal course born by NSVD arrives in the nursery appearing well with initial regular heart rate 120/min and respirations 22/min with saturation of 98% by pulse oximetry. At 8 h of age, he appears mildly tachypneic with rapid pulse maintaining normal perfusion and blood pressure. A stat rhythm strip is obtained (Figs. 14.3 and 14.4).

1. What is the most likely rhythm disturbance?
   (A) Sinus tachycardia with aberrant ventricular conduction
   (B) Supraventricular tachycardia with aberrant ventricular conduction
   (C) Ventricular tachycardia
   (D) Ectopic atrial tachycardia with aberrant conduction
2. What initial intervention is indicated?
   (A) Cardioversion
   (B) Facial ice bag application or other vagal maneuvers
   (C) Propranolol 0.1 mg/kg IV
   (D) Urgent transfer to closest NICU
3. Following initial therapy the rapid heart rate persists without associated cardiovascular symptoms. What is the next treatment step?
   (A) IV adenosine 100 mcg/kg IV.
   (B) Digoxin loading dose followed by IV adenosine.
   (C) Cardioversion.
   (D) Propranolol IV followed by IV adenosine if tachycardia persists after adenosine administration; thus, rhythm strip is obtained.
4. What is the most likely underlying rhythm abnormality?
   (A) Orthodromic reentrant supraventricular tachycardia
   (B) Sinus tachycardia with AV block
   (C) Atrial flutter
   (D) Ventricular tachycardia

Answers: 1B 2B 3A 4C

Except for sinus tachycardia and atrial premature beats, many tachyarrhythmias are potentially symptomatic short-term or progress over time. Sustained ventricular tachyarrhythmias are often a medical emergency. When presenting in the

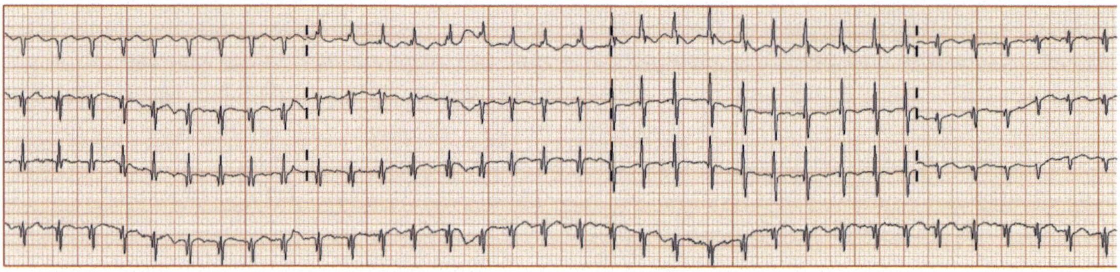

Fig. 14.3 Supraventricular tachycardia with aberrant ventricular conduction

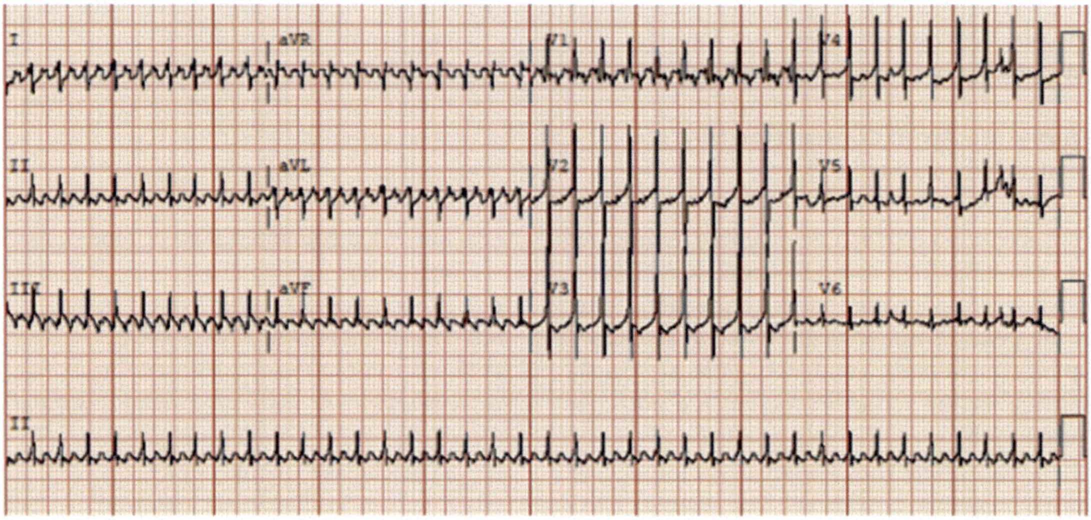

Fig. 14.4 Atrial flutter with AV block

nursery setting, cardiovascular support ranging from physical vagal maneuvers to front-line drug therapy and emergency acute life support intervention should be available.

Sinus Tachycardia

Sinus tachycardia in neonates presents as a regular rhythm with rate ranging from 160 to 230 beats/minute. Sustained heart rates progressively greater than 180 beats/minute increase the likelihood of the existance of an abnormal atrial or AV node-generated ectopic rhythm such as atrial flutter or fibrillation, reentrant supraventricular tachycardia, or an ectopic focus. Unlike most ectopic tachycardias, the EKG will show consistently present and normal P waves. Normal or abnormally oriented P waves may be seen in ectopic atrial tachycardias. Apart from increased sympathetic tone or myocardial dysfunction, sinus tachycardia is often secondary to non-cardiac causes as fever, hypoxemia, hypovolemia, or pain. If non-cardiac factors are resolved and sinus tachycardia is sustained, a 2D echocardiographic examination is indicated to evaluate for myocardial function.

Atrial Flutter/Fibrillation

Unlike older children where atrial flutter and particularly atrial fibrillation is typically associated with structural heart deformities, isolated atrial flutter often occurs in a fetus or newborn with normal heart structure and function. Evidence of persistent fetal atrial tachycardia prior to delivery is indication for high-risk delivery and neonatal ICU support.

In both atrial flutter and re-entry atrial tachycardia, the nursery newborn will typically present with heart rates above 200 beats/minute with atrial flutter rates more likely to approach 300 beats/minute. Higher maximal heart rates greater than 400 beats/minute are constrained by the longer AV node refractory period in neonates. The EKG in atrial flutter, like reentry tachycardia, will typically show narrow QRS complexes with no discernable P waves in the short interval between the rapid ventricular complexes. Sawtooth "flutter" waves are only seen when the ventricular rate slows with vagal maneuvers or drug therapy.

Even if a definitive diagnosis of the specific tachydysrhythmia is not yet established, vagal maneuvers are an appropriate initial response to attempt conversion to sinus rhythm. Since the mechanism of action of a vagal maneuver is to increase parasympathetic tone and incite temporary AV block, these maneuvers are more effective in converting reentrant tachycardias rather than atrial flutter arising from the atrial tissues. The most practical vagal maneuver in neonates is application of an iced cloth to the upper face, gagging maneuvers, or right carotid artery massage. If these efforts fail to convert the tachycardia, then intravenous adenosine should be administered for both diagnostic and possible therapeutic effects. Although adenosine is significantly less effective in converting non-reentrant tachycardias such as atrial flutter, the resultant transient AV block when monitored by rhythm strip will eliminate ventricular depolarization exposing the atrial flutter waves. In reentrant tachycardias no significant atrial depolarizing signal or P waves should be evident.

An initial adenosine dose of 100 mcg/kg should be rapidly infused by bolus intravenously over 1–2 sec increasing every 2 min by 50 mcg/kg until AV block is achieved. Unlike in reentrant tachycardias, further increases are unlikely to result in conversion to sinus rhythm.

If available, ongoing antiarrhythmic therapy and, if unsuccessful, cardioversion or atrial pacing should be managed in an intensive care setting. If ongoing atrial flutter is resulting in impaired perfusion, acidosis, or hemodynamic compromise, then emergency asynchronous cardioversion should be performed in the nursery prior to transfer.

Reentrant Supraventricular Tachycardia

Reentrant SVT is the most common symptomatic arrhythmia seen in neonates with incidence of up to 1:200 live births. Initial presentation after birth is identical to atrial flutter with somewhat lower ventricular rates typically less than 300 beats/minute. First-line management is no different than atrial flutter with use of vagal maneuvers and intravenous adenosine. 2D echocardiogram evaluation is indicated given the possible association with structural heart deformity. Specific defects are, most commonly, Ebstein's anomaly with preexcitation and right-sided accessory pathways in 10% of cases, L = transposition of the great arteries, and atrial septal defects.

The involvement of the AV node in the reentrant circuit increases the dose-dependent effectiveness of intravenous adenosine. As in atrial flutter, an initial IV bolus of 100 mcg/kg of adenosine is administered increasing by 50 mcg/kg sequentially up to 300 mcg/kg until conversion is achieved. At adequate adenosine dosage, up to 90% of reentrant tachycardias involving the SA or AV nodes will convert to sinus rhythm. Following termination of tachycardia, beta-blocker therapy is indicated to prevent recurrence during early infancy. If maximal adenosine dosage does not produce sinus rhythm, then pretreatment with IV beta-blocker can be administered with propranolol 0.1 mg/kg IV at 6-h intervals before repeat adenosine bolus infusion. Continued persistence of tachycardia after blocker treatment and adenosine infusion requires alternative antiarrhythmic drug treatment in an intensive care setting also equipped with atrial pacing and cardioversion capability.

Ventricular Tachyarrhythmia

Tachyarrhythmias of ventricular origin are rare in neonates. Widened QRS complex beats either in isolation or sustained typically represent a supraventricular focus with aberrant conduction though the ventricles. Isolated premature ventricular contractions are rare, asymptomatic, and self-limiting within the first month. In rare cases frequent isolated PVCs increase the risk of sustained tachycardia.

A sustained ventricular tachyarrhythmia in the neonate is a medical emergency capable of inducing progressive impairment in cardiac output and potential cardiac arrest. All tachycardia rhythms with a widened QRS duration greater than 120 ms and typically an abnormal axis should be considered of ventricular origin and trigger emergency management. In rare cases ventricular tachycardia displays a narrow but abnormal QRS configuration. Widened QRS complexes of rapidly varying morphology are seen in "torsade de pointes," with an underlying QT interval prolongation and imminent deterioration to ventricular fibrillation.

Fortunately the majority of wide complex tachycardias are of atrial origin with associated aberrant ventricular conduction due to relative refractory AV node and bundle branch conduction. Although normal perfusion suggests supraventricular origin, it does not eliminate the possibility of a ventricular focus. Adenosine administration is useful in differentiating SVT with aberrant conduction from ventricular tachycardia. Since the AV node does not participate in the ventricular tachycardia pathway, no rate response is seen upon adenosine infusion. A blockade of ventricular conduction with adenosine indicates a supraventricular origin.

Sustained ventricular tachycardia with hemodynamic compromise requires immediate intervention with synchronized cardioversion at 0.5 joules/kg increasing if ineffective to 2 joules/kg. If sinus rhythm is not achieved, then asynchronous cardioversion should be performed. 2D echocardiography is indicated to evaluate cardiac structure and assess for persistent myocardial dysfunction. Lidocaine or procainamide can be used under cardiologist supervision to prevent recurrence of ventricular tachycardia.

Case Presentation

A healthy-appearing full-term female newborn is noted to have a slow pulse on examination with HR 70–80/min; physical examination is normal with good perfusion and no respiratory distress, full oxygen saturation on RA. The parents state that an older sister recently died suddenly at 8 years of age while swimming (Fig. 14.5).

1. Initial management should include:
   (A) Transfer to NICU for electrophysiology consultation
   (B) CBC, electrolytes including NA K Ca Mg
   (C) Head CT scan
   (D) Holter monitoring

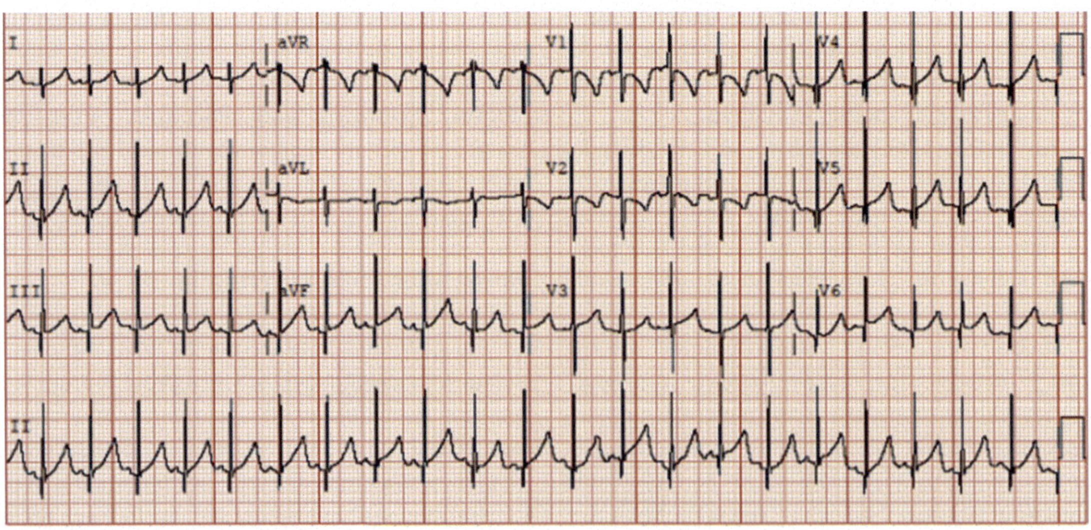

Fig. 14.5 QT interval prolongation

2. Which of the following drugs are contraindicated for future use?
   (A) Digoxin
   (B) Erythromycin
   (C) Gentamicin
   (D) ASA

3. What management is now indicated?
   (A) Start beta-blocker therapy and refer for cardiology evaluation.
   (B) Cardiac monitoring in NICU until discharge home.
   (C) Transfer for immediate cardiology evaluation prior to discharge home.
   (D) Start oral amiodarone and refer for cardiology evaluation.

Answers: 1B 2B 3A

QT Interval Prolongation

Abnormal ionic transport across the cardiomyocyte membrane may manifest as an electrocardiographic prolongation of the QT interval. A high risk of life-threatening tachyarrhytthmia exists in neonates when AV block and extreme QT prolongation is evident.

Every EKG obtained in the nursery whether performed due to the existence of arrhythmia, congenital heart defect, or family history of sudden death should be evaluated for QT interval prolongation. Given the frequent inheritance of QT interval abnormality, a family history of every neonate with arrhythmia should include assessment of familial sudden death and QT interval prolongation.

Most neonates with abnormal QT intervals will be asymptomatic at birth. An underlying QT interval prolongation is more likely in the presence of sustained bradycardia or ventricular ectopy.

The QT interval is measured as the time duration from the onset of the QRS complex to the intersection of the T wave downslope with the EKG baseline. A trailing U wave is excluded from the measurement unless its magnitude is equally prominent as the T wave peak. A corrected QT interval is standardized for heart rate with division by the square root of the R-R interval.

Symptomatic arrhythmias are significantly more likely if the corrected QT interval exceeds 0.60 milliseconds or in the presence of 2:1 AV block, T wave alternans, or sustained bradycardia. Higher risk is seen with coexistent sensory neural hearing loss. In these high-risk cases, propranolol should be started at dosage of 1 mg/kg orally every 8 h. Additional antiarrhythmic medications may be needed if sinus rhythm is not achieved.

QT intervals greater than 0.50 milliseconds or coexistent arrhythmia require beta-blocker therapy. More precise individualized drug therapy may be later substituted under pediatric cardiology supervision with genetic subtyping of the underlying channelopathy. Temporary self-resolving QT prolongation can be seen in the first week of life with initial corrected QT duration greater than 0.44 milliseconds. Electrolyte abnormalities such as hypocalcemia and hypokalemia, macrolide antibiotics, and CNS abnormalities can produce "acquired" QT prolongation. An initial corrected QT interval between 0.44 and 0.50 milliseconds should be re-evaluated by follow-up EKGs in the first week of life before drug therapy is considered.

Case Presentation

A full-term clinically well appearing male infant is noted to have a heart murmur on arrival to the nursery. Prenatally an intermittent tachycardia was suspected with no specific documented arrhythmia. The initial vital signs show a regular heart rate of 120/min, respiratory rate 32/min with right arm blood pressure of 80/60, and pulse oximetry 94% on RA (Fig. 14.6).

1. What is the first initial management indicated?
   (A) Transfer to ICU for murmur evaluation
   (B) Physical examination including four-extremity pulses and blood pressure and pre- and postductal pulse oximetry

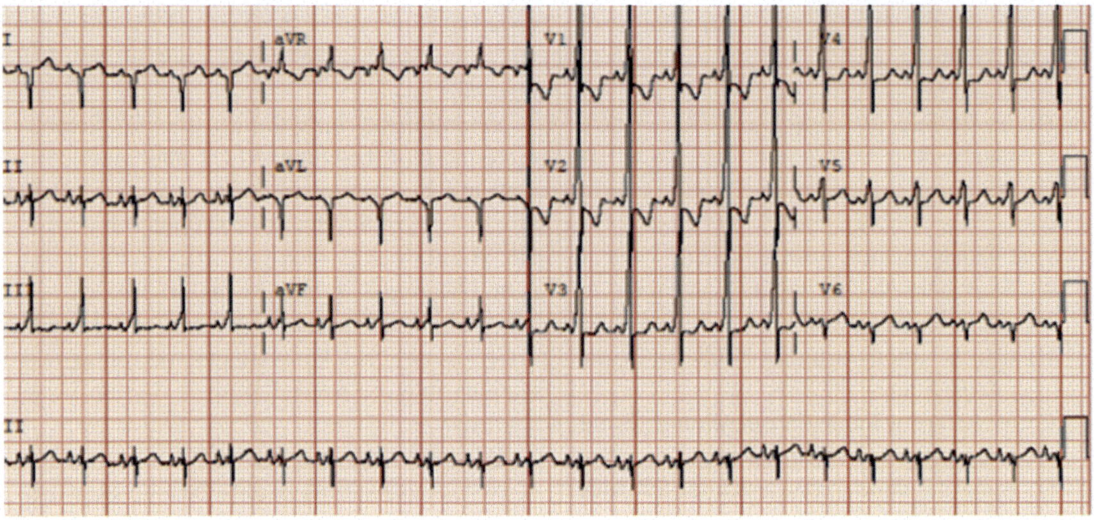

Fig. 14.6 Ventricular preexcitation

(C) EKG and rhythm strip
(D) 2D echocardiogram

The EKG displayed the rhythm as seen, and 2D echocardiogram shows moderate right heart enlargement with a redundant tricuspid valve and moderate tricuspid valve insufficiency.

2. What structural heart abnormality is suspected?
   (A) Ebstein's anomaly
   (B) Congenitally corrected L-transposition of the great arteries
   (C) Pulmonary hypertension
   (D) ASD

3. What cardiac arrhythmia should be anticipated?
   (A) Ventricular tachycardia
   (B) Supraventricular tachycardia
   (C) Premature atrial contractions
   (D) Complete heart block

Answers: 1B 2A 3B

Neonatal Arrhythmia in Congenital Heart Disease

Infants with structural heart defects are more likely to exhibit coexistent cardiac arrhythmias triggered by an abnormal conduction system, altered hemodynamics, or hypoxic stress. Most significant newborn congenital heart disease will present with abnormal physical findings such as heart murmur, abnormal respiration, impaired perfusion, or desaturation. Some asymptomatic neonates with underlying heart defects may initially present with a wide spectrum of arrhythmias. A 2D echo should be obtained in the nursery on recognition of sustained cardiac arrhythmia. Mandatory performance of echocardiography is not required for asymptomatic transient sinus bradycardia or isolated premature atrial beats which are rarely associated with anatomic abnormality.

Most urgent is the recognition of heart defects that will imminently manifest with critical or life-threatening symptoms. Complex heterotaxy is often associated with fragile malpositioned ventricular conduction pathways resulting in impaired AV conduction or heart block. Associated pulmonary outflow obstruction or left-sided obstructive defects in these cases may result in ductal dependency and need to initiate PGE infusion. L-transposition of the great vessels in particular is associated with conduction pathway defects distal to the HIS bundle.

Of particular significance is the frequent association of Ebstein's anomaly with Wolff-Parkinson-White syndrome due to the presence of right-sided accessory AV pathways. Infrequently SVT and atrial ectopy will also be seen in isolated atrial septal defects.

In rare cases focal cardiac tumors may provide the nidus for ventricular automaticity causing frequent or incessant ventricular tachycardia.

Neonatal Arrhythmia and Systemic Disease

Hypoxemia resulting from systemic illness such as sepsis, respiratory failure, and central neurologic abnormalities may induce automaticity of cardiomyocytes with resultant ectopy. In these situations myocardial dysfunction can contribute to altered hemodynamics causing increased cardiac muscle strain and ectopy. Severe congenital hypertrophic cardiomyopathy can lead to inadequate perfusion and oxygen delivery to heart tissues also inducing myocyte irritability. Autoimmune illness such as system lupus erythematosus (SLE) and Sjogren's syndrome can be manifested through production of maternal antibodies, destruction of AV node tissue, and resultant heart block in the fetus and newborn.

Clinical Pearls

1. Neonatal QT interval prolongation may present as profound sinus bradycardia or AV block.
2. Impaired AV node conduction and resultant heart block is a presenting feature of complex congenital heart disease.
3. Bradycardia in the presence of PACs is typically indicative of nonconduction of ectopic atrial beats rather than primary AV node dysfunction.
4. The underlying ectopic basis of sustained tachycardia rhythm is often unmasked upon adenosine-induced AV node blockade.
5. If hemodynamic stability is maintained, sustained wide complex tachycardia is typically of supraventricular rather than ventricular origin.

Suggested References

2015 American Heart Association Guidelines Update for Cardiopulmonary Resuscitation and Emergency Cardiovascular Care. Part 11: Pediatric Basic Life Support and Cardiopulmonary Resuscitation Quality; Part 12: Pediatric Advanced Support; Part 13: Neonatal Resuscitation.

Artman M, Mahony L. Neonatal cardiology. 3rd ed. Philadelphia: Elsevier; 2017.

Galli MA, Danzi GB. A guide to neonatal and pediatric EKGs. New York: Springer; 2013.

Garson AT. Science and practice of pediatric cardiology. 3rd ed. Baltimore: Williams and Wilkins; 2005.

Goldberg I, Moss AJ. Long Qt syndrome. J Am Coll Cardiol. 31(2):229–33.

Kothari DS, Skinner JR. Neonatal tachycardias, an update. Arch Dis Child Fetal Neonatal Ed. 2006;91(2):F138–44.

Park MK. Pediatric cardiology handbook. 4th ed. Philadelphia: Mosby/Elsevier; 2010.

Polin RA, Abman SH, Rowitch D, Benitz W. Fetal and neonatal physiology. 5th ed. Philadelphia: Saunders; 2016.

St. George Hyslop C, Morton C, Daley E. Neonatal and pediatric guidelines for arrhythmia management, what every neonatal and pediatric critical care nurse needs to know. Canada: Pedaitric Cardiology Intensive Care Society; 2014.

Gastrointestinal Problems in the Newborn Nursery

15

Gregory C. Martin

Introduction

Gastrointestinal problems are one of the most common problems in newborn medicine and in the newborn nursery and are the source of numerous phone calls to clinicians daily. These problems can represent an acute emergency or by contrast a nonissue. With the first call received, it may be very difficult to make this distinction.

The challenge is to anticipate what the most common issues are and how to triage the issues appropriately. This is further complicated by the average length of stay in a newborn nursery which is a day and half [1]. Many of the early symptoms that newborns will suffer are similar for both urgent and nonurgent problems. For example, feeding difficulty can be related to poor breastfeeding or intestinal obstruction. In this chapter we will focus on two particular gastrointestinal symptoms, emesis and abdominal distension.

G. C. Martin, MD (✉)
Banner University Medical Center Phoenix, Phoenix, AZ, USA

Department of Child Health, University of Arizona College of Medicine Phoenix, Phoenix, AZ, USA
e-mail: Gregory_Martin@Mednax.com; Gregory.Martin@Bannerhealth.com

Case Presentation

It is Friday morning, and you are examining a new admission from the previous night in the newborn nursery. The patient is a term infant born to a mother who is 27 years old, G1P0, and the pregnancy was uncomplicated other than some reports of mild polyhydramnios. The mother had limited prenatal care, and the child was born via a normal spontaneous vaginal delivery. The child looked well and was sent to the newborn nursery.

The child was doing well in couplet care, but at 5 h of age, the child was noted to have oral secretions and emesis. Additionally, during feeds it is reported that the child appeared to choke and cough.

At this time you:

1. Order a chest x-ray.
2. Order an abdominal x-ray.
3. Order a CBC.
4. Watch the baby feed.

The first step for this child is to observe the child feeding. It is important to discern if the child is having difficulty feeding because of a respiratory issue or a gastrointestinal system issue.

Answer: 4

G. I. Martin, W. Rosenfeld (eds.), *Common Problems in the Newborn Nursery*,
https://doi.org/10.1007/978-3-319-95672-5_15

During your observation of the feeding, the baby started to have non-bloody emesis with choking and cyanosis.

Your differential diagnosis should include the following:

1. Tracheoesophageal fistula with esophageal atresia
2. Duodenal atresia
3. Swallowed maternal blood
4. Neonatal abstinence syndrome
5. Delayed transition
6. Normal/gastroesophageal reflux disease

The next step of the evaluation is directly linked to your differential diagnosis. In this patient with a history of polyhydramnios and feeding difficulties, esophageal atresia needs to be excluded. While all the other diagnoses could be considered, ruling out (or in) esophageal atresia is an appropriate first step. In the first day of life infants breastfeeding minimal amounts may not show immediate symptoms, while others can be profoundly affected if they are unable to handle their own secretions.

Your next step for this patient is?

1. Chest x-ray
2. Chest x-ray, abdominal x-ray
3. Pass an orogastric tube with follow-up chest and abdominal x-ray
4. Upper gastrointestinal study

In this particular patient, symptoms of esophageal atresia are presenting early, and the quickest way to evaluate if there is atresia is to pass an orogastric tube with follow-up chest and abdominal x-ray [2]. The results of the OG tube placement and abdominal x-ray will determine the next steps of treatment. Whether or not the orogastric tube is passed easily and in the stomach will lead to different pathways on the evaluation.

Answer: 3

The orogastric tube is not placed easily:

If the OG tube is not placed easily and is seen to curl or not pass into the stomach on the x-ray, then we know the patient has an esophageal atresia. A typical x-ray for this patient is shown below (Fig. 15.1):

The types of esophageal anatomy and atresia are listed below.

1. Type A: Esophageal atresia with no tracheoesophageal fistula
2. Type B: Esophageal atresia with proximal tracheoesophageal fistula
3. Type C: Esophageal atresia with distal tracheoesophageal fistula

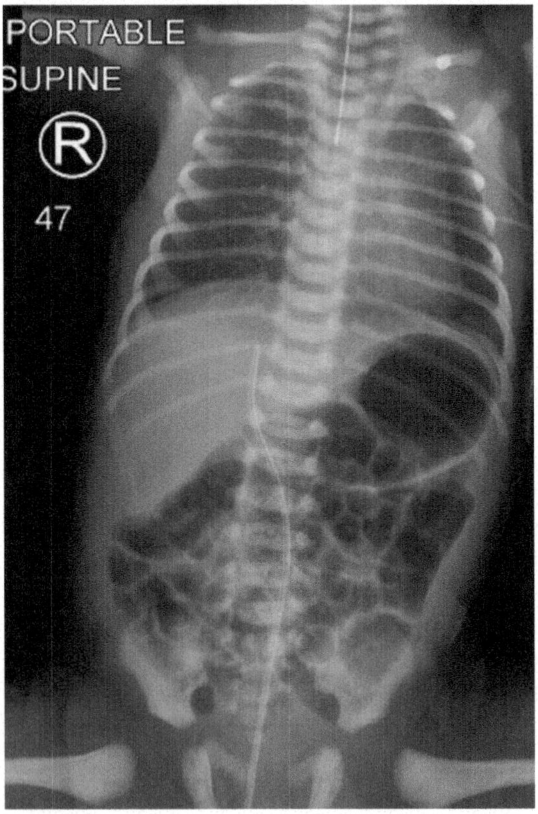

Fig. 15.1 Chest and abdominal film demonstrating esophageal atresia
This x-ray demonstrates a well-aerated lung, gas-filled small and large intestine, and an orogastric tube that stops at the level of T-4. In some cases the tube may seem to pass the appropriate distance needed to reach the stomach but is curled in the esophageal pouch. Confirmation of the tube position with x-ray prevents reaching an inaccurate conclusion. This x-ray also demonstrates an air-filled blind esophageal pouch.

4. Type D: Esophageal atresia with proximal and distal tracheoesophageal fistula
5. Type E: Tracheal esophageal fistula with no esophageal atresia

In Type A (8% of TE fistulas) there is complete esophageal atresia without any connection to the intestine [3]. The result is a complete absence of air in the intestine. In Type B (1%) there is no connection of the trachea to the stomach, but in this defect, there is a proximal connection to the esophagus. However, because there is no distal connection, the intestines would be airless. In Type C (84%) and by far the most common presentation of tracheo-esophageal fistulas, there are a blind esophageal pouch and a distal connection from the trachea to the GI tract. This results in air-filled intestines and highlights the need for the need to pass an OG tube and x-ray to confirm diagnosis. Without the OG tube in the x-ray, the x-ray may be misinterpreted as normal. In Type D (3%), there is an esophageal-tracheal fistula with a blind pouch and a distal connection. This type like Type C results in air-filled intestines. In Type E (4%), there is an H-type connection of the esophagus to the trachea, and without a blind pouch, air is present in the intestine. This type of connection can be difficult to identify and lead to complications if not identified.

An important clinical intervention to order in this situation is?

1. Sepsis work-up.
2. STAT glucose measurement.
3. IV bolus of normal saline.
4. Place a double-lumen nasogastric suction tube.

The most immediate threat to this baby's condition is the possible aspiration of oropharyngeal secretions that may obstruct the child's airway and interfere with normal respiration. The placement of a double-lumen decompression tube rather than a single-lumen orogastric tube is important. In contrast to a single-lumen tube, when the double-lumen tube is connected to suction, blockage of the tube will not occur. Adequate management of secretions will allow the clinician time to arrange and plan care without the child having a secondary respiratory decompensation.

Answer: 4

What is the next step of the evaluation?

1. Neonatology consultation
2. Surgical consultation
3. Radiographic survey that includes vertebrae and limbs.
4. Renal ultrasound
5. Cardiac echocardiogram
6. Transfer to level III NICU
7. All of the above

In this patient you would want to start the process for all of the above. Depending upon the service level of your facility, the first steps may be to arrange a neonatology consultation and transport to a level III NICU, or if your facility has a level III NICU, the general pediatrician may simply consult the neonatologist. This patient also requires a significant evaluation for all of the VACTERL associations. The first step is a complete physical exam.

Answer: 7

What percentage of patients with esophageal atresia/tracheoesophageal fistula have an associated anomaly?

1. 25%
2. 50%
3. 60%
4. 75%

Approximately 50% of patients with esophageal atresia/tracheoesophageal *fistulas have one or more associated anomalies* [2, 4].

Answer: 2

What percentage of patients with esophageal atresia/tracheoesophageal fistula have VACTERL?

1. 10–25%
2. 26–50%
3. 51–75%

The occurrence of VACTERL (3 or more associated anomalies) in this group is far less and has been reported in 10–25% [4]. Although many children have an isolated atresia/TE fistula, investigation of associated anomalies and life-threatening conditions is imperative. A recent study [4] found 54% of patients had a recognizable genetic or malformation sequence. Given that prevalence of additional anomalies is so high, a systematic approach to the evaluation is required.

Answer: 1

The diagnostic process starts with a detailed physical exam looking for visual or auditory anomalies that are detectable. Historically imperforate anus was an anomaly that easily detected by the nurse when the first temperature was routinely taken rectally. Today the diagnosis may be missed because of the move away from rectal temperatures and the frequency of fistulas that may allow the passage of stool. This combination of factors may make the diagnosis less apparent. Therefore there is no substitution for a thorough physical exam when looking for this diagnosis. If the patient has an imperforate anus or other anorectal malformations, the initial treatment is holding feeds, gastric decompression, and surgical consultation [5]. Unfortunately, if the patient has an esophageal atresia, gastric decompression is not initially possible prior to surgical intervention.

The next steps in the process is the review all of the imaging studies that have been ordered. The spine and limb studies need to be reviewed looking for anomalies that may include vertebral or radial defects. The renal ultrasound needs to be evaluated for renal abnormalities, and the cardiac echocardiogram has to be reviewed for structural cardiac pathology. Some of the anomalies (i.e., cardiac defects) may require immediate attention, while others (i.e., bony anomalies) may become relevant in the future.

In patients with VACTERL association, 69% will have some form of renal anomaly [6]. The most common manifestation is vesicoureteral reflux, reflux with a structural defect, followed by unilateral renal agenesis, then dysplastic or multicystic kidney disease. Given the high prevalence of renal anomalies, these patients may require additional imaging and ongoing support from both nephrology and urology services. Renal disease may have a significant impact on neonates undergoing both pediatric and cardiac surgery in the immediate neonatal period.

Cardiac anomalies are also prevalent in patients with VACTERL association. The reported rates vary from 40% to 80% and the anomalies can be subtle or complex [7]. The most common cardiac defect to present is a ventricular septal defect (VSD). This defect is fairly common and in the majority of cases does not need to be addressed in the immediate neonatal period. Many VSD's often close spontaneously. However, if the VSD is large during the child's initial stay, it may be the source of developing congestive heart failure. In addition to VSD, other congenital heart diseases that have been described in patients with VACTERL association include Tetralogy of Fallot (TOF), Hypoplastic left heart syndrome (HLHS), atrial septal defects, and transposition of the great vessels (TGV). HLHS and TGV require immediate attention and intervention. TOF may or may not have the need for immediate intervention depending on the degree of pulmonic stenosis involved. Some patients are "Pink TETS" because they are not cyanotic, while others are "Blue TETS" because of cyanosis. If congenital heart disease is involved, obviously there will be significant implications and timing for all of the needed interventions [7].

The bony abnormalities found on x-rays generally do not require any intervention in the neonatal period. It is important to look for vertebral, rib, radial, and limb anomalies [7]. These anomalies may require additional support in the future and may present challenges. In the neonatal period, these anomalies may lend support to the diagnosis of the VACTRL association.

Once this initial evaluation is complete, the surgical plan can then take place. The comorbid conditions will be taken into account when planning the surgical repair. If the patient has complex cyanotic heart disease, that surgical repair may take priority. The pediatric surgeon during the operative procedure will attempt to identify a tracheoesophageal fistula and repair.

Case Presentation

Same presentation but the OG tube is passed easily and is in the stomach:

If the OG tube is passed easily and reaches the stomach (Fig. 15.2), a completely different diagnostic path should be followed.

This result does not completely rule out a tracheoesophageal fistula, but it does eliminate the possibility of esophageal atresia. As mentioned previously the H-type fistula is still a possibility but is a rare condition. Therefore, we must turn our focus to much more common problems and in general problems that are easier to address.

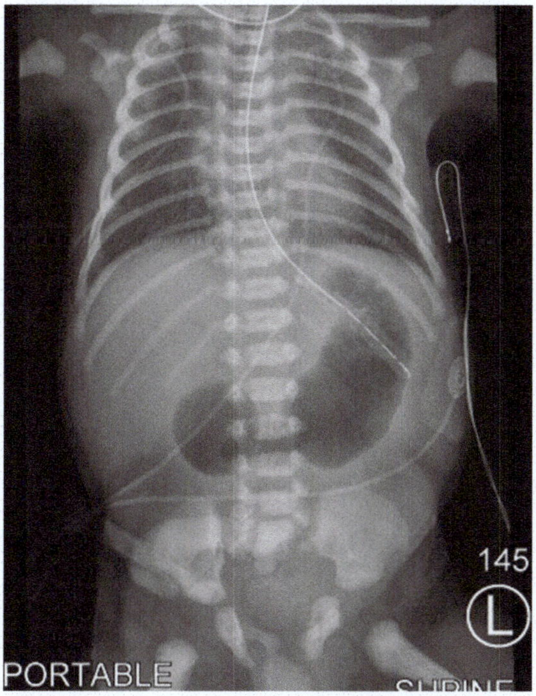

Fig. 15.2 Chest and abdominal film demonstrating a double bubble, a patient with duodenal atresia

Your differential diagnosis now includes the following:

1. Swallowed maternal blood
2. Transient tachypnea of the newborn
3. Neonatal abstinence syndrome
4. Duodenal atresia
5. Normal/gastroesophageal reflux disease

The review of the chest and abdominal x-ray with tube in the stomach will then direct the next steps of the evaluation process. When considering the results of the study, it is important to place them within the context of the differential diagnosis.

Swallowed maternal blood at times becomes a diagnosis of exclusion. Presuming all of your studies are negative and upon OG tube placement some blood is noted in the drainage, it could be enough to make the diagnosis. The maternal blood can be an irritant and lavage may help alleviate some of the symptoms. It is also important to note that bloody stool is also common in these patients. This is a common and simple explanation to poor feeding and emesis.

If the chest x-ray demonstrates retained fetal lung fluid and the patient is tachypneic, this could be the source of the feeding difficulty and emesis. The tachypnea could be the cause of the source of all of the problems. The physical exam should demonstrate a patient with some respiratory distress and a benign abdomen. This patient should be able to gavage feed or receive intravenous fluids pending resolution of respiratory symptoms.

Neonatal reflux can occur in patients in the NICU and couplet care area. Reflux can be either benign or the cause of symptoms. Within the pediatric community, there is significant disagreement on the approach to treatment or even the need for treatment [8]. Prematurity or milk protein allergy can cause more profound reflux. Milk protein allergy does not usually present in the initial nursery stay. Obviously this will not typically present when the mother is exclusively breastfeeding but reports exist of mother's intake of cow milk protein leading to symptoms. In fact it has been demonstrated that exclusively breastfed infants can have IgA antibodies to milk proteins measured in sera [9]. In these cases, if the mother eliminates the protein, then there should be improvement in symptoms. It is also important to note that bloody stool may be seen in these patients, but the abdominal exam is not consistent with a surgical abdomen. The treatment of reflux with antacids in the immediate neonatal period is unnecessary and leads to complications including necrotizing enterocolitis and a change in the typical colonization pattern of the intestine. Given the lack of benefit of antacids and risks of major complications, the routine use in the neonatal period is contraindicated [10]. Mild reflux in the neonatal period is normal.

Neonatal abstinence syndrome (NAS) is an ever-increasing problem within our society. In the United States today, the numbers of mothers being prescribed narcotics are also increasing. The result is that there are large numbers of infants presenting with signs and symptoms of the NAS syndrome. These patients commonly present with irritability, hypertonia, difficulty with feeding, and diarrhea. The timing of presentation is linked to the type of opiates mom was using and the time of last consumption. The exam and history of these patients generally make it easier to document the NAS syndrome as the cause of the child's symptoms.

Duodenal atresia may also present in the couplet care area. In this condition the chest and abdominal film will show the "double bubble" sign which demonstrates the duodenal obstruction. Once this diagnosis is made and surgery is consulted, it is also important to check the patient for signs of trisomy 21 as this occurs in 25–40% of patients with duodenal atresia [11]. If the patient has signs or symptoms of trisomy 21, then it is important to include an echocardiogram looking for congenital heart disease. If the patient has complex congenital heart disease, this may impact surgical planning. The treatment of this patient includes surgery, ICU care, and pain management. Once the repair is complete and bowel function returns, the child should have a complete recovery.

Case Presentation

The patient is a term male born to a mother who is G3P3 of Caucasian ancestry with a history of obesity, diet controlled diabetes mellitus, and hypertension. The mother's medical problems were under control prior to pregnancy, but with the pregnancy, the mother required additional treatment with medications for her hypertension and diabetes. All of mom's maternal laboratory tests were negative and her labor was unremarkable. The infant was delivered via vaginal delivery with Apgar scores of 9 and 9. The infant started to breastfeed during the "golden hour" and was found to have abdominal distension with reported "yellow, green emesis."

What is your differential diagnosis?

1. Duodenal atresia
2. Malrotation/volvulus
3. Ileal atresia/jejunal atresia
4. Hirschsprung's disease
5. Colonic atresia/small left colon syndrome

Answer: All of the answers above are to be considered in this patient.

What is the next step for this patient?

1. Place an IV and give glucose.
2. Chest x-ray and abdominal x-ray.
3. Transfer to NICU.
4. CBC, blood culture, and antibiotics.

Answer: 2

A chest x-ray and abdominal x-ray are ordered, and the following picture is seen (Fig. 15.3):

What findings do you note on this x-ray?

1. Paucity of gas
2. Double bubble
3. Bowel obstruction
4. Normal

Answers: 1 and 3

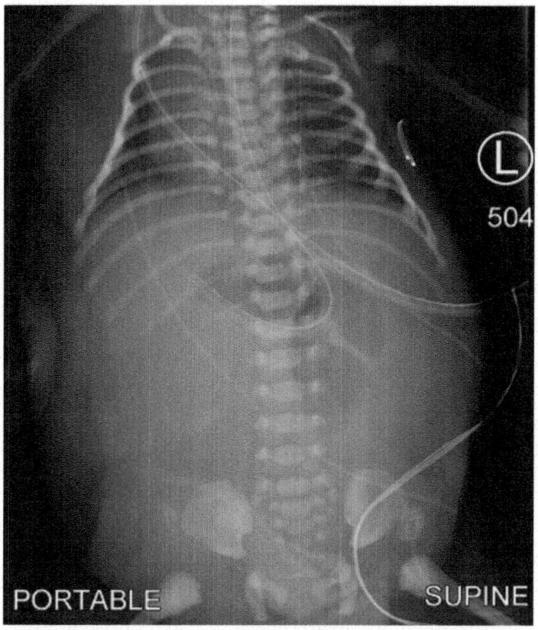

Fig. 15.3 A chest and abdominal x-ray demonstrating bowel obstruction

Diagnoses that might be considered include:

1. Meconium ileus
2. Meconium plugs
3. Hirschsprung's disease
4. Jejunal or ileal atresia
5. Colonic atresia (small left colon syndrome)
6. Malrotation
7. Volvulus
8. Ileus secondary to infection

The differential diagnosis for this condition is taken within the context of this patient's x-ray demonstrating obstruction. Is the obstruction mechanical versus functional? If the obstruction is mechanical, is there a congenital versus acquired cause? There is significance to this patient's history of diabetes. The context is important because a decision needs to be made to determine the most likely location of the obstruction. Is this an upper GI obstruction or a lower track obstruction? The differential needs to reflect the situation.

At this time, the differential is long and does involve many surgical conditions, some of which may be an emergency. The following steps are generally recommended. Given that infection is on the list in the form of an ileus, a sepsis evaluation is generally warranted if the patient has risk factors for infection. In this particular patient, we do not have evidence of infection from history or on physical exam. Once infection is considered, the placement of a double-lumen orogastric tube to suction and the consultation of a surgeon and neonatology are always a good option. The next steps of the evaluation involve contrast studies. If the lower GI tract is of greater suspicion, then a lower GI can be performed first. However, you must be certain that the vomiting is not grossly bilious because malrotation and volvulus are emergencies. Time is critical in this scenario, and if there is a delay in surgical intervention, bowel may be lost.

What are the next steps for this patient?

1. Upper GI
2. Barium/contrast enema
3. Rectal suction biopsy
4. Surgery consult

Answer: 1

The decisions on the next steps for this patient are based upon history and index of suspicion for the location of the obstruction. If the provider does an upper bowel contrast study first, this will prevent doing a lower bowel contrast study until the contrast is cleared. However, if the provider does a lower contrast enema first, there is the possibility of delay of diagnosis of a malrotation and volvulus. If the patient is developing an acidosis and has a grossly bilious emesis, I would suggest starting with an upper bowel contrast study because missing a malrotation can have dire consequences.

The upper bowel contrast study and abdominal x-ray help differentiate duodenal atresia, malrotation, volvulus, and other small intestine atresias. Patients with atresias may have had vascular accidents in utero, exposure to vasoconstrictor medicines and or illicit drugs such as cocaine, or perhaps a significant history of maternal hypertension [12]. The lower contrast studies help identify meconium ileus, meconium plugs, colonic atresia, small left colon syndrome, or Hirschsprung's disease by identifying a transition zone. The maternal history of diabetes in this patient places this child at greater risk for small left colon syndrome [13].

The treatment for these bowel obstruction issues involves surgery for most of these conditions. However, the therapeutic intervention for meconium ileus and meconium plugs is the contrast study itself. The contrast helps clear the meconium plugs making them easier to pass. Cystic fibrosis is associated with patients that have meconium plugs or meconium ileus as well. Cystic fibrosis will dehydrate the meconium in utero, and this may lead to volvulus and intestinal perforation [14]. If a perforation were to occur, this may be identified on plain film by the presence of abdominal calcifications, and that would be the main diagnostic test. Taken as a group, some refer to these syndromes as distal intestinal obstruction syndrome. This syndrome places patients at risk for greater complications and hospitalizations later in life if the patient has cystic fibrosis as well [15].

The treatment for atresia is surgery and ICU care. The acute management prior to surgery is gastric decompression, antibiotics if needed for perforation, and ultimately surgery when the patient is adequately prepared. Preparation involves treatment for any metabolic acidosis and volume resuscitation if needed. If the patient has duodenal atresia, the diagnosis of trisomy 21 needs to be considered, and an echocardiogram would be needed prior to surgery as complex congenital heart disease occurs in a greater percentage of trisomy 21 patients than the background population. Ultimately post repair the care involves recovering from anesthesia, pain control, waiting for bowel function, the reintroduction of feeding, the prevention of nosocomial infection, and coordination of initial follow-up care for the recovery.

If the patient is found to have Hirschsprung's disease, a key notable finding, in addition to distension, is the failure to pass stool within the first 48 h of life [16]. On lower contrast studies, a transition zone would be seen, and this would indicate the need for a rectal suction biopsy. Surgery would perform the rectal suction biopsy, and pediatric pathology would look for the absence of ganglion cells confirming the diagnosis. If this diagnosis is suspected, access to pediatric pathology is needed for the diagnosis and treatment of this condition. Pediatric surgery then resects the aganglionic zones. The zones can be of different sizes and in rare circumstances involve the entire colon. Post repair in the NICU the focus is again recovery from anesthesia, pain control, nutritional support pending bowel function, prevention of nosocomial infection, and coordination of initial follow-up care. If the patient has the ability to stool using enemas, there is the possibility to continue to keep the child decompressed using enemas and delay repair until a later date. The benefit would be delaying anesthesia and surgery within the immediate neonatal period. However, the main risk is the possibility of developing toxic megacolon. The key to determining which pathway to take is based upon the severity of the presentation and the reliability of the family.

Conclusion

Gastrointestinal conditions are common in the nursery. Many of these conditions are benign and transient in nature; however, the potential for severe complications is high. The newborn in the couplet care area is under observation for a brief period of time and the risks are high. Like most areas of medicine, history is the key giving clues where to look for problems or congenital conditions. Resources are needed to care for these neonates if problems are suspected. These resources are not universally available and transfer to a higher level of care may be required. The care of neonates with surgical conditions requires intensive care, pediatric radiology, pediatric surgery, and pathology support. If you suspect these resources may be needed, it is always prudent to move a patient sooner than later. Hypertension, diabetes, and drug use can lead to many complications involving the intestines. Major problems involving the gastrointestinal tract present with the most common of symptoms of emesis and distension; the key for the pediatrician is to not be "lulled to sleep" and discern a common problem from a catastrophic one.

Clinical Pearls

1. Gastrointestinal problems can be benign or a major emergency.
2. Bilious emesis is an emergency until proven otherwise.
3. Many gastrointestinal problems are accompanied by other congenital anomalies.
4. Hypertension, diabetes, and illicit stimulant use can lead to intestinal complications.
5. The care of neonatal surgical patients requires resources; a transport to a higher level of care may be needed.

References

1. Farhat R, Rajab M. Length of postnatal hospital stay in healthy newborns and re-hospitalization following early discharge. N Am J Med Sci. 2011:146–51. https://doi.org/10.4297/najms.2011.3146.
2. Taeusch HW, et al. Structural anomalies of the gastrointestinal tract. In: *Avery's diseases of the newborn*. Philadelphia: Elsevier Saunders; 2005.
3. Clark DC. Esophageal atresia and tracheoesophageal fistula. Am Fam Physician. 1999:910, 919–6, 920.
4. Stoll C, et al. Associated anomalies in cases with esophageal atresia. Am J Med Genet A. 2017;173(8):2139–57. https://doi.org/10.1002/ajmg.a.38303.
5. Levitt MA, Pena A. Anorectal malformations. In: *Fundamentals of pediatric surgery*. New York: Springer; 2010. p. 499–512. https://doi.org/10.1007/978-1-4419-6643-8_64.
6. Cunningham BK, et al. Analysis of renal anomalies in VACTERL association. Birth Defects Res A Clin Mol Teratol. 2014;100(10):801–5. https://doi.org/10.1002/bdra.23302.
7. Solomon BD, et al. An approach to the identification of anomalies and etiologies in neonates with identified or suspected VACTERL (Vertebral Defects, Anal Atresia, Tracheo-Esophageal Fistula with Esophageal Atresia, Cardiac Anomalies, Renal Anomalies, and Limb Anomalies) association. J Pediatr. 2014;164(3). https://doi.org/10.1016/j.jpeds.2013.10.086.
8. Golski CA, et al. Pediatric Specialists' beliefs about gastroesophageal reflux disease in premature infants. Pediatrics. 2009;125(1):96–104. https://doi.org/10.1542/peds.2008-3841.
9. Järvinen KM, et al. Role of maternal elimination diets and human milk IgA in the development of cow's milk allergy in the infants. Clin Exp Allergy. 2014;44(1):69–78. https://doi.org/10.1111/cea.12228.
10. Terrin G, et al. Ranitidine is associated with infections, necrotizing enterocolitis, and fatal outcome in newborns. Pediatrics. 2011;129(1) https://doi.org/10.1542/peds.2011-0796.
11. Pediatric Duodenal Atresia. Background, history of the procedure, problem, 24 August 2016, emedicine.medscape.com/article/932917-overview
12. Dalla Vecchia LK, et al. Intestinal atresia and stenosis: a 25-year experience with 277 patients. Arch Surg. 1998;133(490):490–6.
13. Ellis H, et al. Neonatal small left colon syndrome in the offspring of diabetic Mothers-an analysis of 105 children. J Pediatr Surg. 2009;44(12):2343–6. https://doi.org/10.1016/j.jpedsurg.2009.07.054.
14. Chouikh T, et al. Prenatal intestinal volvulus: look for cystic fibrosis. Br Med J. 2016; https://doi.org/10.1136/bcr-2016-217003.
15. Lavie M. Long-term follow-up of distal intestinal obstruction syndrome in cystic fibrosis. World J Gastroenterol. 2015;21(1):318. https://doi.org/10.3748/wjg.v21.i1.318.
16. Bradnock TJ, et al. Hirschsprung's disease in the UK and Ireland: incidence and anomalies. Arch Dis Child. 2017;102(8):722–7. https://doi.org/10.1136/archdischild-2016-311872.

16 Hypotonia in the Newborn

Ranjith Kamity

Introduction

A newborn presenting with abnormal muscle tone is often a diagnostic and therapeutic challenge to those caring for newborn babies in the general nursery. Hypotonia in a newborn infant can be best defined as the decrease in resistance to passive motion, ideally in an awake infant, as opposed to weakness, which is merely the decrease in active strength [1–3]. While recognizing hypotonia is fairly obvious, the underlying etiology is often not, since neurological dysfunction at various levels can cause hypotonia. Hypotonia without weakness is highly suspicious for central nervous system causes (brain and brain stem/upper motor neuron), while hypotonic infants with weakness tend to have a systemic etiology or a defect in the peripheral nervous system (spinal cord, anterior horn cells, lower motor neurons, neuromuscular junction, peripheral nerves, and muscles) [4]. Higher brain functions are not affected in disorders affecting the peripheral nervous system. In many cases, hypotonia in the newborn might be the initial presentation of a more serious underlying condition, which, if unrecognized, might lead to persistent long-term complications, including seizures, developmental delays, and/or death.

The clinical management of these infants varies from observation to immediate interventions based on the diagnoses identified. The nursery provider is tasked with identifying a possible etiology using a systematic approach, performing a timely workup, as well as transferring to a neonatal intensive care unit or referring to higher centers for treatment when necessary. It is of utmost importance to identify time-sensitive etiologies since they have the most response to therapy.

Case Presentation

You are called from the newborn nursery to evaluate a full-term newborn delivered 3 h ago for decreased activity noted on the nurse's initial assessment on admission to the nursery. The infant is a 4100 gram male at 38 2/7-week gestational age based on first trimester ultrasound. The mother is a 38-year-old primigravida African American woman with negative prenatal labs including human immunodeficiency virus (HIV), hepatitis B, syphilis, and rubella as well as group B streptococcus (GBS). Pregnancy was complicated by gestational diabetes managed with glyburide and preeclampsia managed with labetalol and magnesium sulfate prior to delivery. She

R. Kamity, MD FAAP
Department of Pediatrics, NYU Winthrop Hospital, Mineola, NY, USA

SUNY Stony Brook School of Medicine, Stony Brook, NY, USA
e-mail: ranjith.kamity@nyulangone.org

G. I. Martin, W. Rosenfeld (eds.), *Common Problems in the Newborn Nursery*,
https://doi.org/10.1007/978-3-319-95672-5_16

presented with prolonged rupture of membranes for 20 h and was delivered via cesarean section for breech presentation.

Delivery of the infant was complicated by difficult extraction of the head with a nuchal cord, after delivering the rest of the body from the uterine incision. He was born with a weak spontaneous cry and required vigorous stimulation followed by brief CPAP via face mask with good response. He did not require any further resuscitation and was allowed to room in with the mother. Apgar score was 7 and 8 at 1 and 5 min. respectively (points taken off for tone and color). While in the recovery room, he attempted to breastfeed with some difficulty latching on.

The baby was just admitted to the nursery from the recovery room, and the admitting nurse is concerned that the baby is not very active. The infant's vital signs including heart rate, respiratory rate, oxygen saturations, and axillary temperature are within normal limits. On a brief exam, the baby has truncal hypotonia as evidenced by significant head lag and decreased tone on ventral suspension.

At this time you attempt to obtain a detailed history. What specific prenatal history would be highly suspicious for a congenital neuromuscular disorder in this infant?

1. History of maternal diabetes
2. Decreased fetal movements and abnormal presentation
3. Abnormal fetal heart tracing
4. Large for gestational age fetus

A detailed history and comprehensive neurological exam are the first steps in identifying the etiology of hypotonia in a newborn. A detailed medical history of the mother's general health (e.g., diabetes, hypertension, metabolic disorders, etc.) as well as specific neuromuscular conditions could suggest a possible congenital or genetic etiology (e.g., myotonic dystrophy, myasthenia gravis, seizure disorders, etc.) [5, 6]. Some of this information might not be available immediately and should be addressed when possible. Infants exposed to maternal drugs or medications (e.g., general anesthesia or maternal magnesium sulfate administration) may present with decreased muscle tone and, in severe cases, with respiratory failure. Maternal infections such as chorioamnionitis as well as toxoplasmosis, (Syphilis, etc.), rubella, cytomegalovirus and herpes (TORCH) infections can cause perinatally acquired systemic illness in the newborn. The affected infants may have other signs and symptoms of systemic illness, including abnormal vital signs, respiratory distress, desaturations, apnea, tachypnea, bradycardia, tachycardia, hypotension, decreased peripheral perfusion, hypothermia, as well as feeding intolerance. These infants warrant additional workup geared toward identifying and treating the underlying etiologies.

In addition to the above, antenatal history of fetal malpresentation, decreased fetal movements, polyhydramnios, or oligohydramnios can hint congenital causes of hypotonia including certain genetic conditions [5, 7]. The decreased muscle tone and abnormal movements in these fetuses could result in malposition and malpresentation. Any abnormal swallowing mechanism in these fetuses could present with polyhydramnios [8]. Arthrogryposis is another condition associated with certain congenital neuromuscular disorders with decreased fetal movements and contractures [9].

The newborn's course at delivery and resuscitation history can often point to a possible etiology for systemic compromise in a newborn. While abnormal intrapartum fetal heart tracing is considered a marker for fetal compromise, it often does not point to the etiology. In addition, a need for resuscitation at birth, especially when prolonged, is a well-accepted marker for perinatal distress [10]. While it is not uncommon for an otherwise normal newborn to have delivery complicated by various factors leading to perinatal hypoxia, a newborn with a neuromuscular disorder might be much less able to tolerate the stress of labor and delivery and hence is at higher risk of developing perinatal hypoxia.

Answer: 2

Table 16.1 Key points on a detailed history in a newborn with hypotonia

Maternal medical history	Drug/medications: magnesium sulfate, general anesthetics, opioids Infections: chorioamnionitis, GBS, TORCH Neuromuscular illnesses: muscular dystrophies, myasthenia gravis
Family history	Neurological or metabolic disorders in family members, e.g., congenital myotonic dystrophy, spinal muscular atrophy, metabolic disorders, etc. Fetal and infantile deaths Developmental delays Seizure disorders Race/ethnicity/consanguinity
Pregnancy and delivery history	Prematurity Abnormal fetal presentation, decreased fetal movements Polyhydramnios, oligohydramnios Delivery mode, complications during delivery Resuscitation at delivery, APGAR score Cord gases
Nursery course	Abnormal cry, tone Decreased spontaneous activity Decreased alertness Feeding difficulties, especially poor latch during feeding

To summarize, an accurate history should focus on the key areas, given the broad list of differential diagnoses (Table 16.1).

Case Presentation Continued

Maternal history for this newborn was negative for myasthenia gravis, muscular dystrophies, or seizure disorders, with no known family history of genetic conditions. The infant did not have any risk factors for sepsis other than prolonged rupture of membranes. Information about decreased fetal movements during pregnancy could not be confirmed at this time, but there was reported suspicion of decreased fetal movements prenatally. In addition, the infant had history of polyhydramnios and was in breech position at delivery. The infant is now 3 h old with hypotonia and some difficulty with breastfeeding.

At this time, which one of the following statements is most applicable?

1. Brain imaging should be performed immediately.
2. Transient systemic causes of hypotonia must be ruled out.
3. Infant should obtain a full sepsis workup.
4. Electroencephalography (EEG) is recommended at this time.

The magnitude of differential diagnoses causing hypotonia in a newborn varies from a wide range of transient systemic causes, chromosomal (genetic) causes, inborn errors of metabolism, endocrine causes, as well as central and peripheral neurological and neuromuscular causes [3]. Since systemic causes are by far the most common etiology for hypotonia in a newborn, it is essential to identify the transient and reversible etiologies as soon as possible, given the risk of permanent neurological injury if untreated [11]. A detailed newborn physical exam includes a head-to-toe evaluation for general assessment, including Dubowitz assessment for gestational age (if unclear), evaluation for dysmorphic features, skeletal abnormalities, microcephaly, macrocephaly, as well as a complete neurological exam, including mental status, muscle tone, newborn reflexes, as well as deep tendon reflexes.

Poor perfusion may be seen in infants with hypovolemia, hypotension, hypoxia, and acidosis and can be easily identified on a quick general exam. Infants with transient electrolyte abnormalities like hypoglycemia, hypocalcemia, and hypermagnesemia often present with nonspecific clinical signs and symptoms in the newborn period requiring higher index of suspicion. Infants with sepsis are usually ill-appearing and could deteriorate rapidly if untreated. Hence it would be prudent to assume that a hypotonic infant is septic until proven otherwise [11, 12]. If the infant does not appear well, a sepsis workup is definitely warranted. Infants with a difficult delivery course and complicated resuscitation often have transient acidosis which can be identified on the cord or infant's blood gases. Although most units obtain routine cord blood gases at all deliveries, it is not always available. Cord blood gases, when available, may show evidence of acidosis as a surrogate marker for in utero hypoxia.

Low Apgar scores (especially if prolonged) on the other hand have been linked to increased neonatal mortality and worse neurodevelopmental outcomes [13–16].

Hypoxic-ischemic encephalopathy (HIE) is the most common cause for hypotonia presenting in a newborn soon after birth, resulting from perinatal hypoxia [11], and is associated with other systemic causes like hypoglycemia, hypermagnesemia, hypocalcemia, hypovolemia, and acidosis. The reported prevalence of HIE in full-term infants with Apgar score of 0–3 at 5 min is as high as 70% [10]. Affected infants usually have early signs in the initial newborn period with abnormal cry, tone, activity, alertness, and feeding difficulties, to name a few. Altered mental status is usually noted in encephalopathies, including HIE which needs to be identified as soon as possible. The therapeutic intervention with hypothermia therapy is time-critical and needs to be started within 6 h of birth [17]. Infants with mild HIE present with mild hypotonia, irritability, increased alertness, and normal/increased deep tendon reflexes. The outcomes for these infants are usually favorable [17]. Moderate cases (Sarnat Stage 2 HIE) present with generalized hypotonia with depressed reflexes and depressed mental status. These infants may also present with seizures. Infants with Stage 2 HIE can improve significantly if treated with hypothermia in a timely manner. Infants with severe (Sarnat Stage 3) HIE are severely depressed with severe hypotonia and absent reflexes and may even present with posturing [17, 18]. The details of staging and management of HIE are discussed elsewhere in this book (Chaps. 1 and 17).

Although brain imaging is vital, transient and reversible systemic causes for hypotonia should be ruled out prior to obtaining imaging studies. Brain imaging and EEG are primarily indicated in newborns presenting with signs of focal neurological deficits, e.g., seizures, or if the infant has focal abnormality on neurological exam. Head ultrasound scan is usually the easiest to obtain and does not involve risk of radiation. A brain MRI is indicated if suspecting structural abnormality and is preferred to head CT due to high resolution and low risk of ionizing radiation [19]. Head CT may have better resolution than a brain ultrasound but not used as the first-line investigation due to risk of radiation and limited yield. Imaging may also be obtained to complete the diagnostic workup in infants with hypotonia of unknown etiology [11].

Table 16.2 Transient causes of hypotonia and key diagnostic points

Etiology	Key points
Acidosis	Infant appears sick with depressed strength and reflexes Abnormal cord gases or infant's blood gases Any history of resuscitation at birth
Hypoglycemia	Variable newborn exam; usually subtle neurological findings Hypotonia, jitteriness, seizures in severe hypoglycemia Maternal history of diabetes
Hypermagnesemia	Depressed reflexes, respiratory distress, ileus Maternal treatment with magnesium sulfate
Hypocalcemia	Hypotonia, seizures, myoclonic jerks
General anesthesia	Neonatal hypotonia, respiratory distress/apnea
Congenital hypothyroidism	Hypotonia, decreased activity Large anterior fontanelle Poor feeding, constipation Jaundice
Infections/sepsis	Ill-appearing infant Acidosis, poor perfusion, risk factors present

Answer: 2

The table above lists common transient systemic illnesses in a newborn with hypotonia with key diagnostic points (Table 16.2).

Case Presentation Continued

This infant did not require resuscitation and was stable in room air after delivery with a normal level of alertness. Upon review of the chart, you notice that the infant's cord arterial blood gas showed pH of 7.28, pCO_2 of 48, and pO_2 of 30 with a base deficit of 3. Cord venous blood gas showed pH of 7.36, pCO_2 of 40, and pO_2 of 35, with a base deficit of −3.

While conducting a detailed exam, what laboratory testing would you order first in this infant?

1. Point-of-care glucose
2. Serum calcium
3. Complete blood count
4. Arterial blood gas

Infants with transient electrolyte abnormalities can be identified quickly with simple laboratory testing and can be managed with intravenous fluids and supportive care until the electrolytes normalize. Infants with nuchal cords at birth can present with acute hypovolemia with hypoxemia and acidosis from cord compression and can also present with generalized hypotonia. It is standard practice in many units to observe infants in the recovery room with the mothers after a cesarean section and transfer them to the nursery when the mother is sent to the postpartum floor. However, since this infant has no tachycardia as evidenced by normal vital signs as well as normal cord blood gases, the index of suspicion for hypovolemia and acidosis is low.

Preeclampsia, maternal diabetes, and perinatal stress are associated with increased risk of hypocalcemia early in the neonatal period. Hypocalcemia in the early neonatal period (<3–4 days of life) is largely asymptomatic and is diagnosed incidentally unless severe. In severe hypocalcemia (calcium <7 mg/dL or ionized <4 mg/dL), infants may present with signs of neuromuscular irritability, myoclonic jerks, jitteriness, exaggerated startle, and seizures [20].

Although all the above choices are correct, the most time-critical choice at this time would be a point-of-care test for glucose. Untreated hypoglycemia could rapidly progress to cause neurological injury which may present with worsening hypotonia and seizures. It is vital to monitor for hypoglycemia in a large for gestational age infant of a mother with gestational diabetes, especially in the first 24 h of life [21]. Point-of-care glucose testing can identify hypoglycemia which can then be managed appropriately.

Answer: 1

Case Presentation Continued

The infant's glucose was 65 mg/dL, and serum calcium is 9.2 mg/dL, which are within normal limits.

You then send a serum magnesium level on this infant. What do you expect to find on neurological exam if the baby presented with elevated serum magnesium?

1. Hypotonia with decreased level of alertness
2. Hypotonia with intact level of alertness

Infants born to mothers with preeclampsia or eclampsia who received magnesium sulfate can have hypermagnesemia, presenting with generalized hypotonia, apnea, bradycardia, feeding difficulty, and, in severe cases, respiratory distress and may even mimic septic shock. Magnesium is known to inactivate acetyl choline at the neuromuscular junction, especially in the respiratory muscles, and does not affect the brain directly [22]. Hence the infants' clinical presentation would be similar to peripheral neurological disorders, with intact alertness.

Answer: 2

Case Presentation Continued

The infant's electrolyte panel is normal including a serum magnesium level. Workup has been sent to rule out sepsis and is in progress. The infant was large for gestational age (97th percentile) and measured appropriately for weight, length, and head circumference. On exam, this patient was awake, warm, well perfused, and otherwise well appearing.

You continue to perform a detailed exam on the infant. Which of the following can be best used to differentiate peripheral and central causes of hypotonia?

1. Decreased strength
2. Decreased tone
3. Decreased reflexes

Hypotonia can be caused by neurological dysfunction anywhere from the brain all the way down to the muscles. Central hypotonia results from a defect arising from the brain, brain stem, or spinal cord above the anterior horn cells (AHC), while peripheral causes are the result of a defect anywhere from the AHCs, peripheral nerves, neuromuscular junction (NMJ), and muscles. Central neurologic causes of hypotonia are more common than peripheral causes and account for about 60–80% of the cases, while peripheral causes are seen in 15–30% of the cases with a neurological etiology [11, 23]. It is essential to differentiate the two and narrow down the differential diagnosis.

Central causes affect the brain and brain stem and are associated with altered mental status with a depressed level of consciousness, while peripheral nervous system causes for hypotonia tend to have an intact mental status with normal sleep-wake patterns. The evaluation of higher mental functions in a newborn is limited to alertness and wakefulness. In an older infant, normal sleep-wake cycles should be established. In a newborn however, sleep-wake cycles are not fully established [24].

A complete neurological exam begins with an assessment of the infant's resting posture and tone. Infants with normal tone have flexed posture of all four limbs with active movements of the extremities. Hypotonic newborns do not have the usual flexed posture of all limbs. Instead they tend to present with abducted and extended limbs [25]. Evaluation of axial tone in a newborn is done best by suspending the infant horizontally and vertically. During horizontal (ventral) suspension, the hypotonic infant drapes over the hand of the examiner like an inverted "U" with the head and legs dangling on the side. Poor axial tone also causes these infants to have a significant head lag when pulled to sit off the bed and a positive "shoulder slip-through" sign when picked up vertically by grasping under the arms [24].

Newborns with central hypotonia have predominantly axial hypotonia with intact strength. Strength is more preserved than tone in central lesions, while peripheral lesions tend to present with profound hypotonia and weakness. While hypotonia is described as reduced resistance to passive movements, weakness is the reduction in maximum power [1–3]. Additionally, asymmetry in muscle tone is a red flag and requires further investigation to identify focal neurological lesions, e.g., neonatal ischemic stroke, traumatic myelopathy, brachial plexus injuries, etc. Deep tendon reflexes are usually exaggerated in central lesions, including clonus, while they are normal/depressed in peripheral disorders. Higher brain functions are usually not affected in disorders affecting the peripheral nervous system [24, 26].

On the other hand, a newborn with severe hypotonia, weakness, and intact higher mental functions – e.g., alert, with normal sleep-wake patterns – tends to have a peripheral neurological cause affecting the lower motor neuron and motor unit as well as muscular disorders [27]. Spinal muscular atrophy (SMA) is a good example of a peripheral neuromuscular disorder where a third of the patients can present as early as the neonatal period and eventually progress to develop respiratory failure later in infancy. The SMAs consist of a group of disorders with progressive loss of spinal AHCs, leading to muscular atrophy and weakness. Since the problem is distal to the brain and brain stem, these infants have significant hypotonia and generalized weakness and absent deep tendon reflexes, but the higher functions are spared, giving the classic presentation of alert facies with significant distal weakness. Fasciculations of the tongue are often seen in infants with SMA as weakness starts to develop [5]. Albeit rare, other common peripheral causes include congenital myotonic dystrophies and congenital myopathies, which also present with profound hypotonia and weakness. The rest of the exam should be geared toward identifying additional clues to the etiology and localizing the site of defect (Table 16.3).

Hence, while there are many ways to differentiate central from peripheral causes of hypotonia, intact alertness and decreased strength out of proportion to the degree of hypotonia are strongly suggestive of peripheral hypotonia. However, it is important to note that the level of alertness is

Table 16.3 Key clinical features in hypotonic infants based on site of lesion

	Central hypotonia		Peripheral hypotonia			
	Congenital	Acquired (injury)	Anterior horn cell	Peripheral nerve	Neuromuscular junction (NMJ)	Muscle
Strength	Normal	Normal (decreased in early severe cases)	Decreased	Decreased	Decreased	Decreased
DTRs	Normal	Normal/ increased (decreased in severe cases)	Decreased/ absent	Decreased/ absent	Decreased/normal	Decreased/ absent
Alertness	Decreased (with exceptions)	Decreased (with exceptions)	Intact	Intact	Intact	Intact
Examples	Chromosomal disorders (e.g., PWS), cerebral dysgenesis	HIE, metabolic disorders	SMA, hypoxic-ischemic myelopathy	Hereditary sensory and autonomic neuropathy, congenital hypomyelinating neuropathy	Transient acquired neonatal myasthenia, hypermagnesemia	Muscular dystrophy syndromes, metabolic myopathies

Adapted from Peredo and Hannibal [11]

variable depending the degree of involvement and might not be enough to differentiate congenital and acquired causes of hypotonia in the early newborn stage.

Answer: 1

Case Presentation Continued

A detailed neurological exam was performed and was significant for generalized moderate hypotonia as evidenced with a prominent head lag and hypotonia on ventral suspension, with symmetric muscle tone on all extremities. No focal defects or seizures were identified. However the infant was able to move his limbs against gravity and did not have any obvious weakness on active movements. Deep tendon reflexes were normal.

Which specific findings on exam would you look for in a newborn if you suspect congenital central hypotonia?

1. Dysmorphic features
2. Level of alertness
3. Decreased strength

It is often difficult to differentiate congenital central causes of hypotonia from acquired causes of central hypotonia (e.g., injury). Central causes affect higher brain functions with possible seizure from cerebral cortical involvement. Infants with central hypotonia may be noted to have with dysmorphic features, scissoring of the legs on vertical suspension, as well as fisting of the hands [24]. On the other hand, if the brain stem and cranial nerves are involved, the newborn may present with abnormal or irregular breathing pattern, apnea, and abnormal eye movements. These babies could present with hypotonia and weakness along with depressed deep tendon reflexes. The features of hypotonic infants with central disorders vary with the etiology and, in some cases, with the timing of assessment in relation to the injury. Strength is usually preserved in central causes and cannot differentiate congenital from acquired causes. A focused exam with imaging might be necessary to identify the underlying etiology. Another special group is premature infants who tend to have generalized hypotonia, but reflexes and strength are spared. Since their muscle tone is gestational age dependent, it is important to compare to a normal preterm infant of appropriate gestation.

A detailed exam should help identify congenital central causes from an acute injury, an ongoing injury, and a static or progressive developmental disorder. The best example is HIE which can present with a mild, moderate, or severe encephalopathy [28]. The onset is usually acute, presenting with hypotonia. These infants could progress to develop hypertonia and hyperreflexia in the future as signs of cerebral palsy become more apparent [29]. Congenital developmental causes of central hypotonia tend to have unchanged or worsening hypotonia as in most genetic syndromes [2, 30], while injury-induced central causes develop hypertonia overtime as seen in cerebral palsy [3, 11]. Congenital causes may have associated dysmorphic features specific to the underlying condition as listed in Table 16.4 (e.g., Down syndrome, Prader-Willi syndrome (PWS), etc.).

Answer: 1

Alternative Scenario What would you do if this infant had no dysmorphic features, has severe hypotonia, decreased DTRs and has normal sleep-wake patterns?

1. Obtain EEG
2. Obtain creatine phosphokinase levels
3. Send for neuromuscular testing

A baby in this alternative scenario has features consistent with peripheral causes of hypotonia, narrowing down the defect to the level of the peripheral nerves, neuromuscular junction, or muscles. An EEG would not help in this situation, since this is not a suspected central neurological lesion. Serum creatine phosphokinase (CPK) levels are helpful to further localize the lesion. Significant elevation in CPK levels are often seen in congenital muscular dystrophies, while congenital myopathies and spinal muscular atrophy may have a normal CPK level. Anterior horn cell diseases can have mild elevation in CPK levels [5]. If inconclusive, the next step is to obtain electrophysiological studies for neuromuscular testing using electromyography (EMG) or nerve conduction studies. A normal EMG usually suggests central origin for hypotonia with some exceptions. Muscle biopsies are reserved for differentiating muscular dystrophies and myopathies. If biopsy

Table 16.4 Common findings in selected syndromes presenting with hypotonia

Syndrome	Hypotonia	Other common features
Achondroplasia	Mild	Macrocephaly, prominent forehead, short limbs, low nasal bridge
Acrocallosal syndrome	Mild	Absence of corpus callosum, polydactyly
Cerebro-oculo-facio-skeletal syndrome	Generalized	Neurogenic arthrogryposis, microcephaly, microphthalmia, cataract (later onset)
Down syndrome	Moderate/severe	Congenital heart disease (murmur), flattened facial profile, brachycephaly, short nasal bridge, epicanthal folds, single palmar crease, clinodactyly, loose nuchal folds
Myotonic dystrophy syndrome	Variable/severe	Variable onset from prenatal to adulthood; decreased activity, difficulty swallowing, muscle atrophy, hypogonadism
Organic acidemias, urea cycle defects	Variable	Abnormal odor; findings are variable depending on specific condition
Prader-Willi syndrome	Moderate/severe	Hypogonadism (undescended testes, hypoplastic labia), dysmorphic facial features (almond-shaped eyes with up slanting palpebral fissures, prominent forehead, narrow face, small mouth, thin upper lip, and micrognathia)
Zellweger syndrome	Moderate/severe	Murmur (PDA/septal defects), high forehead, flat facies, hepatomegaly (seen later in infancy and beyond)

shows specific abnormalities on immunohistochemical staining and electron microscopy, it may be indicated to do specific gene testing for definitive diagnosis. It is important to remember that CPK levels may be elevated transiently following these procedures and hence should be checked before the procedures if peripheral neuromuscular disorders are being considered.

Answer: 2

Case Presentation Continued

You complete examining the infant. In addition to the abnormal neurological findings, he was noted to have undescended testes and subtle dysmorphic features including a prominent forehead and a small mouth.

Does the newborn require genetic testing?

1. Yes
2. No

Karyotyping is indicated when multiple specific dysmorphic features are noted to identify any cytogenetic defects. Down syndrome and Prader-Willi syndrome are among the most common genetic conditions that present with hypotonia in the newborn period. This patient has generalized hypotonia with suspicion for a congenital central etiology and warrants a consult with a geneticist as well as focused testing. However given the delivery course, other transient causes of hypotonia had to be ruled out first.

Infants with hypogonadism (undescended testes) on exam with moderate to severe hypotonia and feeding difficulties are highly suspicious for Prader-Willi syndrome. Newborns with Prader-Willi syndrome tend to have typical facial features, including a prominent forehead, narrow face, almond-shaped eyes, small mouth, thin upper lip, and micrognathia [31]. Although older children with Prader-Willi syndrome are often noted to be obese, the infants might not necessarily be large for gestational age at birth. A vast majority of infants with Prader-Willi syndrome have feeding difficulties, leading to failure to thrive until 8–11 months of life. These infants however go on to develop severe hypotonia, insatiable appetites, obesity, and short stature later in infancy [7, 11]. Karyotype testing alone is inadequate for Prader-Willi since the genetic defect involves imprinting defects, affecting a small portion of chromosome 15 (15q11.2). The specific diagnostic tests include comparative genomic hybridization, DNA methylation studies, and fluorescence in situ hybridization (FISH) for Prader-Willi syndrome.

On the other hand, Down syndrome (Trisomy 21) is the most common chromosomal defect causing developmental delay in newborns. Typical newborn presentation includes hypotonia, congenital heart defects, and dysmorphic features. The most common dysmorphic features include flattened facial profile, brachycephaly, short nasal bridge, epicanthal folds, single palmar crease, clinodactyly, as well as loose nuchal folds [11, 32]. Testing for Down syndrome involves karyotype analysis, which is usually diagnostic. In mosaic cases of Down syndrome, FISH testing might be required.

Answer: 1

Case Summary

This is a case of a full-term infant with Prader-Willi Syndrome. The infant in this vignette presented with hypotonia in the early newborn period. The approach to this infant began with a comprehensive history and physical exam. Detailed physical exam of this infant showed a large for gestational age infant (97th percentile) with undescended testes. A hypotonic infant like this case demands a comprehensive neurological exam including a detailed assessment of tone, strength, reflexes, as well as higher mental functions.

The infant in this case had prenatal concerns for congenital etiology, due to abnormal fetal presentation and suggested decreased fetal movements with no other explanation. The presence of dysmorphic features is also suspicious for a congenital/genetic etiology. Despite having a nuchal cord at delivery, the infant did not require any resuscitation, and the cord blood gases did not show any acidosis and hence not likely to have resulted from hypoxic insult. The next course of action involved ruling out transient systemic causes. Given the history of maternal diabetes, the infant was screened with point-of-care glucose testing, which was normal. A baseline electrolyte panel was also normal including normal calcium and magnesium levels. Given the history of normal cord gases, absence of hypoglycemia, and normal calcium and magnesium levels, including the history of lack of resuscitation at delivery, hypotonia in this infant was less likely to be secondary to a transient systemic etiology.

While transient causes of hypotonia were being ruled out, the infant underwent a detailed general and neurological exam to identify the location of neurological dysfunction. On examination, the infant had moderate hypotonia with intact strength as evidenced by normal strength during movements, which was suggestive of central etiology. The next steps involved identifying congenital versus acquired etiology for hypotonia. The infant was awake, alert, and responsive to stimulation. He did not have any clinical features of HIE barring isolated hypotonia. Decreased alertness is not always seen in newborns with Prader-Willi, and some newborns can have intact alertness [33]. Despite the presence of intact alertness in the early newborn period, this infant is suspicious for a congenital central cause of hypotonia.

Absence of any history suggestive of acidosis without encephalopathy goes against acquired causes like HIE. In addition, absence of asymmetric decreased movements ruled out any brachial plexus injuries. Presence of normal DTRs in this infant was also suggestive of possible congenital etiology. To be positive, however, this infant would require close follow-up to monitor the progression of muscle tone or lack thereof. Infants with Prader-Willi syndrome often tend to have significant hypotonia during the newborn period, with significant feeding challenges at times, even requiring tube feedings. Genetic testing with comparative genomic hybridization, DNA methylation studies, and FISH are diagnostic for Prader-Willi syndrome.

Infants with Prader-Willi syndrome are usually normal in birth weight and have poor weight gain in early infancy. However, they go on to develop insatiable appetites later in infancy and develop obesity between 6 months to 6 years. The infant in this vignette was LGA, which is not uncommon in the setting of maternal diabetes. Since these babies are at high risk of feeding problems, it is essential to monitor feeding closely and provide supportive care as needed until their feeding improves later in infancy.

An overview of the approach to a newborn with hypotonia is presented in Fig. 16.1. For the purposes of flow of case discussion, a review of systemic causes was discussed before clinical examination. It is important to note that in most situations, history is being reviewed and point-of-care assessments are done simultaneously, while the newborn is being examined. A detailed history and physical exam can identify up to 50% of the diagnoses without any additional testing. Imaging studies, evaluation by geneticist, and genetic testing can further diagnose about 25% of hypotonic infants [23]. Infants with normal tone at birth and subsequently developing hypotonia could have inborn errors of metabolism usually presenting after at least 1–2 days of life, once the baby accumulates the affected metabolites. These include disorders of carbohydrate metabolism, organic acidemias, urea cycle defects, fatty acid oxidation disorders, and various miscellaneous defects. The remaining infants require expanded biochemical testing for metabolic disorders, neuromuscular testing (EMG, muscle biopsy with immunohistochemical staining, etc.) and other miscellaneous tests. A small portion of these infants with hypotonia remain undiagnosed despite extensive workup. The importance of a detailed history and physical exam cannot be overstated when attempting to diagnose a newborn with hypotonia.

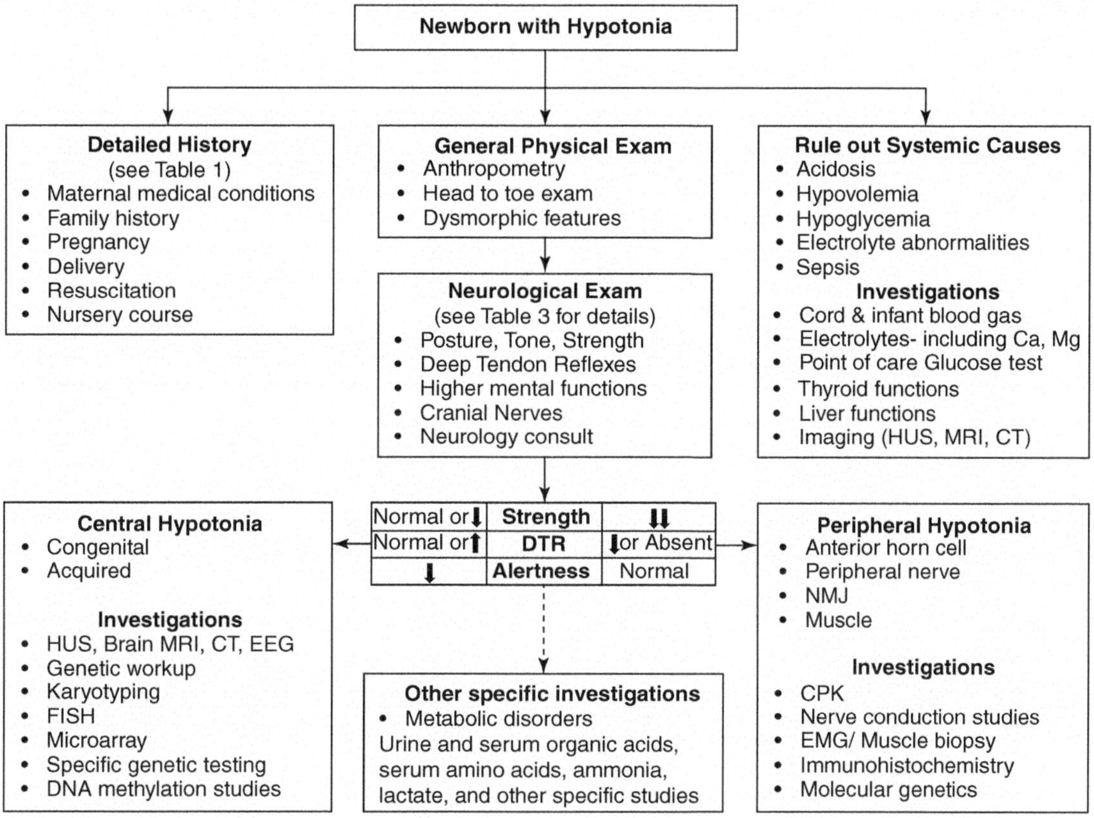

Fig. 16.1 Suggested approach for evaluation of a newborn with hypotonia

Clinical Pearls

1. Infants presenting with hypotonia should be assessed for posture, tone, and strength using ventral suspension, vertical suspension, and pull to sit by traction. It is essential to be able to differentiate normal from abnormal.
2. A detailed history and physical exam can yield a diagnosis in about half of the infants with hypotonia.
3. History of decreased fetal movements, malpresentation, and polyhydramnios are suspicious for congenital neuromuscular disorders. Family history of congenital neuromuscular disorders needs to be investigated.
4. Systemic causes of hypotonia need to be ruled out using history and physical exam of the newborn.
5. Central causes of hypotonia may present with decreased alertness, abnormal sleep-wake patterns, hypotonia, and normal or elevated DTRs, but strength is relatively preserved; peripheral causes of hypotonia present with intact alertness, profound weakness, significant hypotonia, and low or absent DTRs.

References

1. Crawford TO. Clinical evaluation of the floppy infant. Pediatr Ann. 1992;21(6):348–54.
2. Martin K, Inman J, Kirschner A, Deming K, Gumbel R, Voelker L. Characteristics of hypotonia in children: a consensus opinion of pediatric occupational and physical therapists. Pediatr Phys Ther. 2005;17(4):275–82.
3. Dubowitz V. Evaluation and differential diagnosis of the hypotonic infant. Pediatr Rev. 1985;6(8):237–43.
4. Dubowitz V. The floppy infant. 2nd ed. London: Spastics International Medical Publications: in association with W.H. Heinemann/Philadelphia: J.B. Lippincott; 1980. 158 p.
5. Leyenaar J, Camfield P, Camfield C. A schematic approach to hypotonia in infancy. Paediatr Child Health. 2005;10(7):397–400.
6. Fenichel GM. The hypotonic infant. In: Fenichel GM, editor. Clinical pediatric neurology. 4th ed. Philadelphia: WB Saunders Company; 2001. p. 149.
7. Tuysuz B, Kartal N, Erener-Ercan T, Guclu-Geyik F, Vural M, Perk Y, et al. Prevalence of Prader-Willi syndrome among infants with hypotonia. J Pediatr. 2014;164(5):1064–7.
8. Hamza A, Herr D, Solomayer EF, Meyberg-Solomayer G. Polyhydramnios: causes, diagnosis and therapy. Geburtshilfe Frauenheilkd. 2013;73(12):1241–6.
9. Kowalczyk B, Feluś J. Arthrogryposis: an update on clinical aspects, etiology, and treatment strategies. Arch Med Sci. 2016;12(1):10–24.
10. Hogan L, Ingemarsson I, Thorngren-Jerneck K, Herbst A. How often is a low 5-min Apgar score in term newborns due to asphyxia? Eur J Obstet Gynecol Reprod Biol. 2007;130(2):169–75.
11. Peredo DE, Hannibal MC. The floppy infant. Evaluation of hypotonia. Pediatr Rev. 2009;30(9):e66–76.
12. Ahmed MI, Iqbal M, Hussain N. A structured approach to the assessment of a floppy neonate. J Pediatr Neurosci. 2016;11(1):2–6.
13. Moster D, Lie RT, Irgens LM, Bjerkedal T, Markestad T. The association of Apgar score with subsequent death and cerebral palsy: a population-based study in term infants. J Pediatr. 2001;138(6):798–803.
14. Casey BM, McIntire DD, Leveno KJ. The continuing value of the Apgar score for the assessment of newborn infants. N Engl J Med. 2001;344(7):467–71.
15. Nelson KB, Ellenberg JH. Apgar scores as predictors of chronic neurologic disability. Pediatrics. 1981;68(1):36–44.
16. Ehrenstein V. Association of Apgar scores with death and neurologic disability. J Clin Epidemiol. 2009;1:45–53.
17. Cotten CM, Shankaran S. Hypothermia for hypoxic–ischemic encephalopathy. Expert Rev Obstet Gynaecol. 2010;5(2):227–39.
18. Shankaran S, Laptook AR, Ehrenkranz RA, Tyson JE, McDonald SA, Donovan EF, et al. Whole-body hypothermia for neonates with hypoxic-ischemic encephalopathy. N Engl J Med. 2005;353(15):1574–84.
19. Volpe JJ. Specialized studies in the neurological evaluation. In: Volpe JJ, editor. Neurology of the newborn. Philadelphia: Saunders Elsevier; 2008. p. 154–202.
20. Jain A, Agarwal R, Sankar MJ, Deorari A, Paul VK. Hypocalcemia in the newborn. Indian J Pediatr. 2010;77(10):1123–8.
21. Adamkin DH. Postnatal glucose homeostasis in late-preterm and term infants. Pediatrics. 2011;127(3):575–9.
22. Ali A, Walentik C, Mantych GJ, Sadiq HF, Keenan WJ, Noguchi A. Iatrogenic acute hypermagnesemia after total parenteral nutrition infusion mimicking septic shock syndrome: two case reports. Pediatrics. 2003;112(1 Pt 1):e70–2.
23. Paro-Panjan D, Neubauer D. Congenital hypotonia: is there an algorithm? J Child Neurol. 2004;19(6):439–42.
24. Volpe JJ. Neurological examination: normal and abnormal features. In: Volpe JJ, editor. Neurology of the newborn. Philadelphia: Saunders Elsevier; 2008. p. 121–48.
25. Dubowitz LM, Dubowitz V, Palmer P, Verghote M. A new approach to the neurological assessment of the preterm and full-term newborn infant. Brain Dev. 1980;2(1):3–14.
26. Balmakund J. Hypotonia in children: an approach for evaluation and treatment. Resid Staff Physician. 1997;43(9):74–89.
27. Vasta I, Kinali M, Messina S, Guzzetta A, Kapellou O, Manzur A, et al. Can clinical signs identify newborns with neuromuscular disorders? J Pediatr. 2005;146(1):73–9.
28. Sarnat HB, Sarnat MS. Neonatal encephalopathy following fetal distress. A clinical and electroencephalographic study. Arch Neurol. 1976;33(10):696–705.
29. Shankaran S, Woldt E, Koepke T, Bedard MP, Nandyal R. Acute neonatal morbidity and long-term central nervous system sequelae of perinatal asphyxia in term infants. Early Hum Dev. 1991;25(2):135–48.
30. Igarashi M. Floppy infant syndrome. J Clin Neuromuscul Dis. 2004;6(2):69–90.
31. Wang P, Zhou W, Yuan W, Huang L, Zhao N, Chen X. Prader-Willi syndrome in neonates: twenty cases and review of the literature in Southern China. BMC Pediatr. 2016;16:124.
32. Devlin L, Morrison PJ. Accuracy of the clinical diagnosis of Down syndrome. Ulster Med J. 2004;73(1):4–12.
33. McSweeney N, Cowan F, Manzur A, Robb S, Muntoni F. Perinatal dyskinesia as a presenting feature in Prader Willi syndrome. Eur J Paediatr Neurol. 2009;13(4):350–5.

17 The Jittery Baby and Seizures

Lu-Ann Papile

Introduction

The recognition of neonatal seizure activity is one of the most challenging tasks facing providers of newborn care. Neonatal seizures may occur at any time following delivery, although they tend to cluster in the first 3 days after birth. The clinical signs of neonatal seizures are often subtle and have unique characteristics when compared to those of older infants. In addition, because the relative frequency of neonatal seizures is low (1.5–5.5 per 1000 live births), providers may not be familiar with their clinical presentations. However, even when seizure-like activity is identified, the clinician needs to realize that only a small percentage of newborn infants who manifest seizure-like activity, in fact, have seizures [1].

The prolongation of neonatal seizures may increase the extent of brain injury. Thus, it is important to identify seizures early, as well as the underlying cause, in order to provide effective treatment in a timely manner. This is especially relevant for seizures resulting from neonatal hypoxia ischemia where the window for effective treatment is the first 6 h after birth [2, 3]. Conversely, treating newborn infants for seizures, without verifying that, indeed, they do have seizures, may be harmful.

L.-A. Papile, MD
Division of Neonatology, Department of Pediatrics, University of New Mexico Health Sciences Center, University of New Mexico, Albuquerque, NM, USA
e-mail: papile@unm.edu

Case Presentation

You are called to the delivery room for the imminent birth of a term infant who has intermittent bradycardia on a fetal heart race tracing. The mother is a primigravida whose pregnancy was uncomplicated. Prenatal care began early in the first trimester. She has been in active labor for 20 h and received epidural analgesia. The fetal heart rate tracing was unremarkable until she started pushing. At birth the baby is limp and cyanotic with no respiratory effort. The baby does not respond to tactile stimulation. Neonatal resuscitation with bag and mask ventilation is initiated. The Apgar score at 1 min is 3. At 5 min of age, the baby is pink and breathing spontaneously; the Apgar score is 8. Bag and mask ventilation is discontinued, and at 10 min of age, the Apgar score is 9. On clinical examination at 20 min of age, you note a term appropriate for gestational-age infant who is alert with good respiratory effort and a normal heart rate. The Moro and suck reflexes are normal, and the motor exam is unremarkable with normal tone and posture. The pupils are equal in size and react briskly to light. Umbilical artery cord blood gas values reveal a pH of 7.1, a pCO_2 of 80, and a base deficit of −5.

G. I. Martin, W. Rosenfeld (eds.), *Common Problems in the Newborn Nursery*,
https://doi.org/10.1007/978-3-319-95672-5_17

At this time you:

1. Contact a neonatologist and request admission for an infant with presumed hypoxic-ischemic encephalopathy.
2. Admit the infant to the observation nursery to closely monitor vital signs for 24 h and observe for seizure activity.
3. Allow the infant to be placed on the mother's chest in order to breast feed.

Apnea at birth may be primary or secondary. The primary apnea will respond to tactile stimulation, whereas secondary apnea can only be resolved with assisted ventilation. Because primary and secondary apnea is indistinguishable clinically, every baby with apnea at birth is presumed to have secondary apnea and needs to be treated accordingly [4].

The 1 min Apgar score is an evaluation of an infant's transition from the intrauterine to the extra-uterine environment. Later scores measure an infant's response to resuscitative efforts [5, 6]. The hypotonia and the absence of spontaneous respirations at birth are not an indication that the infant has suffered brain injury but rather are a reflection of the infant's condition at birth. The subsequent Apgar scores at 5 and 10 min indicate the effectiveness of the resuscitative efforts and the vitality of the infant. Although the Apgar scores, particularly the score at 5 min, have been associated with an increased risk of neonatal mortality, they are not a predictor of poor neurodevelopmental outcome.

The low pH and high pCO2 noted on the umbilical artery cord blood sample implies that there was a compromise of fetal gas exchange. However the normal base excess value indicates that the infant's vital organs received a sufficient amount of oxygen to maintain aerobic metabolism [7].

The assumption that a baby has hypoxic-ischemic encephalopathy must include clinical evidence that the neurological examination is abnormal. The modified Sarnat staging is the most widely utilized neurologic examination for determining the presence and extent of neonatal encephalopathy (Table 17.1). The infant's neurologic examination shortly after birth falls into the category of normal on the modified Sarnat staging scale [8].

The lack of respiratory effort at birth coupled with the fetal bradycardia shortly before delivery suggests that the baby had secondary apnea. The most probable cause is umbilical cord or fetal head compression during the second stage of labor. The baby responded quickly to resuscitative efforts and by the Sarnat staging does not have clinical evidence of acute hypoxic-ischemic encephalopathy. You might consider close observation of the baby. This can be done at the mother's bedside and is not a sufficient reason to

Table 17.1 Modified Sarnat staging for neonatal encephalopathy

Category	Normal	Mild	Moderate	Severe
Level of consciousness	Normal	Excessively irritable or sleepy but arousable with light stimulation	Lethargic, unarousable	Stuporous, coma
Spontaneous activity	Normal	Normal	Decreased activity	Absent activity
Posture	Normal	Normal or mild distal flexion	Increased flexion	Decerebrate
Tone	Normal	Normal	Generalized mild hypotonia	Flaccid
Suck	Normal	Weak	Weak or absent	Absent
Moro reflex	Normal	Strong	Incomplete	Absent
Pupils	Normal	Normal	Constricted	Nonreactive to light, often unequal
Seizures	None	None	Common	Uncommon

Derived from Sarnat [8], Volpe [9]

separate the baby from the mother. The best option would be to place the baby on the mother's chest in order to facilitate breastfeeding.

Answer: 3

Case Presentation (Continued)

You are called by the mother-baby care provider when the baby is 12 h old because she is concerned that the baby might be having seizures. She describes the baby as being very jittery but alert and active when awake. The vital signs have been stable. The baby has been put to the breast every 2 h but still appears to be hungry. Urine and stool output are adequate.

You ask the mother if she has any concerns regarding her baby. She tells you that the baby is having difficulty breastfeeding. Specifically she has noted that when she strokes the baby's face with her breast to facilitate latching, the baby begins to shake, and the shaking gets worse the more the baby is handled. On observing the baby, you note that the baby is awake and jittery. The jitteriness has a pendulum-like quality with equal back and forth movement. During the physical examination, the baby's jitteriness worsens, but by gently restraining the baby's limbs, you are able to suppress the movement. Neurologic assessment reveals normal tone and reflexes. Pupils are midline and react to light, and no nystagmus is noted.

This type of movement could best be classified as:

1. Seizure
2. Myoclonus
3. Tremor
4. None of the above

The jitteriness noted is most likely neonatal tremors [9]. Although a tremor is a movement disorder, it is not invariably a sign of a seizure. The distinguishing features between jitteriness and seizures are fairly clear. Tremors do not have abnormal gaze or eye movement, while seizures often present with these clinical signs. Tactile stimulation and loud noise provoke tremors but not seizures. If the examiner provides flexion or physical restraint of the affected limb, the tremors will stop, while if there is a true seizure, they will continue.

Tremor is the most common involuntary movement seen in infants. During the first day or two after birth, the majority of healthy infants exhibit some degree of tremulousness. Neonatal tremors usually resolve spontaneously by 2 months of age but may continue until 7 to 9 months of age. Neither the presence nor the duration of tremors places an infant at risk for later neurodevelopmental problems [10, 11].

Answer: 3

At this time you order:

1. Plasma glucose level
2. Serum ionized calcium level
3. Drug screening
4. A consult with the neurologist for evaluation of seizures

Tremors have been associated with several medical morbidities, specifically neonatal hypoglycemia, hypocalcemia, hypoxic-ischemic encephalopathy, and drug withdrawal. Prenatal risk factors for both neonatal hypoglycemia and hypocalcemia include a maternal history of diabetes mellitus or glucose intolerance during pregnancy and intrauterine growth retardation. Neonatal risk factors include preterm birth and large-for-gestational-age infants. Because the mother's pregnancy was uncomplicated and the baby was an appropriate for gestational-age term infant, the baby is not at risk for hypoglycemia or hypocalcemia. However, the AAP clinical report on postnatal glucose homeostasis does recommend that blood glucose concentration be measured in term infants who have clinical signs that have been associated with hypoglycemia, including jitteriness [12]. Hypoxic-ischemic encephalopathy is an unlikely cause, since, with the exception of tremors, the infant's neurological examination remained normal.

Maternal nonmedical substance use during pregnancy is often underdiagnosed even when prenatal screening is performed. Maternal self-reporting underestimates drug exposure, and maternal urine screening during pregnancy fails to identify many cases of drug use [13]. Although the mother does not have any of the characteristics known to be associated with nonmedical substance use during pregnancy, the infant's jitteriness is a clinical sign compatible with intrauterine drug exposure. This fact would justify screening the newborn infant.

Urine for drug screening must be collected as soon as possible after birth, because the duration of urinary excretion of some drugs is relatively short. Alcohol is detectable for up to 16 h after maternal ingestion, and opioids, amphetamines, and cocaine metabolites are detectable for 1–3 days. Thus, a urine sample may be falsely negative in the setting of significant intrauterine drug exposure, especially if collected days after birth. Analysis of meconium, which takes several days to weeks for results, is a more accurate reflection of maternal drug use but is usually not the first test used in determining maternal drug use [14].

Answer: 1, 2, 3

Case Presentation (Alternative Birth Scenario)

At birth, the baby is limp and cyanotic with no respiratory effort. The baby does not respond to tactile stimulation. Neonatal resuscitation with bag and mask ventilation is initiated. The Apgar score at 1 min is 3. Despite good chest movement, the heart rate is still less than 100 beats per minute, and the baby remains cyanotic. Intubation is performed at 2 min of age. At 5 min of age, the baby still is not breathing spontaneously, the heart rate is 80 beats per minute, and the SpO2 is 80%. Spontaneous unlabored respirations are noted at 8 min of age. On clinical examination at 20 min of age, you note a term appropriate for gestational-age infant who has good respiratory effort and a normal heart rate but is lethargic, unarousable, and hypotonic. Axillary temperature is 34.5 °C. The baby has a partial Moro reflex and a weak suck reflex. The pupils are restricted. Umbilical artery blood gas values reveal a pH of 7.00 and a base excess of −16 mmol/L.

At this time you:

1. Warm the baby
2. Assess the baby with the modified Sarnat staging for encephalopathy
3. Admit the baby to the observation nursery to closely monitor vital signs for 24 h and observe for seizures

The only known effective therapy for neonatal encephalopathy is therapeutic hypothermia [15–18]. Because the therapeutic window for cooling is narrow (6 h), it is imperative that any baby who requires neonatal resuscitation be evaluated for encephalopathy immediately after birth in order to determine if the baby has moderate or severe encephalopathy and thus is a potential candidate for cooling.

Answer: 2

Head or total body cooling must be started by:

1. 2 h of life
2. 4 h of life
3. 6 h of life
4. 8 h of life

In addition to having clinical evidence of moderate or severe encephalopathy, an infant must be less than 6 h of age, be greater than 35 weeks of gestational age, and have one of the following criteria [15–18]:

Apgar score ≤5 at 10 minutes after birth
Continued need for resuscitation at 10 minutes of age
pH ≤7.0 or base deficit ≥12 mmol/L on umbilical cord blood sample
pH ≤7.0 or base deficit ≥12 mmol/L on any blood sample obtained within the first hour after birth

Answer: 3

The baby's abnormally low temperature may be an indication that the baby has neonatal encephalopathy. Warming babies with moderate to severe encephalopathy may worsen their condition, whereas allowing them to remain hypothermic may be beneficial [19, 20]. Thus any decision regarding temperature maintenance should be deferred until after the baby has been assessed for encephalopathy. If it is ascertained that a baby has moderate or severe encephalopathy, passive cooling which involves the removal of all external sources of heat should be implemented. Initiating active cooling in a community setting is not advised since there is uncertainty regarding the safety of this practice.

Using the modified Sarnat staging in Table 17.1, what level of encephalopathy does the baby have?

1. Mild
2. Moderate
3. Severe

The baby has all of the clinical characteristics of moderate encephalopathy (lethargy, decreased activity, generalized hypotonia, an incomplete Moro reflex, weak suck, constricted pupils).

Answer: 2

Is the baby a candidate for therapeutic hypothermia?

1. Yes
2. No

The baby meets the criteria for cooling. He is term gestational age, is less than 6 h of age, has moderate encephalopathy, and has two additional criteria: a pH of 7 and a base deficit ≥16 mmol/L on umbilical cord blood sample.

Answer: 1

Approximately 50% of babies with hypoxic-ischemic encephalopathy are born in community hospitals to women with low-risk pregnancies and are not identified until after birth. Thus all delivery services in a community, including birthing centers, need to implement an educational program specifically addressing the awareness and timely identification and assessment of infants at risk for encephalopathy.

Case Presentation

You are called by the mother-baby care provider because she is concerned that a baby might be having seizures. She describes the baby as being very jittery and having a high pitched cry. The baby has been put to the breast every 2 h but still appears to be hungry. In between feeding he sucks frantically on his fist. His stools are loose and watery. The vital signs have been stable. He was born at term and is appropriate for gestational age.

Review of the mother's labor and delivery record indicates that she is a 27-year-old healthy primigravida who received prenatal care starting in the first trimester. Prenatal laboratory values are unremarkable, and she is not colonized with Group B streptococcus. Her labor was spontaneous in onset and lasted 22 h. Her membranes ruptured 10 h prior to delivery. Fetal presentation was vertex, and Apgar scores were 7, 9, and 9 at 1, 5, and 10 min. Analgesia during labor consisted of fentanyl via a patient-controlled pump. She was diagnosed with depression at 20 years of age and has been on a selective serotonin uptake inhibitor since then.

On observing the baby, you note that he is hyperalert and jittery. Physical examination findings include increased muscle tone, an exaggerated Moro reflex, and hyperactive deep tendon reflexes. You discuss your findings with the mother, and during the conversation, she tells you that she had severe back pain during the last month of her pregnancy and was given a prescription for Vicodin at a local urgent care center.

Although all of the following can be considered, the course of action with the highest yield would be:

1. A sepsis work up and place the baby on antibiotic therapy
2. Plasma glucose level

3. Serum ionized calcium level
4. Serial evaluation for signs of neonatal abstinence syndrome

Although neonatal sepsis, hypoglycemia, or hypocalcemia may present with the clinical picture above, the signs the infant is manifesting are more compatible with neonatal drug withdrawal. Common signs of neonatal drug withdrawal are outlined in Table 17.2. Neonatal abstinence syndrome can occur when low-dose prescription opiates are used during pregnancy [21]. The rising prevalence of prescription opioid use during pregnancy, particularly in the third trimester, has resulted in an increase in the number of infants with neonatal abstinence syndrome. In addition, recent evidence indicates that the ingestion of selective serotonin uptake inhibitors or benzodiazepines in addition to an opiate during pregnancy may increase the incidence and severity of neonatal abstinence syndrome [22, 23].

The baby has many of the clinical features of neonatal abstinence and needs to be monitored closely with a scoring tool to assess the severity of his withdrawal. There are several semi-objective tools available for quantifying the severity of neonatal withdrawal signs. The modified Neonatal Abstinence Scoring System is the most widely used tool [14]. Serial scores are helpful in deciding when to treat an infant with pharmacologic therapy.

Answer: 4

Table 17.2 Features of newborn drug withdrawal

Neurologic signs	Somatic signs
Tremors	Poor feeding
Irritability	Uncoordinated and constant suck
Increase wakefulness	Emesis
High pitched cry	Loose stools
Yawning and sneezing	Dehydration
Hypertonicity	Failure to gain weight
Increased deep tendon reflexes	Temperature instability
Exaggerated Moro reflex	Sweating
Seizures	Nasal congestion

The initial treatment of infants with confirmed intrauterine drug exposure who have no or minimal signs of withdrawal should include supportive measures such as minimizing environmental stimuli (e.g., sound and light), swaddling to prevent motor hyperactivity and to facilitate oral feeding, and offering frequent small feedings of hypercaloric (24 Cal/oz.) formula. If needed, padding the elbows, knees, and other pressure points to prevent skin excoriation and liberally applying barrier treatments to prevent diaper dermatitis are indicated.

Pharmacologic treatment is required when moderate to severe signs of NAS are documented; however the optimal threshold score for initiating pharmacologic therapy is unknown. The only clear benefit of pharmacologic treatment is the short-term amelioration of clinical signs. The severity of withdrawal signs, including seizures, after intrauterine drug exposure has not been associated with an increased risk of poor neurodevelopmental outcome [24, 25]. Additionally, there is no evidence that treatment results in improved neurodevelopmental outcome.

Pharmacologic treatment of neonatal abstinence syndrome includes all of the following, except:

1. Morphine
2. Methadone
3. Paregoric
4. Phenobarbital

Primary treatment with the same class of drug as the agent causing the withdrawal is usually successful. In the USA, the most commonly used drugs for neonatal drug withdrawal are oral morphine solution and methadone. If morphine or methadone does not adequately control withdrawal signs, the majority of practitioners use phenobarbital as a second drug [14]. There is emerging evidence that clonidine also is effective either as a primary or adjunctive therapy [26]. Paregoric is no longer used because it contains variable concentrations of other opioids, as well as toxic ingredients such as camphor, anise oil, alcohol, and benzoic acid. Additionally, diazepam is no longer recommended because it is less efficacious compared to other agents.

Answer: 3

If pharmacologic treatment is deemed necessary, initial dosing can be tailored to the severity of the signs of withdrawal. In most cases, maintenance doses of 0.2–0.3 mg/kg/day of oral morphine (divided every 3–4 h) or methadone (divided every 8–12 h) can be initiated with higher initial doses used for more severe signs of withdrawal. Because methadone has a longer half-life than morphine (12–24 h vs. 3–4 h), a loading dose of 0.4–0.5 mg/kg may be appropriate. In general, clinicians should wait 12–24 h to reach steady-state drug levels before increasing the dose. Infants who are not responsive to maximal doses of opioid therapy can be treated adjunctively with clonidine or phenobarbital. Once an infant has responded to treatment, the opioid dose can be weaned 10–20% every 1–2 days based on average withdrawal scores. Adjunctive therapy can be weaned once the opioid is discontinued. Opioid weaning can continue even if neonatal abstinence scoring is in the higher range of normal. Developing and adhering to a treatment protocol likely has a greater effect on reducing length of stay than does the choice of a particular drug.

Now that you have determined that the baby has neonatal abstinence syndrome. Which of the following actions are appropriate?

1. Drug screening
2. Discontinuation of breast feeding
3. Referral to child protective services
4. Transfer to a higher level of care

Drug screening is appropriate when there is a question regarding substance use during pregnancy. In the above example, you know what medications the mother took during her pregnancy; therefore drug screening is not needed. Because there is minimal transfer of opioids into breast milk, the American Academy of Pediatrics recommends that breastfeeding be encouraged, as long as the woman is not presently using illicit drugs [27]. Breastfeeding has been associated with decreased severity of neonatal abstinence syndrome symptoms, less need for pharmacotherapy, and a shorter hospital stay for the infant [23]. Breastfeeding contributes to the attachment between a mother and her baby, facilitates skin-to-skin care, and provides immunity to the infant. Breastfeeding should be encouraged and supported, not discouraged.

A referral for a social work assessment is appropriate to assess family, environmental, and social risk factors and the adequacy of support systems at home and to plan for discharge and subsequent follow-up care. Although it is recognized that the legal requirements to report neonatal abstinence syndrome vary from state to state, it is prudent, if possible, to refer to child protective services only if there is a legitimate concern about the future well-being of the infant.

Referral to a higher level of care will result in the separation of the mother and infant and, in many instances, limits the time the mother and family can spend with the baby. Institutions that have a delivery service should have an evidence-based written policy in place to assess and treat infants with neonatal abstinence syndrome. In addition, healthcare providers and staff caring for newborns should be trained in the correct use of an abstinence assessment tool. The ability to score the severity of signs of withdrawal with minimal interobserver variability enables decisions about the institution of pharmacologic therapy to be more objective and allows a quantitative approach to increasing or decreasing medications. Adoption of a weaning protocol has been associated with shorter duration of treatment, a shorter length of hospital stay, and a lower rate of adjunctive drug therapy [28].

Answer: 1, 3, 4

Case Presentation

You are seeing a 2-week-old infant in the clinic. The baby was born at term gestation and was appropriate for gestational age. Apgar scores were 8, 9, and 9 at 1, 5, and 10 min, respectively.

Bilirubin screening in the hospital placed the baby at low risk for hyperbilirubinemia.

The baby is breastfeeding for 15 min 8 times a day. Elimination includes six stools and six wet diapers daily. The infant is alert, active, and well hydrated. There is no evidence of clinical jaundice. Neurologic assessment reveals normal tone and reflexes. Pupils are midline and react to light and no nystagmus is noted.

The mother is concerned that the baby might be having seizures, because the baby has repetitive jerking movements when asleep. The movements occur on both sides and involve the arms and legs. She has noticed that the jerkiness stops when she wakes the baby.

At this point, you:

1. Admit the baby to the hospital for observation.
2. Order an electroencephalogram and make a referral to a pediatric neurologist.
3. Start the baby on phenobarbital.
4. Ask the mother to videotape the baby when asleep.

A history of jerking movements during sleep that stop when the baby is aroused is a hallmark of benign neonatal sleep myoclonus [29]. Characteristically, benign neonatal sleep myoclonus consists of repetitive myoclonic jerks that occur only during sleep and stop abruptly and consistently when the baby is awake [30, 31]. The movements typically begin in the first few weeks after birth and usually resolve spontaneously by 3 months of age [30–32]. The myoclonic jerks can involve the whole body, trunk, or limbs, but typically they are bilateral and symmetrical movements of the arms and/or the legs [29]. They do not stop with restraint, mimicking neonatal seizures. The myoclonus is thought to represent a transient disorder of the neurotransmitter system, possible serotonergic, in the neonatal period [30, 31].

The association with sleep is important in differentiating myoclonus from seizures, since the onset of clinically evident seizures usually occurs in the awake state. Infants with benign neonatal sleep myoclonus who have a normal neurological examination are not at risk for later neurodevelopmental problems [32].

Asking the parents to make a video of the infant's activity during sleep and arousal is helpful in deciding if benign neonatal sleep myoclonus is the most likely diagnosis [33]. If this is not feasible, an electroencephalogram while the infant is asleep is invaluable in distinguishing between benign neonatal sleep myoclonus and seizure activity. Whether you order the electroencephalogram or initially make a referral to a pediatric neurologist will depend on local practices and the timeliness of an appointment with the pediatric neurologist. Admission to the hospital for monitoring and observation is not optimal, because this process invariably results in extensive diagnostic testing, including brain imaging, and a great deal of anxiety for the family. Finally, antiepileptic medication is contraindicated in infants with benign neonatal sleep myoclonus, because it may actually worsen the myoclonus [29]. Because this form of myoclonus is a self-limited and benign condition, treatment is not indicated.

Answer: 4

Clinical Pearls

1. Assume that babies who are not breathing at birth have secondary apnea and need assistance with breathing.
2. Screen all newborn infants who undergo neonatal resuscitation with the modified Sarnat staging score for neonatal encephalopathy.
3. It is important to distinguish true seizures from clinical tremors and/or jitteriness.
4. Remember that the majority of abnormal movements noted in the newborn period are not epileptiform seizures.
5. There are strict criteria required for the initiation of cooling in newborn infants.
6. Carefully question mothers of babies with abnormal movements regarding

drug use, including prescription drugs, during pregnancy.
7. Use a neonatal abstinence scoring tool to assess the presence and severity of neonatal withdrawal signs and to decide when treatment is needed.
8. Don't warm a baby who is hypothermic before screening for neonatal encephalopathy.

References

1. Visser AM, Jaddoe VW, Arends LR, Tiemeir H, Hofman A, Moll HA, Steegers EAP, Breteler MMB, Arts WFM. Paroxysmal disorders in infancy and their risk factors in a population-based cohort: the generation R study. Dev Med Child Neurol. 2010;52:1014–20.
2. Gunn AJ, Gluckman PD, Gunn TR. Selective head cooling in newborn infants after perinatal asphyxia: a safety study. Pediatrics. 1998;102(4 pt 1):885–92.
3. Azzopardi D, Robertson NJ, Cowan FM, Rutherford MA, Rampling M, Edwards AD. Pilot study of treatment with whole body hypothermia for neonatal encephalopathy. Pediatrics. 2000;106(4):684–94.
4. Weiner GM, editor. *Textbook of neonatal* resuscitation. 7th ed. Elk Grove Village: American Academy of Pediatrics; 2016.
5. Apgar V. A proposal for a new method of evaluation of the newborn infant. Curr Res Anesth Analg. 1953;32(4):260–7.
6. Apgar V. The newborn (Apgar) scoring system: reflections and advice. Pediatr Clin North Am. 1966;13:645–50.
7. Pomerance J. Interpreting umbilical cord blood gases. 2nd ed. Pasadena: BNMG; 2004.
8. Sarnat HB, Sarnat MS. Neonatal encephalopathy following fetal distress: a clinical and electroencephalographic study. Arch Neurol. 1976;33(10):696–705.
9. Volpe JJ. Neurology of the newborn. 5th ed. Philadelphia: Saunders Elsevier; 2008.
10. Parker S, Zuckerman B, Bauchner H, et al. Jitteriness in full-term infants: prevalence and correlates. Pediatrics. 1990;85(1):17–23.
11. Parks D, Yetman RJ. The jittery newborn. J Pediatr Health Care. 2001;15(3):147–9.
12. Adamkin D. Postnatal glucose homeostasis in late-preterm and term infants. Pediatrics. 2011;127(3):575.
13. Kilpatrick SJ, Papile LA, editors. *Guidelines for perinatal care*. 8th ed. Washington, DC/Elk Grove Village: American College of Obstetricians and Gynecologists/American Academy of Pediatrics; 2017.
14. Hudak ML, Tan RC. Neonatal drug withdrawal. Pediatrics. 2012;129(2):e540–938.
15. Shankaran S, Laptook AR, Ehrenkranz RA, et al. National Institute of Child Health and Human Development neonatal Research Network. Whole body hypothermia for neonates with hypoxic-ischemic encephalopathy. N Engl J Med 2005;353(15):1574–84.
16. Gluckman PD, Wyatt JS, Azzopardi D, et al. Selective head cooling with mild systemic hypothermia after neonatal encephalopathy: multicenter randomized trial. Lancet. 2005;365(9460):663–70.
17. Azzopardi DV, Strohm B, Edwards AD, et al. TOBY Study Group. Moderate hypothermia to treat perinatal asphyxial encephalopathy. N Engl J Med. 2005;361(14):1349–58.
18. Jacobs SE, Morley CJ, Inder TE, et al. Infant Cooling Evaluation Collaboration. Whole-body hypothermia for term and near-term newborns with hypoxic-ischemic encephalopathy; a randomized clinical trial. Arch Pediatr Adolesc Med. 2011;165(8):692–700.
19. Wyatt JS, Gluckman PD, Lui PY, et al. Cool-Cap Study Group. Determination of outcomes after head cooling for neonatal encephalopathy. Pediatrics. 2007;119(5):912–21.
20. Laptook A, Tyson J, Shankaran S, et al. National Institute of Child Health and Human Development Neonatal Research Network. Elevated temperature after hypoxic-ischemic encephalopathy: risk factor for adverse outcomes. Pediatrics. 2008;112(3):491–9.
21. DeSai RJ, Huybrechts KF, Hernandez-Diaze S, Moqun H, Patomo E, Kaltenbach K, Kertzner LS, Bateman B. Exposure to prescription opioid analgesics in utero and risk of neonatal abstinence syndrome: a population based cohort study. BMJ. 2015;350:h2102.
22. Huybrechts KF, Bateman BT, Desai RJ, Hernandez-Diaz S, Rough K, Mogun H, Kerzner LS, Davis JM, et al. Risk of neonatal drug withdrawal after intrauterine co-exposure to opioids and psychotropic medications: cohort study. BMJ. 2017;358:j3326.
23. Bagley SM, Wachman EM, Holland E, Brogly SB. Review of the assessment and management of neonatal abstinence syndrome. Addict Sci Clin Pract. 2014;9(1):19.
24. Kaltenback K, Finnegan LP. Neonatal abstinence syndrome, pharmacotherapy and developmental outcome. Neurobehav Toxicol Teratol. 1986;8(4):353–5.
25. Doberczak TM, Shanzer S, Senie RT, Kandall SR. One-year follow-up of infants with abstinence-associated seizures. Arch Neurol. 1988;45(6):649–53.
26. Kraft WK, Adeniyi-Jones SC, Chervoneva I, Abatemarco D, Kaltenbach K, Ehlirch ME. Buprenorphine for the treatment of neonatal abstinence syndrome. N Engl J Med. 2017;376(24):2341–8.
27. Sachs HC. The transfer of drugs and therapeutics into human milk: a update on selected topics. Pediatrics. 2013;132:e796–809.
28. Hall ES, Wexelblatt SL, Crowley M, Grow JL, Jasin LR, Klebanoff MA, McClead RE, Meinzen-

Derr J, Mohan VK, Stein H, Walsh MC, OCHNAS Consortium. Implementation of a neonatal abstinence syndrome protocol weaning protocol: a multicenter cohort study. Pediatrics. 2016;136(4):e803–10.
29. Mauer VO, Rizzi M, Bianchetti MG, Ramelli GP. Benign neonatal sleep myoclonus: a review of the literature. Pediatrics. 2010;125(4):e19–24.
30. Huntsman RJ, Lowry NJ, Sankaran K. Nonepileptic motor phenomenon in the neonate. Peadiatr Child Health. 2008;13:680–4.
31. Cohen R, Shuper A, Straussberg R. Familial benign neonatal sleep myoclonus. Pediatr Neurol. 2007;36(5):334–7.
32. Cross JH. Differential diagnosis of epileptic seizures in infancy including the neonatal period. Semin Fetal Neonatal Med. 2013;18:192–5.
33. Di Capua M, Fusco L, Ricci S, Vigevano F. Benign neonatal sleep myoclonus: clinical features and video-polygraphic recordings. Mov Disord. 1993;8(2):191–4.

18 Developmental Dysplasia of the Hip

Lincoln Ferguson

Introduction

Developmental dysplasia of the hip (DDH) in broad terms refers to abnormal growth of the hip joint which can occur anywhere on the continuum from conception to full skeletal maturity. The term teratologic dislocation of the hip includes those cases where the hip did not develop normally in utero and usually presents as a fixed dislocation at birth. These are usually associated with other congenital abnormalities or neuromuscular disorders, the commonest of which are arthrogryposis, myelodysplasia, and myelomeningocele. The focus of this chapter will not be on these conditions but on newborns with congenital instability of the hip joint. This includes frank dislocation, subluxation (partial dislocation), or instability of the hip where there may be movement of the femoral head in and out of the acetabulum.

The incidence of DDH is presumed to be 1–1.5/1000 live births annually [1]. It is extremely important to make an early diagnosis and prompt treatment initiated as failure to do so may lead to lifelong consequences and chronic hip problems. The earlier the detection, the better the outcome. Every newborn should have a careful examination of the hip looking for abnormalities as part of the newborn physical examination. Hip examination should be done at all visits during the first year of life.

There is wide variability with the degree of dysplasia and instability present in DDH. More recent literature has shown that many mild forms of DDH resolve spontaneously without treatment [2, 3]. It is thought that the majority (up to 88%) of patients with mild disease resolve spontaneously by 2 months of age. However those with frank dislocation or more severe instability most often progress with worsening dysplasia [4]. This may lead to leg length discrepancies, abnormal gait, arthritis of the hip and knee joints, and chronic back pain among other long-term problems.

Case Presentation

An 8 lb. 2 oz. female is born at 40 weeks gestation via Cesarean section due to frank breech presentation. On examination at 12 hours of age, the baby's legs are still in hyperextension, and a "hip click" is elicited on examination.

All of the following increase the risk of having DDH in this patient except?

1. Female
2. Breech presentation
3. Presence of hip click
4. Family history of DDH

L. Ferguson, MD, MPH
Department of Pediatrics, Mount Sinai South Nassau Medical Center, Oceanside, NY, USA

NYIT College of Osteopathic Medicine, Glen Head, NY, USA
e-mail: Lincoln.ferguson@snch.org

G. I. Martin, W. Rosenfeld (eds.), *Common Problems in the Newborn Nursery*,
https://doi.org/10.1007/978-3-319-95672-5_18

Most cases of developmental dysplasia of the hip do not occur in patients with known risk factors [5]. It is therefore important that all babies are screened with a proper examination. Patients with certain risk factors may warrant further evaluation even with a negative exam. The incidence of DDH is found to be increased in breech presentation which appears to be the single most important risk factor. Family history of DDH in a first-degree relative has been shown to be associated with a 12-fold increased risk of DDH in the newborn. Also 80% of patients are usually female, and the left hip is affected in about 60% of cases, compared to 20% in the right hip and the other 20% bilateral [6]. The left hip is thought to be more commonly associated because of the left occipito-anterior position of most fetuses with the hip against the mother's spine adducted and little space available for abduction [1, 7]. Girls are thought to be more susceptible to the effects of the hormone relaxin which is produced during ovulation and usually declines in the absence of pregnancy. However during pregnancy, relaxin peaks during the first trimester and again at delivery. Relaxin appears to soften the pubic symphysis and relax the pelvic ligaments which can lead to instability of the hip joint. Other risk factors include family history, firstborns, and cultures with large-scale practice of swaddling.

The presence of a hip click does not increase risk but the presence of a hip clunk would. A hip click is an audible "click" or "pop" when a baby's hip is being examined and is not necessarily related to hip instability but rather the movement of tendons and ligaments adjacent to the hip joint. Hip clicks should be followed and if persistent can be a cause for concern warranting further evaluation. A clunk is a palpable "jerk" or sensation caused by the passage of the femoral head over the posterior lip of the ischium and is a sign of dislocation or dislocatability. This is usually felt during the Barlow maneuver, while the Ortolani test is a reductive maneuver (see Table 18.1).

Answer: 3

Table 18.1 Risk factors for developmental dysplasia of the hips

Risk Factors for Developmental Dysplasia of the Hip
Breech presentation
Female
Family history in first-degree relative
Oligohydramnios
Firstborn
Birthweight >4 kg
Swaddling
Monozygotic twin with other twin having DDH

What is the approximate percentage of babies with breech presentation having developmental dysplasia of the hip?

1. 30%
2. 20%
3. 10%
4. 5%

The hip joint consists of the femoral head and the acetabulum. They develop from the primitive mesenchyme, and their development is usually complete by the 11th week of gestation [1]. By the 12th week of gestation, medial rotation of the lower limbs occurs which can cause dislocation to the hip joint. By about the 18th week of gestation, the hip musculature develops. Hence conditions affecting the development of the hip muscles can lead to easy dislocations of the joint. These early dislocations are commonly called teratologic dislocations and can occur in conditions such as arthrogryposis and myelodysplasia [1].

The typical developmental dysplasia of the hip occurs in late pregnancy but can also occur postnatally. The last month of pregnancy can significantly affect the hip joint if there exist abnormal conditions in the environment in utero. Conditions such as frank breech presentation, uterine fibroids, and oligohydramnios can affect the positioning of the fetus in utero, thereby increasing the risk of hip dysplasia. Breech presentation occurs in about 3% of births, and developmental dysplasia of the hip occurs in more than 20% of these babies [1].

Answer: 2

Postnatally, tight swaddling restricting movement and causing abnormal positioning of the lower extremities can lead to DDH. Studies have shown that the incidence of DDH in cultures with this practice is significantly higher. Studies done in Native Americans showed that with interventions such as teaching "safe swaddling," the prevalence decreased from six times more to equal the prevalence in the general population in the United States [8]. Similar findings were found in studies done in other countries including Japan and Turkey. Although the frequency of traditional swaddling has been reduced in Turkey, traditional swaddling during infancy still is the greatest risk factor for hip dysplasia compared to breech birth, family history, or gender [9].

The most significant screening tool for DDH in the newborn is?

1. Physical examination
2. X-ray
3. Ultrasound
4. CT

Screening programs have been shown to be valuable in early diagnosis [10]. Physical examination remains the most significant screening tool in diagnosing DDH. While there are no tests pathognomonic for hip dislocation, the examiner must look for findings associated with increased risk for DDH. These include a positive Ortolani or Barlow test, leg length discrepancy, asymmetric skin folds, and restricted hip abduction.

Assessment of the hip joint should start with observation for asymmetry. This may be suggested by abnormal skin folds and leg length discrepancies. The Ortolani and Barlow tests are the most useful clinical examination tools to evaluate for developmental dysplasia of the hip in newborns. Less useful in the newborn is the Galeazzi sign which is elicited by laying the infant supine with the knees flexed and the feet placed flat. Unequal height of the knee is then observed. This is due to "apparent shortening" of the femur because of displacement from the acetabulum. Bilateral dislocations can thus be misleading. It may also be difficult to achieve the correct positioning to evaluate for Galeazzi sign in the newborn.

X-rays are not useful in the newborn as the ossification centers in the femoral head do not develop until 4–6 months. Ultrasound evaluation may be more helpful but is not always accurate before 3–4 weeks. Significant joint laxity in the newborn tends to produce abnormalities causing a high false-positive rate with early sonograms. This could lead to unnecessary treatment and unwarranted complications. Computerized tomography scans are not very useful at this time and expose the newborns to excessive and unnecessary radiation exposure.

Despite the focus on physical exam, it must be borne in mind that the incidence of late presentation of DDH has not significantly decreased and remains in the same range as those without screening. This is why ultrasound is recommended even in patients with normal exam if they are at high risk.

Answer: 1

During physical examination of the patient, the Barlow maneuver should be performed by?

1. Gentle adduction with posterior pressure on the femur
2. Gentle abduction with posterior pressure on the femur
3. Gentle adduction with anterior pressure on the hip
4. Gentle abduction with anterior pressure on the hip

The Barlow's maneuver (Fig. 18.1) is commonly used. Here the examiner dislocates an unstable hip joint. With the infant is lying supine, the thigh is grasped with the examiner's thumb on the medial aspect of the thigh and the middle finger along the greater trochanter. The hip and knees are flexed. The thigh is adducted while applying posteriorly directed pressure on the femur in the line of the femur shaft. This causes the femoral head to dislocate posteriorly from the acetabulum. Dislocation is palpable as the femoral head slips out of the acetabulum.

Answer: 1

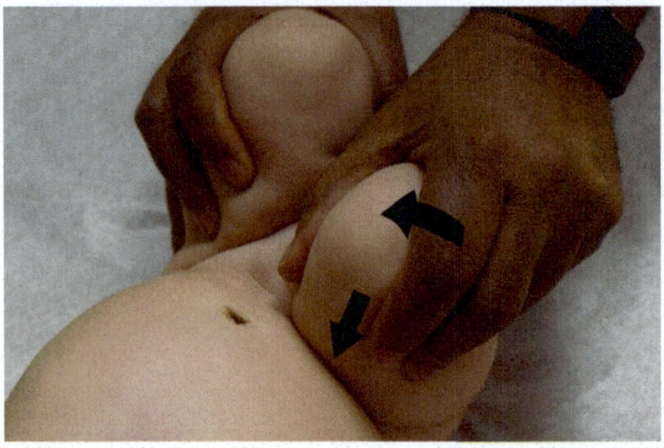

Fig. 18.1 Barlow maneuver. With the baby in the supine position, the hip is adducted while a posterior force is being applied on the thigh promoting dislocation (Photography by A. Agarwal, MD and E. Lewit)

During physical examination, how should the Ortolani maneuver be performed?

1. Gentle adduction with posterior pressure on the femur
2. Gentle abduction with posterior pressure on the femur
3. Gentle adduction with anterior pressure on the hip
4. Gentle abduction with anterior pressure on the hip

Ortolani maneuver (Fig. 18.2) is largely considered to be the most important clinical test used to detect DDH. The examiner relocates a dislocated femoral head into the acetabulum. Here the patient is lying supine. The examiners' index and middle fingers are placed along the greater trochanter and the thumb placed along the inner thigh. The infant's hip and knee are flexed to 90 degrees. The thigh is then gently abducted with gentle anterior pressure on the proximal femur bringing the femoral head from its posterior position to opposite the acetabulum. If positive, there is a palpable and audible clunk as the hip reduces.

Answer: 4

With both tests, each hip should be examined independently. Soft tissue clicks are commonly felt during these maneuvers but are not considered significant if no other abnormality is found.

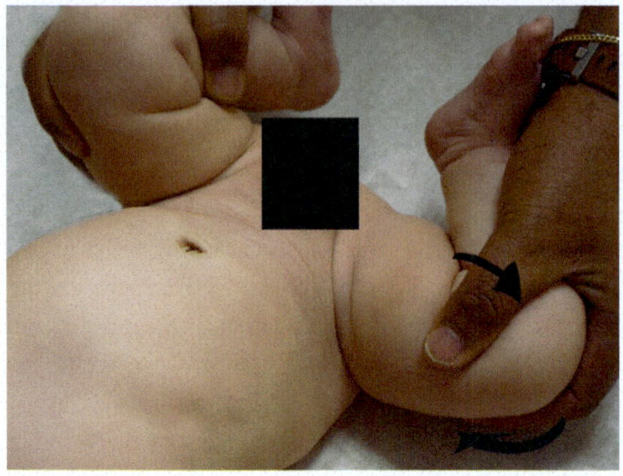

Fig. 18.2 Ortolani maneuver. With the baby in the supine position, the hip is adducted and an anterior force is applied on the femur with the fingers promoting reduction (Photography by A. Agarwal, MD and E. Lewit)

Remember DDH is a dynamic process, and a normal initial physical examination does not exclude a subsequent diagnosis. Patients should be fully evaluated at all health maintenance visits during the first year of life. By 3 months, the Ortolani and Barlow test may become unreliable, and limited abduction of the hip becomes more reliable. The accuracy of the Ortolani and Barlow maneuvers depends largely on the training and experience of the examiner [11].

The patient referred to in the first question was a term gestation, female, and frank breech presentation and had hip click on physical examination. How would you best manage the patient?

1. Reassure the parents.
2. Reassure the parents and reexamine in 2 weeks.
3. X-ray hips in frog leg position.
4. Ultrasound of hip.
5. Refer to orthopedics.

Reassurance only is unacceptable as this patient has multiple risk factors and could have DDH. X-rays at this early age are not likely to be useful since the femoral head is entirely composed of cartilage. As the ossification center in the femoral head develops by 4–6 months of age, X-rays become more useful at that time. Ultrasound can be very helpful but during the first month of life may result in many false positives, thus causing unnecessary treatments. Ultrasound should be used as an adjunct to clinical assessment and not as the sole diagnostic tool. Though most practitioners will tend to refer to orthopedics, this is not the preferred answer as the diagnosis is inconclusive and the orthopedist will most likely have to depend on the same modalities such as ultrasound to make a decision. The finding of a "click" on examination is fairly common among newborns. It is not necessarily related to hip instability but rather the movement of tendons and ligaments adjacent to the hip. A "clunk" which is felt is more likely to be a sign of DDH as it represents the passage of the femoral head over the posterior lip of the ischium. Patient should be reexamined in 2 weeks and if positive for a clunk or equivocal should be referred to orthopedics. If exam is negative, patient should have an ultrasound at 4–6 weeks [1].

Answer: 2

When do X-rays become most useful for diagnosing DDH?

1. During first week of life
2. After 1 month
3. After 2 months
4. After 4 months

Imaging should be used as an adjunct to physical examination after an abnormal exam. Plain radiography has not been proven useful in the first few months of life to diagnose DDH. The ossification center of the femoral head appears by the age 4–6 months [4]. Hence during this time, plain X-rays become more useful. X-rays have the advantage of being more available and having lower costs.

Answer: 4

Radiologists commonly utilize well-established lines on plain radiography to determine subluxation or dislocation. The more important ones are Hilgenreiner's, Perkin's, and Shenton's lines (see Fig. 18.3). Hilgenreiner's line is a horizontal line drawn on AP radiograph of the pelvis running between the inferior aspects of both triradiate cartilages of the acetabulum. Perkin's line is a line drawn perpendicular to Hilgenreiner's line intersecting the lateral-most aspect of the acetabular roof. Shenton's line is an imaginary curve line drawn along the inferior border of the superior pubic ramus (superior

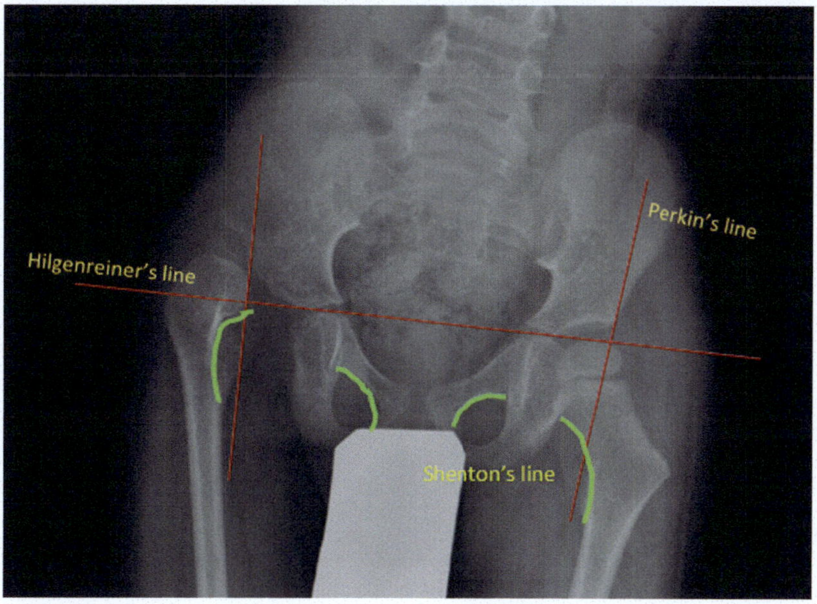

Fig. 18.3 X-ray showing Hilgenreiner's, Perkin's, and Shenton's lines. The right femoral head is in the upper outer quadrant, hence dislocated

border of the obturator foramen) and along the inferior medial border of the neck of the femur. The line should be smooth and continuous [12, 13]. Disruptions may be due to DDH or fracture of the neck of the femur.

Hilgenreiner's line and Perkin's lines divide the pelvis into four quadrants. The ossified capital femoral epiphysis should lie entirely within the inner lower quadrant. In subluxation or dislocation, the medial aspect of the ossified proximal femoral metaphysis usually lies within the superior lateral quadrant. In patients without ossification of the capital femoral epiphysis, the medial metaphyseal beak should lie within the inner lower quadrant of the lines.

Ultrasonography has been beneficial in the management of developmental dysplasia of the hip. Two methods are commonly available. In 1980 Graf described a method of static ultrasound imaging in the coronal plane [14, 15]. The Graf method (Fig. 18.4) uses static ultrasound imaging in a coronal plane assessing the position of the femoral head, the acetabulum, and the acetabular labrum and calculating alpha and beta angles. A normal alpha angle is at least 60 degrees. Less than 60 degrees suggests developmental dysplasia (Fig. 18.5). A Graf scale is used grading the abnormality from a grade I to grade IV where grade I represents no abnormality and grade IV complete dislocation. More institutions are now using a dynamic form of ultrasonography where the actual subluxation/dislocation can be seen in real time while performing the Ortolani and Barlow maneuver. In 1993 a North American standard was agreed upon which makes use of both methods combining one coronal Graf view with a transverse view with and without a modified Barlow maneuver [16]. Ultrasonography is however very user dependent and, though having a high negative predictive value, may cause a large amount of false-positive cases which in many instances lead to overtreatment. Ultrasonography ideally should not be done before the first 3–4 weeks of life as the significant

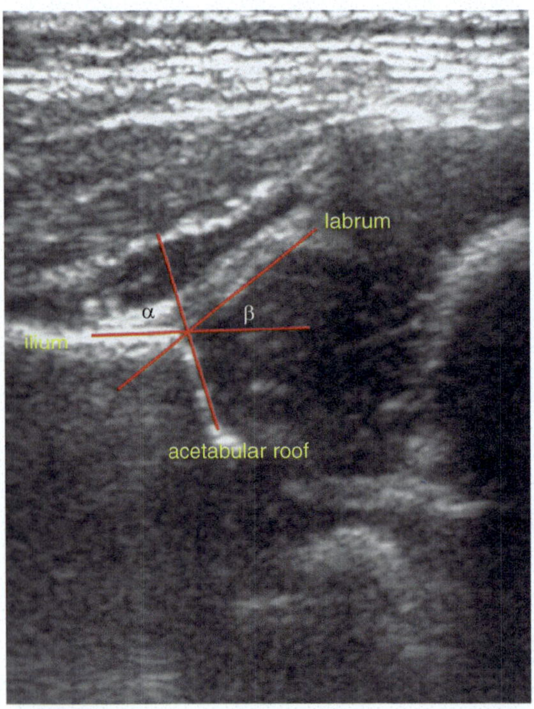

Fig. 18.4 Coronal view of hip ultrasound showing the normal positioning of the femoral head in acetabulum and the normal alpha angle. The beta angle also shown

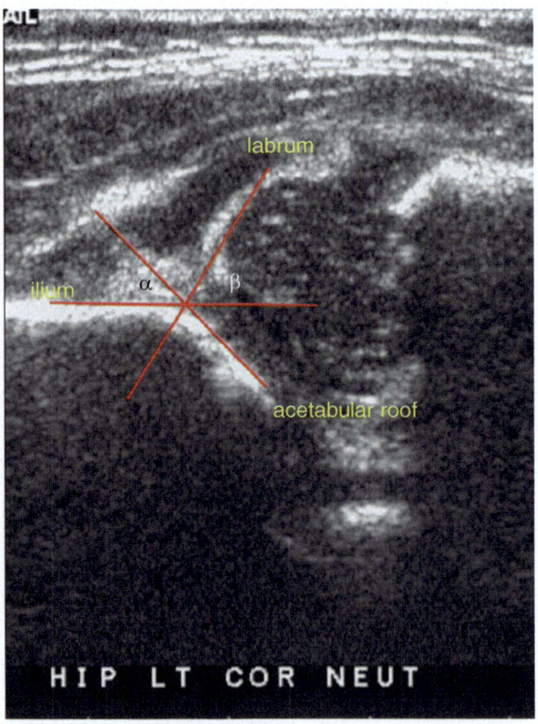

Fig. 18.5 Coronal view of hip ultrasound showing the abnormal positioning of the femoral head and a decreased alpha angle in a subluxated hip

joint laxity in the newborn will produce abnormalities on ultrasound that would not be detected by clinical exam, the vast majority of which will resolve by 6 weeks [4, 17]. The usefulness of ultrasound decreases as the femoral head ossifies, and so between 6 months and 1 year of age, radiography becomes more reliable, and by 1 year old, the ossification prevents good visualization of the acetabulum with ultrasound [17].

Computed tomography magnetic resonance imaging can be useful for evaluation after hip surgery, in complex cases especially those with complications such as avascular necrosis, and for follow-up. The significant radiation exposure with computed tomography is problematic hence limiting its widespread use. It is more used in adolescents and young adults for determining severity and procedure selection for treatment [18].

Magnetic resonance imaging (MRI) can be useful in evaluating the bony and soft tissue anatomy. At least one study showed that the presence of high signal intensity areas on MRI may correlate with risk for poor acetabular growth which could indicate the need for surgical correction. MRI may require a significant length of time to be performed and in most cases require sedation making it more tedious.

Arthrography involves injecting a radiopaque dye into the joint and a fluoroscopic examination. Hence this is a dynamic study. This can be useful in the operating room for showing the cartilaginous anatomy of the head of the femur and the acetabulum and whether there is interposition of soft tissue between the femoral head and the acetabulum. It is therefore useful in helping to determine whether closed reduction can be done or open reduction is needed [7].

Case Presentation

A female patient who was born via Cesarean section due to frank breech presentation at 40 weeks gestation, weighing 4100 g and found to have a hip click on physical exam at birth, now has normal hip examination at her 1-month visit.

How would you further manage this patient?

1. Order X-ray of the hip at 4–6 weeks.
2. Order hip ultrasound at 4–6 weeks.
3. Refer to orthopedics for further evaluation.
4. Continue to reexamine during the first year of life.

Breech presentation, female sex, and a family history of developmental dysplasia of the hip are the most important factors that determine the risk for newborns to develop hip dysplasia (Fig. 18.6). Breech presentation may be the most important single risk factor [3, 4]. If this was a male patient and breech presentation, ordering subsequent imaging would be optional, and follow-up periodic exam could be done. If the exam is abnormal, then the patient should be referred to orthopedics. This being a female patient and breech presentation, an ultrasound at 4–6 weeks is recommended [1]. With the risk factors, DDH may still develop, hence the need to screen with ultrasonography. X-rays would not be helpful at 4–6 weeks because the ossification center in the femoral head is unlikely to appear this early. An orthopedic evaluation would not be necessary at this time since examination is normal.

Answer: 2

The patient had the ultrasound done at 2 months old and was found to have mild instability of the hip joint. She was referred to orthopedics for further treatment. How should the patient be treated?

1. Apply a Pavlik harness.
2. Open reduction and hip Spica.
3. Use double/triple diapers.
4. Continue to monitor with bimonthly evaluations.
5. Reassure parents, no need for further management.

Developmental dysplasia of the hip can be treated surgically or nonsurgically. This is largely dependent on age of diagnosis, severity, and response to previous treatment. The aim is to achieve and maintain a reduced hip joint at the

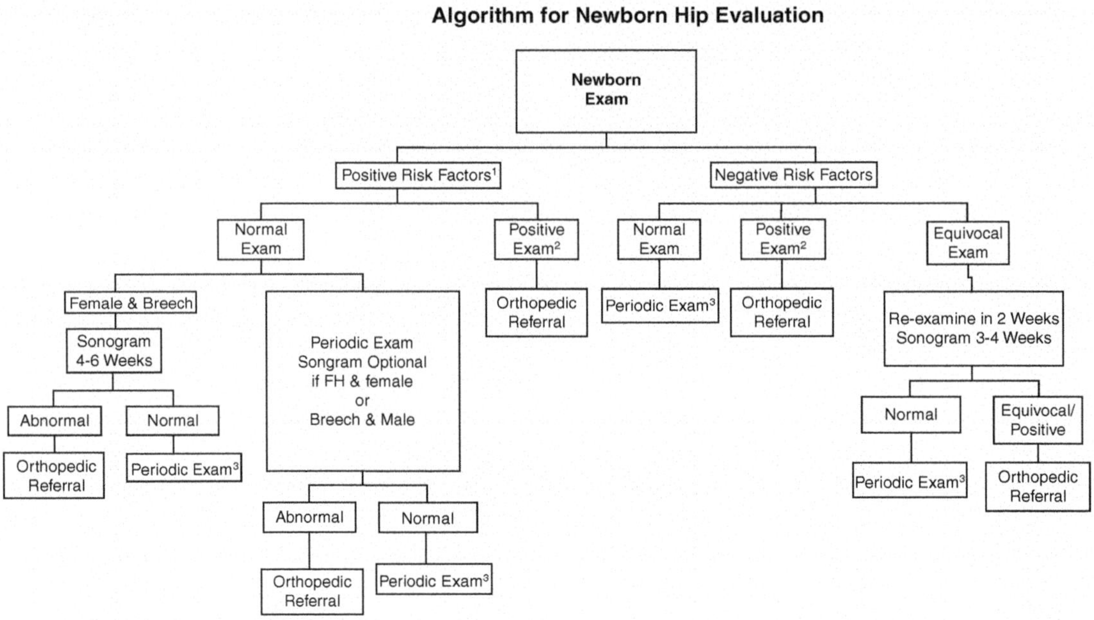

Fig. 18.6 Algorithm for screening for congenital developmental dysplasia of the hip
¹ – Risk factors: breech, family history (FH)
² – Positive exam: abnormal Ortolani/Barlow, decreased hip abduction
³ – Periodic exam: hip evaluation at all well visits <1 year old

youngest possible age with little or no complications. This will reduce the likelihood of later severe osteoarthritis and the chances of requiring hip replacement at an early age.

Patients younger than 6 months with overt dislocation or dislocatable hips are usually treated with a harness or brace. The Pavlik harness, which is the most popular choice, is a soft positioning device which holds the hip in the proper position while allowing movement of the legs and enables easy diaper care. Patient usually wears this device for 1–2 months allowing normal formation of the acetabulum. The main features include a frontal leg strap that flexes the hip and a posterior leg strap that prevents adduction though extreme abduction should be avoided. Close follow-up in most cases at weekly intervals is needed to monitor progress. The Pavlik harness has been found to have >90% success rates [4, 19]. Other devices include the Craig splint and the Von Rosen splint which are used less frequently.

Patients 6 months to 2 years can be treated by closed reduction and Spica casting. This is usually done under general anesthesia and is also indicated for patients who failed to achieve stable reduction using the Pavlik harness. Spica casting is more restrictive and more cumbersome for patient during cleaning and diaper change. Parents should be taught by the healthcare team how to perform their regular task in caring for the child. The use of the Pavlik harness after the age of 6 months is not recommended by most authors [4]. However studies are showing usefulness and good results in certain types of dislocations in patients up to 24 months [20].

In patients with mild instability of the hip, watchful waiting can be done with reexamination twice monthly. If the instability continues for longer than 3–6 weeks, patients should see orthopedics so that a harness can be placed. Review studies have shown that treatment and surgery rates have been reduced by postponing treatment in these patients for 2–8 weeks without any significant increase in dysplasia diagnosed later [21].

The use of double/triple diaper is not recommended as studies have not shown any significant improvement compared to not giving any treatment.

Answer: 1

In patients 6 months to 2 years where closed reduction procedures have been unsuccessful, open reduction is usually done. Open reduction is also considered in patients older than 18 months. These children usually require surgery to realign the hip joint and a hip spica cast placed postsurgery to keep the hip in place. This is worn for 6 weeks to 3 months followed by physical therapy. The outcome is generally better, the earlier the treatment is done, but even with treatment, complications such as osteoarthritis, abnormal gait, and hip deformity may still occur later in life.

Children with diagnosis of developmental dysplasia of the hip should have orthopedic follow-up until skeletal maturity [22, 23]. However, there is wide disagreement regarding the frequency of follow-up, the necessity for radiologic monitoring, and the types of studies that should be used. Many argue close follow-up, and frequent radiologic monitoring is necessary, while others argue against frequent X-ray studies due to the effect of radiation exposure.

Long-term complications of treatment of developmental dysplasia of the hip are:

1. Avascular necrosis of the femoral head
2. Psychological effects on patients
3. Osteoarthritis of the hip joint
4. 1 and 3 only
5. All of the above

The most important adverse effect of developmental dysplasia of the hip treatment is avascular necrosis of the femoral head (AVN) [2, 11]. This can occur with both surgical and nonsurgical treatment. This leads to severe joint dysfunction, pain, growth arrest, osteoarthritis, and eventual destruction of the hip joint. Most patients will eventually require joint replacement. Other complications include femoral nerve palsy which can resolve, joint stiffness, musculotendinous contractures, skin irritation, pressure ulcers, infection, anesthesia complications, and possible psychological effects on patient and parents.

Answer: 5

Clinical Pearls

1. The stability of the head of the femur in the acetabulum during fetal life and postnatally is necessary for normal hip development.
2. Despite the major focus on screening by hip examination from birth, the incidence of late diagnosis of DDH has not significantly fallen.
3. Clinical examination remains the most important screening method and is recommended by the American Academy of Pediatrics.
4. Clinical assessment of the hips should be done at all well visits through the first year of life.
5. Ultrasound is the study of choice in detecting and confirming DDH in early infancy, but routine screening is controversial because of the likelihood of overtreatment.
6. Ultrasound screening is recommended in all high-risk infants at 4–6 weeks of age whether or not positive findings are present.
7. Universal ultrasound screening is not recommended in North America because of inconsistency, subjectivity, and high false-positive rates, given an overall population disease prevalence of 1–2% [24].
8. The use of imaging and imaging techniques are evolving and likely to involve a greater role for MRI and CT scan in the future.
9. Postdelivery cases due to swaddling are preventable and have significantly decreased with education of certain populations.
10. Follow-up imaging is recommended for patients diagnosed and treated for DDH at least in the first year.
11. Early diagnosis and management yield the best result.
12. Unnecessary treatment can have negative consequences such as avascular necrosis.

References

1. American Academy of Pediatrics. Clinical practice guideline: early detection of developmental dysplasia of the hip. Committee on quality improvement, subcommittee on developmental dysplasia of the hip. American Academy of Pediatrics. PediatErics 2000 April;105:896–905.
2. Shipman SA, Helfand M, Moyer V, Yawn B. Screening for developmental dysplasia of the hip: a systematic literature review for the US preventative services task force. Pediatrics. 2006;117(898):e557.
3. Shaw BA, Seegal LS, AAP Section on Orthopaedics. Evaluation and referral for developmental dysplasia of the hip in infants. Pediatrics. 2016;138(6):e20163107.
4. Kotlarsky P, Haber R, Bialik V, Eidelman M. Developmental dysplasia of the hip: what has changed in the last 20 years? World J Orthop. 2015 Dec 18;6(11):886–901.
5. Schwend RM, Schoenecker P, Richards BS, Flynn JM, Vitale M. Pediatric orthopedic Society of North America. Screening the newborn for developmental dysplasia of the hip: now what do we do? J Pediatr Orthop. 2007;27(6):607–10.
6. Storer SK, Skaggs DL. Developmental dysplasia of the hip. Am Fam Physician. 2006 Oct 15;74(8):1310–6.
7. Guille JT, Pizzutillo PD, MacEwen GD. Developmental dysplasia of the hip from birth to six months. J Am Acad Orthop Surg. 2000;8:232–42.
8. Yamamuro T, Ishida K. Clin Orthop Relat Res. 1988;184:34–40.
9. Dogruel H, et al. Int Orthop. 2008;32:415–9.
10. Darmonov AV, Zagora S. Clinical screening for congenital dislocation of the hip. J Bone Joint Am. 1996 Mar;78(3):383–8.
11. Jackson JC, Runge MM, Nye NS. Common questions about developmental dysplasia of the hip. Am Fam Physician. 2014 Dec 15;90(12):843–50.
12. Campbell SE. Radiography of the hip: lines, signs and patterns of disease. Semin Roentgenol. 2005;40(3):290–319.
13. Jones DH. Shenton's line. J Bone Joint Surg Br. 2010;92(9):1312–5.
14. Karmazyn BK, Gunderman RB, Coley BD, Blatt ER, Bulas D, Fordham L, Podberesky DJ, Prince JS, Paidas C, Rodriguez W. ACR appropriateness criteria on developmental dysplasia of the hip-child. J Am Coll Radiol. 2009;6:551–7.
15. Graf R. The diagnosis of congenital hip-joint dislocation by compound treatment. Arch Orthop Trauma Surg. 1980;97:117–33.
16. American College of Radiology. ACR practice guideline for the performance of the ultrasound examination for detection of developmental dysplasia of the hip. In: Practice guidelines and technical standards. Reaston: American College of Radiology; 2007. p. 997–1001.
17. American Institute of Ultrasound in Medicine. American College of Radiology. AUIM practice guideline for the performance of an ultrasound examination for detection and assessment of developmental dysplasia of the hip. J Ultrasound Med. 2009;28:114–9.
18. Grissom L, Harcke HT, Thacker M. Imaging in surgical management of developmental dislocation of the hip. Clin Orthop Relat Res. 2008;466:791–801.
19. Cashman JP, Round J, Taylor G, Clarke NM. The natural history of developmental dysplasia of the hip after early supervised treatment in the Pavlik harness. A prospective, longitudinal follow up. J Bone Joint Surg Br. 2002;84:418–25.
20. van de Sande MA, Melisie F. Successful Pavlik treatment in late-diagnosed developmental dysplasia of the hip. Int Orthop. 2012;36:1661–8.
21. Shorter D, Hong T, Osborn D. Cochrane review: screening programmes for developmental dysplasia of the hip in newborn infants. Evid Based Child Health: A Cochrane Review Journal. 2013 Jan;8(1):11–54.
22. Schwend RM, Shaw BA, Segal LS. Evaluation and treatment of developmental dysplasia in the newborn and infant. Peadiatr Clin North Am. 2014;61:1095–107.
23. AAOS developmental dislocation(dysplasia) of the hip(DDH) http://orthoinfo.aaos.org/topic.cfm?topic=a00347.
24. American Academy of Orthopaedic Surgeons. Detection and nonoperative management of Pediatric Developmental Dysplasia of Hip in infants up to six months of age, Evidence-Based Clinical Practice Guideline. Rosemont: American Academy of Orthopaedic Surgeons; 2014.

Ambiguous Genitalia and Problems with Sexual Differentiation

19

Moris Angulo

Ambiguous Genitalia and Problems with Sexual Differentiation

Ambiguous genitalia is a rare condition in which an infant's external genitals do not appear to be clearly either male or female. The incidence of genital ambiguity that results in the child's sex being uncertain is 1 per 4500 [1], although some degree of male under-virilization or female virilization may be present in as many as 2% of live births [2]. Parents and doctors may not be able to immediately determine the newborn's sex. For example, a baby can have an enlarged clitoris that looks more like a small penis and fusion of the labia so that they look more like a scrotum. Ambiguous genitalia is not a disease but a sign of a condition that affects sexual development. Practically, sexual development can be divided into three separate areas: chromosomal, gonadal, and anatomical sex (Fig. 19.1).

A problem in any one of these three areas may lead to issues with sex determination or differentiation. Understanding the cascade from genetic (sex chromosomes), gonadal (ovaries and testicles), and anatomical sex (female or male phenotype) is essential to understanding "sex determination and differentiation." Collectively, conditions resulting in discordance between genetic, gonadal, and anatomic sex are referred to as disorders of sex development (DSD) and may affect up to 1:1000 individuals in the population [3–5].

Genetic factors as well as hormonal production and action are essential for normal sex development (Table 19.1).

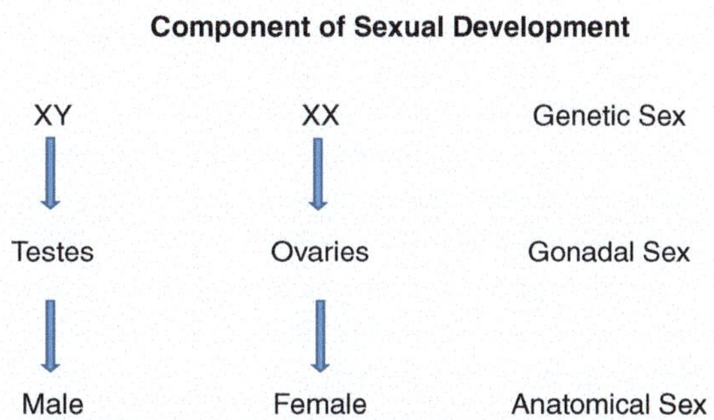

Fig. 19.1 To simplify understanding of sexual development and abnormalities, it should be divided into genetic, gonadal, and anatomical sex (phenotype). Genetic sex is determined from the moment of conception and determines the differentiation of the gonad. The differentiation of the gonad in turn determines the development of both the internal genital tracts and the external genitalia and thus phenotypic sex, which occurs later in development (from about 5–6 weeks of gestation). Both male and female genitalia differentiate from the same structures along the urogenital ridge that contains the cells that are the precursors for follicular, Sertoli, theca, and Leydig cells. DSDs are congenital conditions in which development of the chromosomal, gonadal, or anatomic sex is atypical

M. Angulo, MD
SUNY/Stony Brook School of Medicine, Stony Brook, NY, USA

Division of Genetics, NYU Winthrop Hospital, Mineola, NY, USA
e-mail: mangulo@nyuwinthrop.org

G. I. Martin, W. Rosenfeld (eds.), *Common Problems in the Newborn Nursery*,
https://doi.org/10.1007/978-3-319-95672-5_19

Table 19.1 Major steps involved in development of internal and external genitalia

Steps in sex determination and differentiation	
Sex determination	Formation of a 46 XY or 46 XX zygote
Sex differentiation: gonadal differentiation	Formation of either testes or ovary
Sex differentiation: ductal differentiation	Maintenance of Wolffian structures with regression of Müllerian structures or vice versa
Sex differentiation: differentiation of external genitalia	Masculinization of external genitalia under the influence of dihydrotestosterone (DHT) in a male

Genetic factors on both sex and autosomal chromosomes are required to have normal gonadal development in either sex. Early in gestation, the tissue that will become the gonads is undifferentiated and has the potential to become either ovaries or testes. The sex-determining region of the Y gene (*SRY* gene) on the short arm of the Y chromosome initiates male sex differentiation of this gonadal tissue to develop as a testis [6] around the 6th week of fetal life. In turn, the testes produce testosterone, which stimulates the growth of Wolffian structures (internal male genitalia), and anti-Müllerian hormone (AMH), which suppresses the development of Müllerian structures (uterus, cervix, and the upper one third of the vagina). Müllerian structures do not require hormonal stimulation but rather develop when there is an absence of AMH.

Phenotypic females with normal external genitalia but who have a XY chromosomes are either the result of complete androgen insensitivity syndrome (CAIS) or complete gonadal dysgenesis. Partial androgen insensitivity syndrome (PAIS) and partial gonadal dysgenesis however could result in ambiguous genitalia in a 46 XY newborn. The enzyme 5-α-reductase-2 is needed for conversion of testosterone (T) to dihydrotestosterone (DHT), the final step of male masculinization. 5-α-Reductase-2 deficiency therefore can also result in ambiguous genitalia. Some enzymes required for androgen production from cholesterol are shared by testis and adrenal cortex. Enzyme deficiencies in adrenal cortisol synthesis will divert accumulated cortisol precursors to androgen biosynthesis and result in ambiguous genitalia in otherwise normal genetic XX female with congenital adrenal hyperplasia (CAH).

Usually, ambiguous genitalia are obvious at or shortly after birth, and it can be very distressing for families and health-care providers as well. A medical team of specialists will determine the cause of ambiguous genitalia and provide information and counseling that can help guide decisions about the baby's gender and any necessary treatment. However, nursery providers are often the first ones to meet the parents and provide information about the health and newborn's sex. The parents should receive adequate education and counseling and participate in making the decision concerning their child's sex assignment. The main objective of this chapter is to discuss the basic knowledge necessary to understand normal and abnormal sexual development.

Case Presentation

You are called to see an infant shortly after birth with ambiguous genitalia: enlarged clitoris that looks like a small penis, with a single urethral/vaginal opening and almost complete fusion of the labia without any other dysmorphic features. Parents are waiting to hear about their first newborn's condition.

In order to provide the best and most accurate information as quickly as possible, you should?

1. Order chromosome analysis and wait until genetic sex has been determined before assigning sex.
2. Order STAT serum 17-hydroxyprogesterone levels.
3. Send off state metabolic screen sample on day 2 of life.
4. Order pelvic sonogram.

In infants born with ambiguous genitalia or any other abnormality of external genitalia, sex assignment is never based on the genetic sex alone; therefore, we should not wait for chromosome analysis to inform the parents about their infant's sex. Chromosomal analysis helps to determine genetic sex, 46 XX or 46 XY, but it could be discordant with anatomical sex; therefore, further testing including hormone levels in the blood and possibly urine and/or ultrasound in addition to the chromosome and molecular analysis will be necessary. While state screening can be helpful, it takes many days to be analyzed and results returned. If there is suspicion of a metabolic cause, then immediate testing should be performed.

Answer: 2, 4

The parents are very concerned and are waiting to talk to you after you examine the baby.

Your approach might include the following, except?

1. Tell them all the data must be collected before you can talk.
2. Reassure them a sex will be assigned.
3. They did nothing wrong and the problem was not preventable.
4. The problem is treatable.
5. You may be able to give them answers after blood tests and sonogram.

Parents require reassurance that either a male or female gender will definitely be assigned. However, the outcome of some of the investigations may take few days or even weeks, and registration of the child's birth should be occasionally deferred until gender has been assigned. It is also helpful (if appropriate) to reassure the parents that their child is otherwise healthy. Keeping in mind that the normal source of sex hormones is the gonads (ovaries and testes) and adrenal glands, parents should be informed that infants born with ambiguous genitalia are usually over-virilized female or under-virilized male infants. The good news is that the majority of these infants born with ambiguous genitalia are the results of female virilization in uterus by excessive androgen (male hormone) production by the adrenal gland with excellent prognosis. Congenital adrenal hyperplasia (CAH) is the most common cause of ambiguous genitalia in newborn infants. CAH includes a group of autosomal recessive diseases resulting from mutations of genes for enzymes mediating the biochemical steps of production of cortisol (stress hormone), aldosterone (salt-retaining hormones), or androgens from cholesterol by the adrenal glands. The most common form of CAH is associated with excessive androgen production and ambiguous genitalia in female infants.

For the most part, these effects of CAH can be treated with hormone replacement therapy which counteracts the overproduction of androgens. Serum hormone level results can be obtained in 2 days and newborn screening a few days later. Due to the high incidence of CAH in infants with ambiguous genitalia, pediatric endocrinologists may start medical treatment even before hormonal results are available. Once the condition is confirmed and stable, the female infant can be discharged on hormonal replacement therapy and followed by pediatric endocrinologists and pediatric surgeon if surgery were necessary. Parents should be reassured that they did not do anything wrong and there is nothing they could have done to prevent it.

Answer: 1

After informing parents about the condition, they accepted that "something was wrong" and they asked what caused it to occur. What will be an appropriate response?

1. Abnormal chromosome
2. Genetic condition is unlikely
3. Defect of sex determination or differentiation
4. Most likely abnormal internal organs
5. Sex cannot be determined

Conditions resulting in discordance between genetic, gonadal, and anatomic sex are the result of defective sex determination or differentiation and are now referred to as disorders of sex development (DSD) with good prognosis. This includes chromosomal abnormalities, failure of sexual organs to develop, excessive androgen exposure, and failure of end-organ responsiveness to androgens.

Answer: 3

Children who are born with ambiguous genitalia may have which of the following karyotypes?

1. 46 XX
2. 46 XY
3. 46 XX/46 XY
4. 45 X/46 XX
5. All of the above

While there are a number of different genetic causes of ambiguous genitalia, many patients will have normal karyotypes. The cause in many cases is not known and the disorder appears to occur by chance.

Children with ambiguous genitalia and 46 XX karyotype will have normal internal female structures (uterus, ovaries, fallopian tubes) but masculinized external genitalia. The most common cause of 46 XX DSD is congenital adrenal hyperplasia (CAH). 46 XX DSD can also result from exposure of the fetus to high levels of androgens while in utero in conditions such as maternal virilizing ovarian tumor.

Children with 46 XY karyotype can have normal female external genitalia. Basically, the defect could be in "determination and differentiation" (Fig. 19.1), such as XY gonadal dysgenesis and complete androgen insensitivity syndrome (CAIS), respectively. The loss of the *SRY* or a mutation of the SRY gene that does not allow it to function will result in 46 XY gonadal dysgenesis. As a result, the testis will not develop, and internal and external female genitalia will develop. In CAIS, the testes are anatomically normal, but the end organs are not responsive to normal testicular androgens (testosterone). Without testosterone, the baby will have female external genitalia. Both, complete XY gonadal dysgenesis and CAIS are associated with normal female external genitalia, whereas their partial form can result in ambiguous genitalia.

Ovotesticular DSD is characterized by the presence of both ovarian and testicular tissue in the same individual. An ovotestis (combination of ovary and testis in the same gonad) is present in approximately 2/3 of affected individuals. The most affected individuals have a 46 XX chromosomal makeup followed by XY and mosaicism. If a uterus is present, it is usually underdeveloped (hypoplastic). The external genitalia are usually ambiguous with an abnormal vagina. If a penis is present, it is usually very small with hypospadias. Ovotesticular DSD is diagnosed by a combination of tests including chromosome and genetic analysis, hormonal testing, ultrasound or MRI, and gonadal biopsy. Gender assignment is recommended in the neonatal period and is based on the appearance of the external genitalia, the formation of the internal reproductive glands, and the potential for fertility. Children with 45 X/46 XX or any other sex chromosome mosaicism have undeveloped gonads with female internal structures. Their external genitalia, however, may vary from female, ambiguous, to male phenotype due to residual hormonal production.

Answer: 5

What is the most common cause of ambiguous genitalia?

1. Partial androgen insensitivity syndrome.
2. Congenital adrenal hyperplasia (CAH)
3. Sex chromosome DSD
4. Disorders of gonadal development
5. Ovotesticular DSD

Ninety percent of infants born with ambiguous genitalia have CAH. Approximately 95% of all CAH cases have 21-hydroxylase deficiency, characterized by decreased cortisol and aldosterone production and simultaneous increased production of adrenal androgens that result in masculinization of female infant's genitals [7, 8]. Male infants, however, may have normal-appearing genitalia. CAH is a group of autosomal recessive disorders with an incidence between 1:10,000 to 1: 20,000 births [9–12]. The cortisol synthetic block leads to corticotropin stimulation of the adrenal cortex, with accumulation of cortisol precursors that are diverted to sex hormone biosynthesis (Fig. 19.2). If the disorder is not recognized and treated, both girls and boys undergo rapid postnatal growth and sexual precocity or, in the case of severe enzyme deficiency, neonatal salt loss and death. About 75% of classic CAH cases suffer aldosterone deficiency with

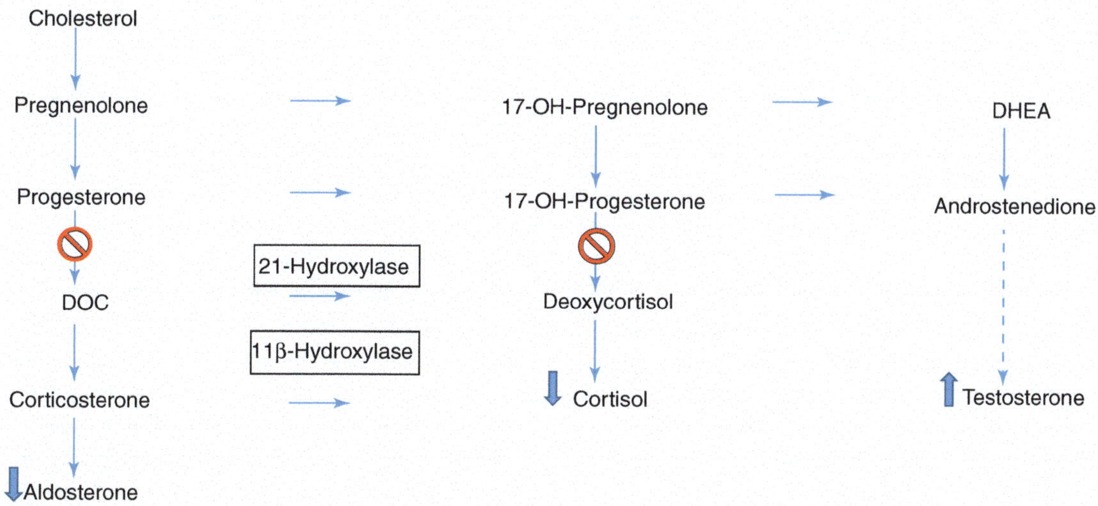

Fig. 19.2 Fetal adrenal steroidogenesis with 21-hydroxylase deficiency (21-OHD). This enzyme deficiency leads to cortisol and mineralocorticoid (aldosterone) deficiency. Corticotropin (ACTH) stimulation of the adrenal cortex leads to accumulation of cortisol precursors which are diverted to androgen biosynthesis with ambiguous genitalia in females but normal genitalia in males. One of the precursors, 17-OH-progesterone level, is used in the newborn screening for CAH due to 21-hydroxylase deficiency

salt wasting, failure to thrive, and potentially fatal hypovolemia and shock [13]. The second most common cause of CAH is 11β-hydroxylase (5–8%) [14]. Both ovarian and testicular tissues are present in ovotesticular DSD (formerly termed true hermaphroditism), an uncommon cause of genital ambiguity.

Answer: 2

The following is true for CAH, except?

1. Treatment may include glucocorticoids.
2. Boys with 21-hydroxylase deficiency (21-OHD) have less glucocorticoid and mineralocorticoid deficiency than affected girls.
3. 21-hydroxylase deficiency is the most common form of CAH.
4. Newborn screening for CAH is assessed by 17-hydroxyprogesterone.

CAH due to a 21-hydroxylase enzyme defect is the most common form and occurs equally often in XX and XY individuals. This form of CAH, however, does not cause ambiguous genitalia in XY individuals because their testes already produce enough testosterone that the added virilizing adrenal hormones do not make a significant difference. Newborn girls with genital ambiguity often come quickly to medical attention, but boys with normal genitalia can have the same medical emergency due to mineralocorticoid and glucocorticoid deficiency. Surgery should only be considered in girls with severe virilization (Prader stage $\geq$ 3) with emphasis on functional outcome rather than a strictly cosmetic appearance. Without newborn screening for CAH by assessing the level of 17-hydroxyprogesterone, affected XY infants could be missed at birth and readmitted later on in adrenal crisis. Molecular testing can be performed in affected individuals, suspected carriers, and prenatally.

Answer: 2

In congenital adrenal hyperplasia (21-OHD CAH)?

1. A genetic male develops ovaries.
2. A genetic male is born with both fallopian tubes, a prostate, and seminal vesicles.
3. An excess level of androgens results in external genitals that are partly or completely male in appearance in a genetic female.

4. A genetic male is likely to be identified as female at birth.
5. Undertreated children may have decreased growth rate.

Males born with classic form of 21-OHD CAH will have normal internal and external genitalia.

Prenatal androgen exposure in females, howfever, has a virilizing effect on the external genitalia. Undertreated boys and girls will have enough androgens to accelerate skeletal maturation and growth velocity. Early complete fusion of the bones, however, can result in lower adult potential height.

Answer: 3

In affected untreated individuals with 21-hydroxylase deficiency (21-OHD CAH), the following is true, except?

1. Diagnosis of 21-OHD CAH is confirmed by biochemical findings, such as an unequivocally elevated serum concentration of 17-OHP.
2. Measurement of 17-OHP concentration in paper blood spot sample is used for newborn screening.
3. If the parents of a proband are both obligate heterozygotes, the risk for an affected child is 25%.
4. Samples taken in the first 24 hours of life are low in all infants and may give false-negative results.
5. In the classical 21-OHD CAH, 25% of affected individuals have simple virilizing and 75% salt-wasting form.

Increased concentration of 17-hydroxyprogesterone (17-OHP) seen on paper blood spot (newborn screen) and serum is required for screening and diagnosis of 21-OHD CAH, respectively.

If the parents of a proband are both obligate heterozygotes, each sib has a 25% chance of inheriting both altered alleles and being affected, a 50% chance of inheriting one altered allele and being an unaffected carrier, and a 25% chance of inheriting both normal alleles and being unaffected. Samples for serum 17-OHP taken in the first 24 hours of life are elevated in all infants and may give false-positive results [15, 16]. False-positive results may also be observed in low-birth-weight infants [16] or premature infants [17]. CAH can be divided in classic and nonclassic. The classic form is further divided into the simple virilizing form (~25% of affected individuals) and the salt-wasting form, in which aldosterone production is inadequate (>75% of individuals). Newborns with salt-wasting 21-OHD CAH are at risk for life-threatening salt-wasting crises. Treatment for CAH principally involves glucocorticoid replacement therapy and mineralocorticoid (9α-fluorohydrocortisone) in individuals with the salt-wasting form of 21-OHD CAH. Individuals with the nonclassic form of 21-OHD CAH have only moderate enzyme deficiency and present postnatally with signs of hyperandrogenism; females with the nonclassic form are not virilized at birth. The use of an algorithm (Fig. 19.3) provides additional help in diagnoses, counseling, and management of an infant with ambiguous genitalia with 46 XX DSD.

Answer: 4

Case Presentation

An anxious 34-year-old pregnant mother requested prenatal diagnosis with serum cell-free DNA at 10-week gestation. Results revealed 46 XY genetic sex without any chromosomal abnormalities. Immediately after delivery, she was informed about her healthy-appearing female infant. The mother has another older daughter without any problem at all.

What would be appropriate?

1. Repeat chromosome analysis in blood from the infant to confirm genetic sex.
2. Pelvic sonogram to visualize uterus.
3. To check for the presence of an inguinal mass.
4. Regardless of genetic sex, the child should be raised as a female.
5. All the above.

Fig. 19.3 Algorithm for evaluation of ambiguous genitalia in 46 XX DSD

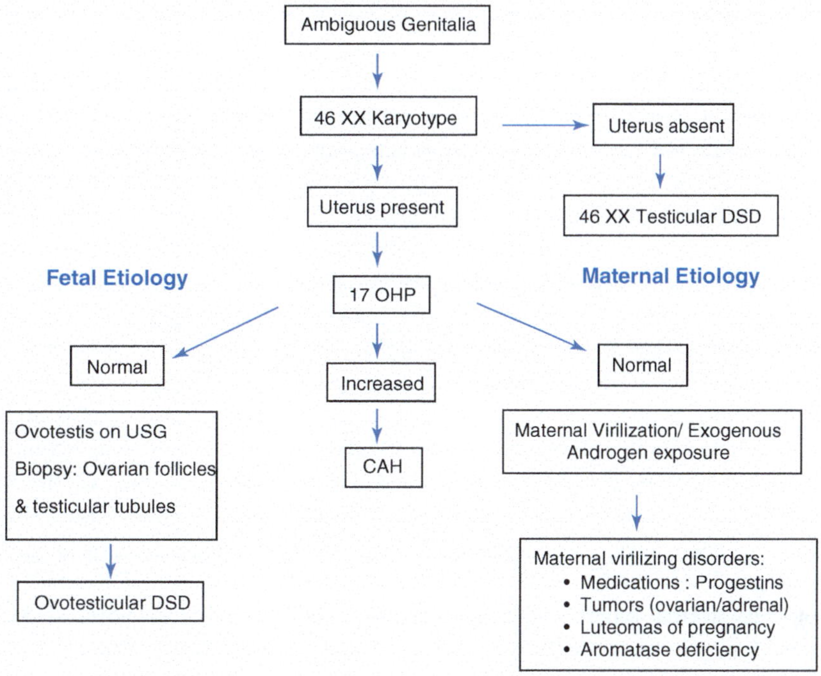

Results of autosome and sex chromosome from cell-free DNA, chorionic villi sample, or amniocyte analysis must be confirmed by peripheral blood lymphocytes analysis. 46 XY genetic sex with female external genitalia is either the result of complete gonadal dysgenesis (CGD) or complete androgen insensitivity syndrome (CAIS). In 46 XY CGD, the lack of hormonal production and function affects the development of internal and external genitalia, resulting in a female phenotype. In CAIS, the testes are normal and produce androgens and AMH. End-organ resistance to androgens will prevent normal masculinization, and AMH will prevent uterus formation. The presence of uterus could be detected by sonogram or genitogram. Sex assignment is based on anatomical sex appearance and functionality rather than genetic sex.

Answer: 5

In the absence of uterus and 46 XY chromosomal complement, the most likely diagnosis in this female infant is?

1. Congenital adrenal hyperplasia due to 21-hydroxylase deficiency
2. XY gonadal dysgenesis
3. Complete androgen insensitivity syndrome (CAIS)
4. Turner syndrome
5. None of the above

CAH with XY chromosomal complement has normal internal and external male genitalia. Androgen insensitivity syndrome (AIS) is a genetic condition that affects sexual development before birth and during puberty. AIS represents a spectrum of defects in androgen action in 46 XY genetically males. There is a wide variation in the degree of under-masculinization, ranging from infertility in an otherwise normal male (mild AIS) to ambiguous genitalia (partial AIS) to a completely female external phenotype [complete AIS (CAIS)].

In an individual with CAIS and karyotype 46 XY, testes develop during gestation. The fetal testes produce AMH and testosterone. However, because cells fail to respond to testosterone, the genitals differentiate into female, rather than the male pattern. AMH function is not impaired at all and causes the fetal Müllerian ducts to regress; therefore, the fetus lacks the uterus, fallopian tubes, and cervix plus the upper part of vagina. In other words, individuals with this condition have male internal and female external genitalia and therefore do not menstruate and are unable to conceive a child [18, 19].

Individuals with CAIS are often not identified at birth and typically raised as females and have a female gender identity. They typically present either before puberty with masses in the inguinal canal that are subsequently identified as testes or at puberty with primary amenorrhea and sparse to absent pubic or axillary hair but normal breast development due to lack of unopposed androgenic effect to the normal estrogen production.

In the female infant or toddler with CAIS, no immediate therapy is needed or warranted. These patients have normal female hormonal levels and have, in fact, never been exposed to elevated androgen levels, so they will develop into phenotypically normal females with scant axillary and pubic hair. Undescended testes (pelvis or abdomen), however, have a small chance of becoming cancerous later in life if they are not surgically removed in CAIS. The risk of malignant tumors is small prior to age 25, and after age 25 it is about 2–5% [20, 21]. The earliest reported malignancy in CAIS is at 14 years of age [22]. In CAIS, some testosterone is converted (aromatized) to estrogens. Orchiectomy therefore is recommended, usually after age 14 to allow normal breast development and genetic potential height. Both XY gonadal dysgenesis and AIS are now classified as 46 XY DSD. Sex assignment in partial gonadal dysgenesis (PGD) and partial androgen insensitivity (PAIS) is based on the phenotype after counseling and direct participation of the parents. The use of an algorithm (Fig. 19.4) provides additional help in diagnoses, counseling, and management of an infant with ambiguous genitalia with 46 XY DSD.

Turner syndrome (TS) is a genetic condition in females with gonadal failure and short stature as result of complete or partial absence of one of the two X chromosomes. The most common sex chromosomal abnormality found in TS is 45 X. The term "45 XO" should be avoided in TS because there is no "O" chromosome and, in addition, it can occur as a result of structural defect of one of the two X chromosomes or mosaicism. The short stature homeobox (*SHOX*) gene is a gene, located on both the short arm of X and Y chromosomes, which is associated with short stature in humans if mutated or present in only one copy (haploinsufficiency). Short stature in TS is the result of SHOX gene haploinsufficiency. XY gonadal dysgenesis has normal height.

Both TS and females with XY with gonadal dysgenesis will need hormonal therapy for secondary sexual characteristic development and oocyte donation as an effective option to conceive a child. Individuals with complete gonadal dysgenesis (CGD) have a particular high germ cell carcinoma (GCC) risk profile, with reported risks varying between 8 and 54%, making early diagnosis particularly relevant [23–25] to consider surgical management.

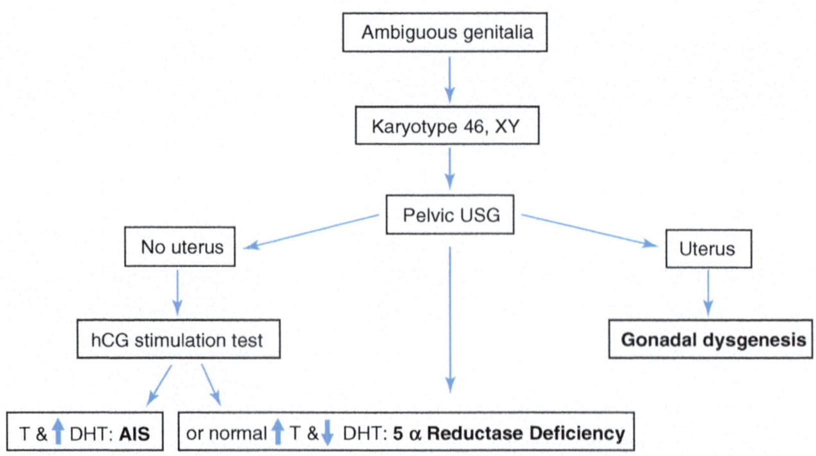

Fig. 19.4 Algorithm for evaluation of ambiguous genitalia in 46 XY DSD. (T = testosterone; DHT = Dihydroxytestosterone)

Answer: 3

Laboratory evaluation revealed:

- Karyotype 46 XY.
- Ultrasound showed the presence of testes.
- Normal 17-OH-progesterone level.
- Normal testosterone/DHT ratio.
- Increased LH and testosterone.

Based on those results, the correct assigned sex will be male?

1. Yes
2. No

Complete androgen insensitivity is the classical example of discordance between genetic and anatomical sex. Sex assignment should be female regardless of the genetic sex.

Answer: 2

Should the older sister be evaluated?

1. Yes
2. No

Androgen insensitivity syndrome (AIS) is inherited in an X-linked recessive pattern. A condition is considered X-linked if the mutated gene that causes the disorder is located on the X chromosome, one of the two sex chromosomes in each cell. In genetic males (who have only one X chromosome), one altered copy of the gene in each cell is sufficient to cause the condition. In genetic females (who have two X chromosomes), a mutation must be present in both copies of the gene to cause the disorder. Males are affected by X-linked recessive disorders much more frequently than females. If the mother is a carrier, there is a 50% chance that she will pass on the gene mutation to each of her children. The older sister therefore should be tested for *AR* receptor mutations. Mutation in the androgen receptor (*AR*) gene is located at the long arm of X chromosome, Xq11–12 [26, 27].

Answer: 1

All of the following are possible causes of ambiguous genitalia in a genetic male (XY) except?

1. Impaired testicle development caused by genetic abnormalities or unknown causes
2. Incomplete XY gonadal dysgenesis
3. Partial androgen insensitivity syndrome
4. 5-α-Reductase-2 deficiency
5. The mother's ingestion of substances with male hormone activity

Production of testosterone from cholesterol involves five enzymatic steps, and defects have been identified at each step. Of these five enzymes, three are shared with the adrenal glands, and their deficiency leads to ambiguous genitalia and symptoms of CAH.

As previously mentioned, both incomplete XY gonadal dysgenesis and partial androgen insensitivity syndrome exhibit ambiguous genitalia.

5-α-Reductase-2 deficiency is an autosomal recessive, sex-limited condition resulting in the inability to convert testosterone to the more physiologically active dihydrotestosterone (DHT). Because DHT is required for the normal masculinization of the external genitalia in utero, genetic males with 5-α-reductase-2 deficiency are born with ambiguous genitalia [28].

Diagnosis of this deficiency can be confirmed in a patient with a 46 XY karyotype by the presence of a high ratio of serum testosterone to DHT. Basal unstimulated T/DHT levels are not usually high enough to make a definitive diagnosis. Human chorionic gonadotropin (hCG) stimulation is needed in order to obtain adequate levels of testosterone and DHT for diagnosis. Normal patients respond with ratios from 8 to 16, while patients with 5-α-reductase-2 deficiency exhibit T/DHT ratios from 35 to 84 [29]. Decreased enzyme activity in cultured skin fibroblasts has been found in these patients [30, 31]. Steroid 5-α-reductase-2 deficiency (SRD) is caused by mutations of the SRD5A2 gene, which can be in addition sequenced in peripheral blood leukocytes to confirm diagnosis [32, 33]. Gender assignment in these patients has been debated because of the major virilization that occurs at puberty. Maternal ingestion of substances with female hormone activity can cause ambiguous genitalia. As in the case of CAH in male infants, other sources of excessive androgen exposure in uterus will not cause ambiguity of genitalia at all.

Answer: 5

In regard to development of female gonads, the following statements are true, except?

1. Requires 46 XX chromosomal complement.
2. Rather than the *SRY* gene, ovarian development requires other genetic factors.
3. 45 X chromosomal complement is associated with gonadal dysgenesis and normal female genitalia.
4. In the absence or inactivation of the *SRY* gene, female gonad will occur by default.
5. 46 XX chromosomal complement carrying *SRY* gene results in XX male phenotype (46 XX male syndrome).

Historically, the development of the female phenotype was thought to occur "by default" when the *SRY* gene and downstream signaling pathways were not activated. Normal ovarian development also requires active genetic pathways (*WNT4, RSP01, FOXL2*). A defect or mutation in any of the genes governing differentiation into a male or female phenotype can result in ambiguous genitalia [34, 35]. 46 XX male syndrome usually is caused by unequal crossing over between X and Y chromosomes during meiosis in the father, which results in the X chromosome containing the normally male SRY gene. When this X combines with a normal X from the mother during fertilization, the result is an XX male. Ninety percent of these patients have Y chromosomal material including the SRY gene. Y sequences are usually located on the distal tip of the short arm of the paternal X chromosome [36]. According to a proposed revised nomenclature [37], the diagnosis of XX male or XX sex reversal is renamed as 46 XX testicular disorder of sex development (46 XX testicular DSD). The XX males have hypogonadism and infertility [38].

Answer: 4

Clinical Pearls

1. Ambiguous genitalia are considered a rare event but are common enough to be seen by clinicians, not only in academic position but general practice.
2. Basic knowledge is necessary to provide helpful information to parents after birth of an infant with ambiguous genitalia.
3. Genetic counseling provided by geneticists/genetic counselors is essential during genetic crisis to reassure parents that there is nothing that they did or anything that they could have done to prevent this diagnosis. Parents eventually have to be informed of any risk of recurrence for future pregnancies, and prenatal diagnosis is available.
4. Diagnosis and management should be orchestrated by a medical team of specialists.
5. Remember that sex assignment should not be based on sex chromosome but phenotype, e.g., in gonadal dysgenesis and complete androgen insensitivity syndrome with XY sex chromosomal complement, their gender assignment is female.
6. Ambiguous genitalia could be the result of different chromosomal anomalies or genetic mutations, but the majority of these infants born with this condition are the results of female virilization in the uterus by excessive adrenal androgen (male hormone) production with excellent prognosis.
7. Based on frequency, congenital adrenal hyperplasia (CAH) should be suspected first in any infant with ambiguous genitalia.
8. Most cases of CAH are due to 21-hydroxylase deficiency, and therefore parents can be informed shortly after hormonal and imaging testing about their infant's gender. This particular condition is now part of the newborn screening program.

9. Some infants may need surgery in addition to hormonal replacement therapy.
10. The goals of treatment should be to ensure the child's long-term emotional well-being, sexual function, potential for fertility, and a stable gender identity.

References

1. Hamerton JL, Canning N, Ray M, et al. A cytogenetic survey of 14,069 newborn infants. I. Incidence of chromosome abnormalities. Clin Genet. 1975;4:223–43.
2. Blackless M, Charuvastra A, Derryck A, et al. How sexually dimorphic are we? Am J Hum Biol. 2000;12:151–66.
3. Jost A, Vigier B, Prépin J, Perchellet JP. Studies on sex differentiation in mammals. Recent Prog Horm Res. 1973;29:1–41.
4. Lee PA, Houk CP, Ahmed SF, Hughes IA. Consensus statement on management of intersex disorders. International consensus conference on intersex. Pediatrics. 2006;118:e488–500.
5. Eggers S, Sinclair A. Mammalian sex determination–insights from humans and mice. Chromosom Res. 2012;20:215–38.
6. Ono M, Harley VR. Disorders of sex development: new genes, new concepts. Nat Rev Endocrinol. 2013;9:79–91.
7. Krone N, Dhir V, Ivison HE, Arlt W. Congenital adrenal hyperplasia and P450 oxidoreductase deficiency. Clin Endocrinol. 2007;66:162–72.
8. White PC, Speiser PW. Congenital adrenal hyperplasia due to 21-hydroxylase deficiency. Endocr Rev. 2000;21:245–91.
9. Nordenström A, Ahmed S, Jones J, Coleman M, Price DA, Clayton PE, Hall CM. Female preponderance in congenital adrenal hyperplasia due to CYP21 deficiency in England: implications for neonatal screening. Horm Res. 2005;63:22–8.
10. Pang S, Shook MK. Current status of neonatal screening for congenital adrenal hyperplasia. Curr Opin Pediatr. 1997;9:419–23.
11. Therrell BL. Newborn screening for congenital adrenal hyperplasia. Endocrinol Metab Clin N Am. 2001;30:15–30.
12. van der Kamp HJ, Wit JM. Neonatal screening for congenital adrenal hyperplasia. Eur J Endocrinol. 2004 Nov;151(Suppl 3):U71–5.
13. NNSIS 2009 National Newborn Screening Information System. Available at http://www2.uthscsa.edu/nnsis.
14. Zachmann M, Tassinari D, Prader A. Clinical and biochemical variability of congenital adrenal hyperplasia due to 11β-hydroxylase deficiency: a study of 25 patients. J Clin Endocrinol Metab. 1983;56:222–9.
15. Therrell BL Jr, Berenbaum SA, Manter-Kapanke V, Simmank J, Korman K, Prentice L, Gonzalez J, Gunn S. Results of screening 1.9 million Texas newborns for 21-hydroxylase-deficient congenital for 21-hydroxylase-deficient congenital adrenal hyperplasia. Pediatrics. 1998 Apr;101:583–90.
16. Allen DB, Hoffman GL, Fitzpatrick P, Laessig R, Maby S, Slyper A. Improved precision of newborn screening for congenital adrenal hyperplasia using weight-adjusted criteria for 17-hydroxyprogesterone levels. J Pediatr. 1997;130:128–33.
17. al Saedi S, Dean H, Dent W, Stockl E, Cronin C. Screening for congenital adrenal hyperplasia: the Delfia screening test overestimates serum 17-hydroxyprogesterone in preterm infants. Pediatrics. 1996 Jan;97:100–2.
18. Oakes MB, Eyvazzadeh AD, Quint E, Smith YR. Complete androgen insensitivity syndrome—a review. J Pediatr Adolesc Gynecol. 2008 Dec;21(6):305–10. https://doi.org/10.1016/j.jpag.2007.09.006.
19. Hughes IA, Deeb A. Androgen resistance. Best Pract Res Clin Endocrinol Metab 2006;20(4):577–598. PMID 17161333. https://doi.org/10.1016/j.beem.2006.11.003.
20. Cools M, Van Aerde K, Kersemaekers AM, et al. Morphological and immunohistochemical differences between gonadal maturation delay and early germ cell neoplasia in patients with undervirilization syndromes. J Clin Endocrinol Metab. 2005 Sep;90(9):5295–303.
21. Hannema SE, Scott IS, Rajperts-De Meyts E, Skakkebaek NE, Coleman N, Hughes IA. Testicular development in the complete androgen insensitivity syndrome. J Pathol. 2006;208:518–52.
22. Hurt WG, Bodurtha JN, McCall JB, Ali MM, Hurt WG, Bodurtha JN, McCall JB, Ali MM. Seminoma in pubertal patient with androgen insensitivity syndrome. Am J Obstet Gynecol. 1989;161:530–1.
23. Page DC. Hypothesis: a Y-chromosomal gene causes gonadoblastoma in dysgenetic gonads. Development. 1987;101:151e5.
24. McCann-Crosby B, Mansouri R, Dietrich JE, McCullough LB, Sutton VR, Austin EG, et al. State of the art review in gonadal dysgenesis: challenges in diagnosis and management. Int J Pediatr Endocrinol. 2014;2014:4.
25. Verp MS, Simpson JL. Abnormal sexual differentiation and neoplasia. Cancer Genet Cytogenet. 1987;25:191e218.
26. Lubahn DB, Joseph DR, Sullivan PM, et al. Cloning of human androgen receptor and complementary DNA and localization to the X chromosome. Science. 1988;240:327.
27. Brinkmann AO, Faber PW, Rooij v, et al. The human androgen receptor: domain structure, genomic organization and regulation of expression. J Steroid Biochem. 1989;34:307.

28. Houk CP, Lee PA. Consensus statement on terminology and management: disorders of sex development. Sex Dev. 2008;2(4–5):172–80.
29. Esoterix endocrinology syllabus. hCG stimulation testing. www.essoterix.com. Available at http://www.esoterix.com/files/Endocrinology_Syllabus_3.22.11.pdf. Accessed 13 May 2014.
30. Imperato-McGinley J, Peterson RE, Gautier T, Sturla E. Androgens and the evolution of male-gender identity among male pseudohermaphrodites with 5alpha-reductase deficiency. N Engl J Med. 1979 May;300(22):1233–7.
31. Saenger P, Goldman AS, Levine LS, et al. Prepubertal diagnosis of steroid 5 alpha-reductase deficiency. J Clin Endocrinol Metab. 1978 Apr;46(4):627–34.
32. Hiort O, Sinnecker GH, Willenbring H, Lehners A, Zöllner A, Struve D. Nonisotopic single strand conformation analysis of the 5 alpha-reductase type 2 gene for the diagnosis of 5 alpha-reductase deficiency. J Clin Endocrinol Metab. 1996;81:3415–8.
33. Okeigwe I, Kuohung W. 5-alpha reductase deficiency: a 40-year retrospective review. Curr Opin Endocrinol Diabetes Obes. 2014;21(6):483–7.
34. Hersmus R, Kalfa N, de Leeuw B, et al. FOXL2 and SOX9 as parameters of female and male gonadal differentiation in patients with various forms of disorders of sex development (DSD). J Pathol. 2008;215(1):31–8.
35. Barbaro M, Wedell A, Nordenström A. Disorders of sex development. Semin Fetal Neonatal Med. 2011;16(2):119–27.
36. Abbas N, McElreavey K, Leconiat M, Vilain E, Jaubert F, Berger R, Nihoul-Fekete C, Rappaport R, Fellous M. Familial case of 46,XX male and 46,XX true hermaphrodite associated with a paternal-derived SRY-bearing X chromosome. C R Arcad Sci III. 1993;316:375–83.
37. Hughes IA, Houk C, Ahmed SF, Lee PA. LWPES consensus group, ESPE consensus group consensus statement on management of intersex disorders. Arch Dis Child. 2006;91:554–63.
38. Vorona E, Zitzmann M, Gromoll J, Schüring AN, Nieschlag E. Clinical, Endocrinological, and epigenetic features of the 46,XX male syndrome, compared with 47,XXY Klinefelter patients. J Clin Endocrinol Metab. 2007;92:3458–65.

20 Dilemmas: Eye Problems in the Newborn

Walter M. Fierson

Evaluation of the Newborn's Eyes

Examination of the eyes of a newborn infant and making a diagnosis and prescribing treatment for any disorders that are present represent a significant problem for physicians and others covering the nursery. This is due to several factors:

1. Ophthalmology is poorly taught, if taught at all, in medical school, internships, and pediatric residency programs across the United States.
2. The examination of the newborn baby's eyes is challenging even to experienced practitioners because of the baby's lack of ability to cooperate or fixate and because of anatomic factors like the presence of perinatal lid swelling and the small size of the palpebral fissure in most neonates.
3. The lack of familiarity with the use of the instrumentation used in ophthalmology for the examination of newborn infants.

The most useful instruments for obtaining a good ophthalmic examination of the newborn are the indirect ophthalmoscope and the slit lamp; however, these are instruments rarely available or utilized. The instrument which is usually available is the direct ophthalmoscope, which, paradoxically, is the most difficult one to use in neonates. There are, however, several techniques that will make the job easier:

1. An attempt should initially be made to determine whether vision is present. In most cases, the best that can be done to make this determination in a newborn is to determine if the baby exhibits avoidance behavior, including squeezing the eyelids closed, in response to a strong light (pocket CREE LED flashlights are strong enough for this testing). If the baby is awake and alert, one can determine if the baby can fixate and follow best by using a small translucent toy with a strong flashlight inserted to make an attractive target.
2. The anterior segment of the eye can be examined using the direct ophthalmoscope and focusing on the anterior structures using the power wheel on plus settings. For example, using the +10 lens gives a 2.5× magnification of anterior structures being examined, but one must be close to those structures being examined; in this example, at about 3 inches distant.
3. While red reflex testing should preferably be done after pupil dilation, dilation is rarely done in the newborn nursery. This examination should be done in a manner in which both eyes are viewed simultaneously in order to compare the color, intensity, and character of the light reflection between the two eyes. Ordinarily, there should be no difference between the two eyes [1].

W. M. Fierson, MD, FAAO, FAAP
Arcadia, CA, USA

G. I. Martin, W. Rosenfeld (eds.), *Common Problems in the Newborn Nursery*,
https://doi.org/10.1007/978-3-319-95672-5_20

Case Presentation: Absent or Diminished Red Reflex

An initial physical examination is being performed on a 39-week gestation infant female, product of an uncomplicated gestation and vaginal delivery. General physical examination is normal, and there are no dysmorphic features present. Inspection of the eyes reveals no apparent abnormalities, but a brief look at the red reflex using a direct ophthalmoscope shows a normal orange glow from the right eye but no light reflection from the left.

At this point, the best course is to:

1. Assume that the asymmetry of reflex is an artifact due to inability of the baby to cooperate and proceed with discharge planning.
2. Perform another red reflex examination after dilating the pupils with 1% tropicamide.
3. Request a stat pediatric ophthalmology consultation.
4. Place the infant on topical antibiotics for presumed infection.

Although #3 is always a temptation and ultimately might be required, the need for a stat consultation is questionable. Routinely ordering ophthalmology consultations for any suspected eye problem results in little education of the pediatrician or staff regarding how to recognize the nature of a problem.

Answer: 2

Examination before pupil dilation showed that the pupils were round and equally reactive to light, with no relative afferent pupillary defect. Vision testing showed that the infant reacted to light by blinking equally with either eye, an indication that vision was present and roughly equal in each eye. The lids, lashes, conjunctiva, and sclera appeared normal. After dilation the red reflex was again present and clear in the right eye but was diminished in the left eye, with a corona of reflected orange light surrounding the dark center in the left eye.

A provisional diagnosis might be:

1. Toxoplasmosis with vitreal inflammatory cells
2. Corneal opacity due to mucopolysaccharidosis
3. Hyphema due to forceps injury
4. Congenital cataract

The classic appearance of a central opacity with a clear circular surrounding zone is characteristic for central lenticular opacity, the usual type of congenital cataract. A family history for congenital or infantile cataract is very important, since if there is a family history of childhood cataracts, the child has no other medical problems, and the parents have lens opacities, then systemic and laboratory evaluations may not be needed unless the parental cataracts were due to a metabolic disorder. If there is no family history of cataracts, a pediatric systemic evaluation is required because these cataracts may be associated with systemic or metabolic disease. Since the cataract is unilateral, a laboratory workup for the cause of this cataract should include TORCH titers and a VDRL. For bilateral cataract, a urine test for reducing sugars (especially galactose), TORCH (toxoplasmosis, rubella, cytomegalovirus, varicella) screening, a Venereal Disease Research Laboratory (VDRL) test for syphilis, and a blood test for calcium, phosphorus, glucose, and galactokinase levels can be checked. Some experts suggest that the more extensive battery of tests should be performed for all congenital cataracts, whether unilateral or bilateral.

Answer: 4

The incidence of congenital cataract is between 1.6 and 6 cases per 10,000 [2]. Congenital cataracts are present at birth but may be insignificant in size and density and are thus not identified until later in life. Prenatal and family history is helpful, since many types of congenital cataract, especially when bilateral, are genetic. Some cataracts are static, especially anterior polar cataracts, but others may be progressive. The less the size and density of cataract at birth, the better the visual prognosis, assuming prompt diagnosis and treatment of visually significant cataracts. However, if these are not removed in a timely manner, permanent visual loss due to dense amblyopia is usually the result.

Not all cataracts are visually significant. If a lenticular opacity is in the visual axis, it usually is considered visually significant, especially if it is of significant density and size.

The most common cause of congenital, bilateral cataracts is:

1. Metabolic disease
2. Herpes simplex
3. Zika virus
4. Down syndrome
5. Cause unknown

The most common identifiable etiologies include intrauterine infections, metabolic disorders, and genetically transmitted syndromes. Metabolic and/or systemic diseases may be found in up to 60% of the patients presenting with bilateral congenital cataract [3]. One third of pediatric cataracts are sporadic; they are not associated with any systemic or ocular diseases. However, they may be spontaneous mutations and may lead to cataract formation in the patient's offspring. As many as 23% of congenital cataracts are genetic, with the most frequent mode of transmission being autosomal dominant with complete penetrance. This type of cataract may appear as a total cataract, polar cataract, lamellar cataract, or nuclear opacity. All close family members and subsequent children in the family should be examined when an infant is discovered to have a congenital cataract, especially if the cataracts are bilateral.

Infectious causes of cataracts include rubella (the most common), rubeola, chicken pox, cytomegalovirus, herpes simplex, herpes zoster, poliomyelitis, influenza, Epstein-Barr virus, syphilis, Zika, and toxoplasmosis.

Congenital cataracts are frequently associated with multi-system disorders. The list of these disorders is quite lengthy and beyond the scope of this chapter [4].

Answer: 5

The differential diagnosis [5] of an absence of the red reflex in one eye is very important. Some very significant diseases may present initially in this manner. These diagnostic entities may arise from all levels of the ocular media and retina. As with considering any problem in ophthalmology, it is helpful to consider the level within the eye at which the pathology occurs and proceed systematically from anterior to posterior:

1. Cornea [6]: the mnemonic "STUMPED" is helpful in remembering the causes of congenital corneal opacity:
   (a) Sclerocornea
   (b) Tears in Descemet's membrane – forceps injury
   (c) Metabolic disorders: mucopolysaccharidoses, cystinosis, tyrosinosis, fetal alcohol syndrome
   (d) Peters anomaly, a developmental defect of anterior chamber development with central corneal opacity
   (e) Edema, congenital glaucoma; congenital dystrophies, congenital hereditary endothelial dystrophy, congenital hereditary stromal dystrophy, posterior polymorphous dystrophy
   (f) Dermoid
2. Lens: any lenticular opacity is called a cataract.
   (a) Familial, inherited – usually autosomal dominant inheritance pattern
   (b) Chromosomal abnormalities
   (c) Systemic metabolic syndromes: galactosemia, cystinuria
   (d) Systemic syndromes: Alport syndrome, Lowe syndrome
   (e) Infectious disease: TORCH entities
   (f) Trauma
   (g) Unknown cause
3. Vitreous.
   (a) Persistent hyperplastic primary vitreous – persistent fetal vasculature, often associated with cataract
   (b) Vitreous hemorrhage
4. Retina.
   (a) Retinoblastoma (white reflex)
   (b) Retinopathy of prematurity

(c) Coat's disease
(d) Retinal infections, including toxoplasmosis, toxocariasis

This listing is not exhaustive, and it is beyond the scope of this textbook to discuss all of these entities and those not mentioned. It is clear, however, that a great number of problems at many levels can result in the disruption of the red reflex.

Figure 20.1 shows differential diagnosis of leukocoria.

Comment

It should always be remembered that anatomically clearing the visual axis from any opacity, whether corneal, lenticular, or vitreal, does not ensure a good visual outcome. Conditions for development or persistence of amblyopia remain, that is, a difference between the two eyes with the visual system on the previously affected side that is at a functional disadvantage. Prophylactic treatment for amblyopia, optical correction of any refractive disparity and patching or the use of atropine penalization on the "good" side is mandatory until the child reaches the age where vision can be assessed numerically by standardized testing and found to be satisfactory. This implies that the child should be under the care of a pediatric ophthalmologist until reaching the age of visual maturity, usually 8–9 years of age.

Case Presentation: Ocular Discharge

A nurse informs you that one of the babies that she has been caring for appears to have some whitish discharge from the left eye, first noticed about 28 hours after birth. The baby is a 40-week gestation infant female, product of an uncomplicated gestation and vaginal delivery.

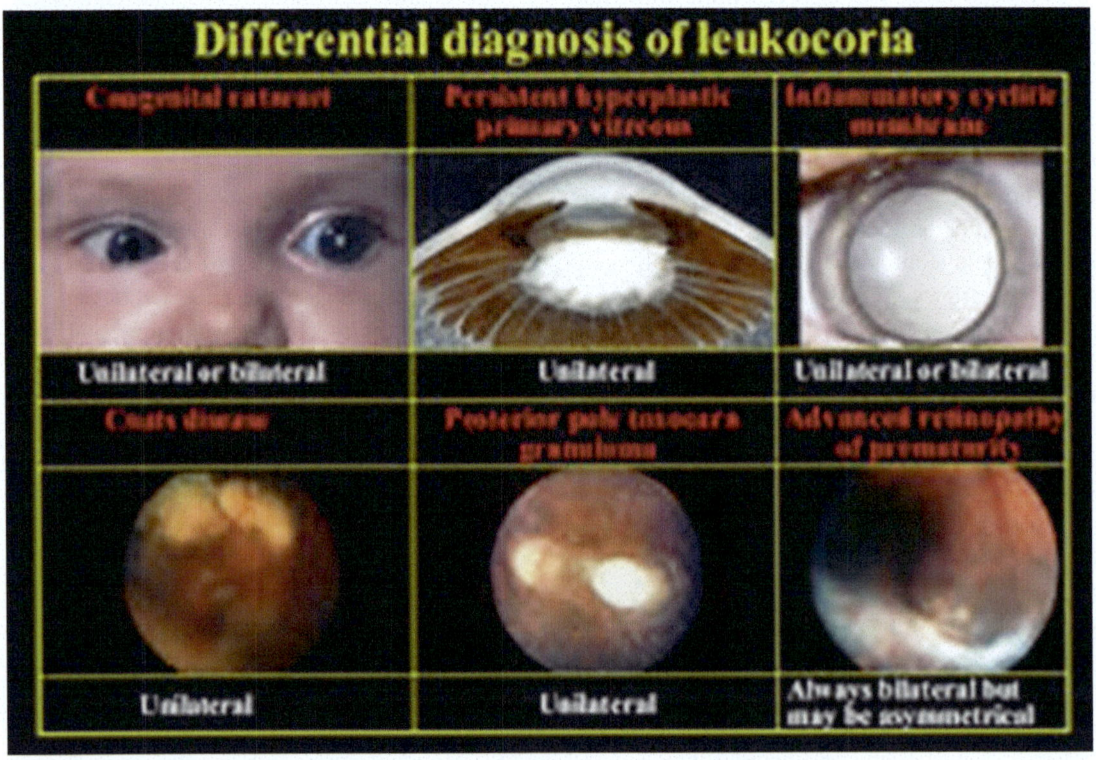

Fig. 20.1 Differential diagnosis of leukocoria

General physical examination is normal, and there are no dysmorphic features present. Inspection of the eyes reveals structurally normal eyelids, normal anterior segment, and red reflex but a small amount of whitish discharge from the left eye with some dried exudate on the eyelid margins.

At this point you:

1. Start the baby on systemic antibiotics.
2. Start the baby on topical antibiotics for the left eye.
3. Take blood cultures.
4. Careful inspection of the eyes, followed by performance of nasolacrimal sac massage to determine if nasolacrimal duct obstruction is present.

The differential diagnosis in a case like this one is largely between neonatal conjunctivitis and congenital nasolacrimal duct obstruction. The former is an infection of the periocular tissue and/or the conjunctiva. The latter is usually not a true infection; rather, it is usually the colonization of the tear fluid within the nasolacrimal drainage system, mostly the nasolacrimal sac, by opportunistic local normal flora with no invasion of any of the periocular tissues.

Answer: 4

The differential can usually be made between these two entities at the bedside by:

1. Inspection of the conjunctiva to determine if any inflammation is present
2. Pressure over the area of the nasolacrimal sac to determine if any nasolacrimal sac reflux of purulent material or tears takes place through the lacrimal punctae
3. Culture and sensitivity studies of any discharge present
4. Numbers 1 and 2

The combination of careful examination of the anterior segment with magnification (direct ophthalmoscope on high plus power and close focal distance or even a magnifying glass and a hand-held light) and pressure over the nasolacrimal sac on the involved side will, in most cases, determine whether infection or nasolacrimal duct obstruction, indicated by purulent reflux from the lacrimal punctae, is present. Possibilities for infection include conjunctivitis, i.e., infection of the conjunctiva, infectious keratitis, infection of the cornea, and intraocular infection. In order of frequency, conjunctivitis is by far most likely, followed by keratitis, and then intraocular infection.

Answer: 4

In this case, pressure over the nasolacrimal sac gave no reflux through the punctae, and inspection with magnification showed conjunctival hyperemia with some purulent discharge present. The corneas were clear and the interior of the eye appeared to be normal. It can logically be concluded that the most likely diagnosis is:

1. Congenital glaucoma
2. Endophthalmitis
3. Neonatal conjunctivitis
4. Nasolacrimal duct obstruction with dacryocystitis

Congenital glaucoma, while it does cause tearing, does not cause purulent discharge, and the cornea is usually cloudy. Endophthalmitis usually causes pronounced inflammation of all the periocular tissues but usually is not accompanied by purulent discharge. Nasolacrimal duct obstruction, as mentioned previously, is accompanied by positive nasolacrimal sac reflux.

Answer: 3

The most common cause of neonatal conjunctivitis is:

1. Chemical irritation
2. Gonorrhea
3. Chlamydia
4. Herpes simplex.

The etiology of neonatal conjunctivitis, defined as conjunctivitis occurring within the first 30 days of life, can be divided into chemical (now rare), bacterial, or viral [7, 8]. The etiological distribution of neonatal conjunctivitis in Western nations has shifted radically in from the early twentieth century, when "ophthalmia neonatorum" was most frequently caused by gonorrhea, to a much wider spread of causation. For many years the most common cause was the use of silver nitrate solution instillation into the eyes at birth, which prevented most cases of gonorrheal conjunctivitis, but led to the creation of chemical conjunctivitis. This chemical conjunctivitis has, in turn, been eliminated by the use of erythromycin ointment in place of silver nitrate; this latter treatment has proven to be as effective as silver nitrate in the elimination of gonorrheal neonatal conjunctivitis.

It must be emphasized that gonorrheal neonatal conjunctivitis has not been completely eliminated in western countries and is still frequent in third world countries. Additionally, it must be emphasized that erythromycin prophylaxis is only effective against gonorrhea, not against *Chlamydia* or *Herpes* viruses.

Bacterial conjunctivitis is most commonly caused by *Chlamydia trachomatis* in developed countries because of higher prevalence of *Chlamydia* as a sexually transmitted disease. This is due to the fact that 60–80% of genital infections with *Chlamydia* in females are asymptomatic. The Center for Disease Prevention and Control (CDC) estimates 3 million cases of chlamydial infections occur per year. It is more prevalent than gonococcal infection and approximately four to six times as common as herpes virus infection. It has a later onset than gonococcal conjunctivitis. The incubation period is 5–14 days, and the colonization of the eye after birth does not always result in infection. Almost 40% of the infected neonates develop watery conjunctivitis, which becomes more copious and purulent later. Most of the cases are mild and self-limited but occasionally may be severe with eyelid swelling, chemosis, papillary reaction, pseudo-membrane, peripheral pannus, and corneal involvement. If left untreated, 10–20% of the cases will develop infantile pneumonia. Other extraocular involvement of *Chlamydia* includes nasopharyngeal, rectal, and vaginal colonization and other form of diseases such as infant pneumonia syndrome. For treatment of *Chlamydia* neonatal conjunctivitis, the American Academy of Pediatrics recommends a 14-day course of systemic erythromycin (50 mg/kg/d, divided in 4 doses) [9].

Although gonococcus is the second most common organism responsible for ophthalmia neonatorum, it is the most virulent infectious agent of neonatal conjunctivitis. It was previously the most common cause of blindness within the first year of life, necessitating the use of prophylaxis at birth. Gonococcal ophthalmia neonatorum had been eradicated in the United States in the 1950s. However, it has now resurfaced following the increasing incidence of adult gonococcal infections and the development of antimicrobial resistance. The incubation period is 2–5 days. It can occur earlier in cases of premature rupture of membranes. It is usually bilateral. The conjunctivitis is characterized by severe hyper-acute purulent discharge, eyelid edema, and chemosis. Gonococci have the capacity to penetrate intact corneal epithelium, leading to corneal epithelial edema and corneal ulceration, which can progress to corneal perforation and endophthalmitis if unrecognized. Hence in all cases of neonatal conjunctivitis, the infant has to be screened for gonococci to prevent these serious consequences. Gonococcal infection of the newborn can also give rise to systemic complications like stomatitis, arthritis, rhinitis, septicemia, and meningitis. Infants with gonorrheal neonatal conjunctivitis should be retained in hospital or readmitted, treated with frequent irrigation of the conjunctiva and intravenous or intramuscular administration of ceftriaxone (25–50 mg/kg, to a maximum dose of 125 mg), and evaluated for disseminated gonococcal disease (e.g., arthritis, sepsis, meningitis). The infant's mother and her sexual partners should be treated for gonorrhea.

Other bacterial causes of ophthalmia include *Staphylococcus aureus*, *Staphylococcus epidermidis*, *Streptococcus pneumoniae*, *Streptococcus viridans*, *Haemophilus influenzae*, *Escherichia coli*, *Klebsiella* sp. and *Pseudomonas aeruginosa.*

Viral neonatal conjunctivitis is usually due to Herpes simplex infection. It often includes infection of the cornea. Herpes simplex keratoconjunctivitis in an infant usually presents with generalized herpes infection. Vesicles around the eye and corneal involvement are also common. Treatment includes systemic acyclovir (60 mg/kg in divided doses 3 times a day) for 14 days, coupled with topical ophthalmic solution (i.e., 1% trifluridine, 0.1% iododeoxyuridine, or 3% vidarabine).

Less commonly, adenovirus may cause a largely self-limited conjunctivitis in the newborn period. This is usually accompanied by adenovirus infection elsewhere systemically. There is no effective treatment at present for adenoviral conjunctivitis.

Answer: 3

Laboratory diagnosis is of paramount importance in establishing the correct diagnosis and initiating the best treatment. Conjunctival scrapings for Gram stain and Giemsa stain should be obtained from the palpebral conjunctiva of all the infants with neonatal conjunctivitis. The presence of intracellular gram-negative diplococci (IGND) has a high sensitivity and specificity and predictive value. Blood agar, chocolate agar, and/or Thayer-Martin media can be used to isolate *Neisseria gonorrhoeae* and other bacteria.

Chlamydia trachomatis can be isolated by the presence of intracytoplasmic inclusion bodies in the Giemsa stain in 60–80% of all infants. Conjunctival swab, smeared onto a microscopic slide and stained with *Chlamydia trachomatis*-specific fluorescent monoclonal antibody (direct immunofluorescence test), often shows the presence of an impressively large number of punctate, fluorescing chlamydial elementary bodies and resembling "star-spangled sky at night." This antigen detection test is still considered the "gold standard" for the diagnosis of chlamydial infections. Polymerase chain reaction (PCR) analysis for diagnosing chlamydial conjunctivitis has an advantage of early diagnosis and higher specificity compared to cell culture. The other laboratory studies for diagnosing chlamydial infections include micro-immunofluorescence assay (MIF) for detection of *Chlamydia trachomatis* IgG and IgM antibodies and ELISA tests [16].

The other major diagnosis in the differential diagnosis of ocular discharge in the newborn period is nasolacrimal duct obstruction [10]. Congenital nasolacrimal duct obstruction, frequently mislabeled dacryostenosis, occurs when the lacrimal duct has failed to open shortly before at the time of birth.

Estimates vary, but it is thought that 5% of infants have nasolacrimal duct obstruction at the time of birth [10]. Most of these open spontaneously during the first 9 months of life. Symptoms of this obstruction include epiphora, which result from overflow of tears due to blockage of the duct, and periocular crusting and discharge due to colonization of the stagnant tears in the nasolacrimal drainage system. Pressure over the lacrimal sac, adjacent to the medial canthus just lateral to the nose, often produces reflux of mucopurulent material through the lacrimal punctae.

Since the overwhelming majority of obstructions of the nasolacrimal duct will resolve spontaneously during the first 9 months, usually thought to be over 90%, there is little reason to employ anything other than conservative measures to treat this problem during that time period. These include gentle cleansing of the eyelids with warm water and cotton or a clean, soft cloth, pressure over the nasolacrimal sac to empty the sac of its content of mucopurulent material, and, if the discharge becomes copious and purulent, the use of topical antibiotics to decrease the amount of discharge. It must be recognized that antibiotics do not treat the cause of the problem, and, consequently, will not cure it, and so should be used sparingly. I have found that topical antibiotic ointment, usually erythromycin, gives superior results in holding down the amount of discharge to antibiotic drops. It is probably unnecessary to use advanced generation antibiotics, like moxifloxacin or ofloxacin, for this problem. If spontaneous clearing does not occur, the primary surgical procedure to eliminate this problem is a nasolacrimal duct probing. In the rare cases where simple probing is followed by recurrent obstruction and the re-emergence of symptoms, a second probing, a nasolacrimal duct dilation with a Lacricath™ (similar to the balloon catheter used for dilation of the coronary arteries in stenosis of the coronary arteries), or insertion of stents in the nasolacrimal drainage system, later removed, can be employed.

A very important differential diagnosis of nasolacrimal duct obstruction is congenital glaucoma, because in cases of congenital glaucoma, there is usually copious tearing, but not discharge, from the affected eye(s). In these cases, the cornea of the eye affected with congenital glaucoma is usually enlarged, usually cloudy and may display Haab striae, lines within the cornea representing Descemet's membrane breaks. These patients are usually very photophobic. Rarely, an eye with congenital glaucoma can appear to be perfectly normal. A pediatric ophthalmology consultation would be required to adequately make this diagnosis.

Case Presentation: The Cloudy Cornea

During your routine examination of a full-term infant, product of an apparently normal gestation, labor and delivery with no significant past medical history in the mother, you note an absence of the red reflex in both eyes. A brief observation with a flashlight and then closer observation using magnification show clouding of the cornea of both eyes and some mild tearing. You have the impression that the eyes may be larger than usual. The baby seems unusually light sensitive. At this point you should:

1. Dim the room lights, and make sure that the baby's eyes are usually covered to avoid retinal damage.
2. Call for a pediatric ophthalmology consultation.
3. Assume that the nasolacrimal ducts are obstructed, and institute a program of "watchful waiting."
4. Treat for neonatal conjunctivitis with topical erythromycin ointment.

There is no reason to assume retinal damage will occur, even if the cornea is clouded, so #1 is not a useful maneuver. Assuming that the tearing is due to nasolacrimal duct obstruction, as implied in #3, neglects all other possibilities and assumes that the most benign entity in the differential diagnosis is the correct response, always a dangerous course in any clinical situation. #4 is incorrect since it makes the same illogical assumption as #3 and ignores the presence of corneal clouding and light sensitivity. It is most likely, in this case, that the pediatric ophthalmologic consultant will find that congenital glaucoma is present.

Answer: 2

Glaucoma can be loosely defined as elevated intraocular pressure leading to damage of the structures of the eye and vision loss. By definition, primary, as opposed to glaucoma associated with some other systemic or ophthalmologic disease, is present at birth, although its manifestation in signs and symptoms may take weeks or months to develop. Usually, however, the worst cases occur in utero *and* manifest at birth. The incidence of primary congenital glaucoma has been estimated at 1 in 10,000 live births. This disorder can cause complete blindness, and the earlier its recognition and effective treatment is accomplished the better the visual prognosis.

Primary congenital glaucoma is probably caused by a defect in the development of the trabecular meshwork, the 360° structure in the peripheral angle of the anterior chamber where fluid is filtered out of the eye into the bloodstream. The precise nature of this defect is not yet entirely clear, but operationally the trabecular network appears and behaves as if it is covered by a thin, relatively impermeable membrane. The disease is bilateral in 75% of cases, although its severity can be asymmetrical. Primary congenital glaucoma is usually genetically determined and inherited as an autosomal recessive [11, 12].

The presentation of primary congenital glaucoma is classic: symptoms include tearing and photophobia, usually severe enough to simulate blepharospasm, with the infant not opening his/her eyes in any but the dimmest of light conditions. Signs include increased corneal diameter, corneal edema resulting in a cloudy appearance of the cornea, and Haab striae (usually horizontal whitish lines within the cornea) which are actually breaks in Descemet's membrane, presumably due to stretching of the eye. If the optic nerve can be visualized, it may be seen to be damaged, appearing usually cupped at time of diagnosis if the previous signs are present. Intraocular pressure can be measured at the bedside with a Tono-Pen™ or iCare™ or Perkins™ tonometer, although more accurately with the infant sedated or undergoing an examination under anesthesia, and is usually elevated.

The differential diagnosis of primary congenital glaucoma includes:

1. Birth trauma
2. Nasolacrimal obstruction
3. Congenital clouding of the cornea due to metabolic disorders may be superficially confused with glaucoma. These disorders include:
   (a) Mucopolysaccharidoses (MPS)
   (b) Sphingolipidoses
   (c) Mucolipidoses
4. Peters anomaly (a rare anterior segment developmental cleavage disorder)
5. Congenital hereditary endothelial dystrophy (CHED)
6. Infection
7. Congenital megalocornea
8. Structural lesions of the cornea, like limbal dermoids, Goldenhar-Gorlin syndrome, corneal keloids, and sclerocornea
9. Rare causes of corneal clouding, including:
   (a) Harboyan syndrome
   (b) Congenital hereditary stromal dystrophy
   (c) Fryn syndrome

The presumptive diagnosis of primary congenital glaucoma is usually made at the bedside by a pediatric ophthalmologist, but the definitive diagnosis is usually made in the operating room by an examination under anesthesia carried out just before surgery for this condition is performed.

Treatment of congenital glaucoma is primarily surgical. Medical treatment, including the use of topical or systemic carbonic anhydrase inhibitors to lower aqueous humor production, may be used to attempt to lower the pressure of the involved eye(s) prior to surgery, especially if prompt surgery cannot be performed due to a precarious general condition of the infant, such as prematurity, cardiorespiratory disease, sepsis, etc. The primary surgical procedures are those attempting to promote greater aqueous outflow through the angle of the anterior chamber where the trabecular meshwork is located. In many cases of congenital glaucoma, more than one surgical procedure per eye must be performed for adequate control. If angle surgery is unsuccessful, a filtering procedure including the implantation of a valve to allow for the egress of aqueous may be performed. When all other surgical approaches have failed, ablation of the ciliary body posterior to the iris, the place where aqueous humor is made, can be performed; Nd:YAG laser, diathermy, or cryotherapy may be used.

It should be noted that even if complete control of the glaucoma is achieved by surgical or surgical/medical means, late-developing open-angle juvenile glaucoma develops in a significant percentage of these children, so that all children with congenital glaucoma should be under the care of a pediatric ophthalmologist or glaucoma specialist all throughout childhood, adolescence, and adulthood. The pediatrician should facilitate this care wherever possible [13, 14].

Case Presentation: Misalignment (Strabismus)

A nurse in the newborn nursery notifies you that a baby you are to see for a routine post-admission physical examination has eyes that "look funny." This baby is the product of an apparently normal labor and delivery with no history in her mother of any medical difficulties during pregnancy. You examine the baby, and note that the eyes do not appear equal, and the pupil of the right eye is deviated to the left.

1. Call for a stat pediatric ophthalmology consult
2. Make sure that TORCH titers have been drawn
3. Perform the routine physical examination as described at the beginning of this chapter
4. Request an MRI scan of the brain to rule out central nervous system malformation

An examination should be performed as part of the general physical examination of any newborn infant. However, this scenario presents a very difficult problem for the pediatrician because, aside from many other reasons, experts may reasonably disagree over what the proper course should be in this setting. However, certain logical steps can be taken and conclusions drawn which will help in working through this problem.

Answer: 3

The first matter to be settled is whether there is ocular misalignment present. There is no greater source of misdiagnosis in referrals to pediatric ophthalmologists than the presence or absence of misalignment of the eyes. Even before examination, certain factors should be noted:

1. The relative position of a newborn baby's eyes is somewhat variable, depending on their level of consciousness. A very alert baby is much more likely to be properly aligned than a baby who is just about to fall asleep or who has just awakened. This means that the best time to check for alignment is when the baby is awake and alert; with busy schedules of the examining physician, this is sometimes difficult to arrange.
2. A baby's eyes' relative position can be accurately determined if it can be assured that the baby is gazing at a known object, something which is difficult to ascertain. The best method is to have the examination performed in an area where the lighting can be dimmed, use a small illuminated toy as a fixation object, and then determine if the light reflection from each cornea is in the same relative position (not if it is centered on each cornea). If it is the eyes are straight at that time. This should be followed by the binocular simultaneous red reflex examination; if this is equal in the two eyes, this is another indicator of the absence of misalignment.
3. It must be borne in mind that pseudo-esotropia is present in a large proportion of the newborn population; this is especially true of infants of Asian, Latino, or Native American ethnicity. Pseudo-esotropia is the impression, but not the fact, of esotropia caused by the presence of epicanthal folds, resulting in seeing more "white" temporally than nasally in a baby with those folds, especially when they are wide. In some cases, there is also an entity known as pseudo-exotropia, where the eyes are straight with respect to fixation of light onto the fovea of each eye, but the appearance of the eyes is exotropic, because the position of the fovea in one or both eyes is displaced from its usual position.
4. It has been reported that almost 1/3 babies who are later found to have straight eyes are actually exotropic during the first few days to weeks of life [15]. This is especially true for premature babies but may also be found in term babies.
5. In cases of true primary strabismus, this strabismus frequently starts after 2 months of age and is not present at birth [16].

When all these factors are considered, it may appear to be a difficult task and one more likely to produce an erroneous conclusion about the state of position of a newborn's eyes than a true one. To this problematic state of affairs must be added another, very significant, complicating factor; anything that seriously leads to decreased vision in one eye very frequently leads to the development of strabismus. This includes any opacities, any unilateral or asymmetrical defect of the retina or optic nerve, or optic nerve hypoplasia or atrophy if unilateral or asymmetrical. Great inequality of the refractive status of the two eyes can cause strabismus. Finally, diseases or defects of the central nervous system, whether prenatal or postnatal, such as hypoxic injury, infection, congenital anomaly from any cause, metabolic defect, etc., are associated with a much higher incidence of strabismus than in neonates with no such problems.

Faced with all these complicating factors, the provider might be excused for being unable to conclude whether strabismus is present, and if present whether it should be ignored. A much better course would be to add the possible presence of strabismus to the infant's problem list and re-examine the situation during the first and second postnatal visit, unless leukocoria or absent red reflex is noted on initial examination. In these latter cases of abnormal red reflex findings, a prompt pediatric ophthalmology evaluation is indicated. If the red reflex is normal bilaterally on initial and early office examination, a referral to a pediatric ophthalmologist can be made if the misalignment of the eyes is felt to persist beyond the third postnatal office visit as recommended by the American Academy of Pediatrics at 2 months.

Clinical Pearls

1. Use of a lid speculum to open the eyelids wide enough for good inspection is quite valuable and easy. It can be made painless for the baby if a drop of Pontocaine or tetracaine ophthalmic solution is instilled into the eye a minute or so before insertion.
2. The anterior segment of the eye can be examined using the direct ophthalmoscope and focusing on the anterior structures using the power wheel on plus settings. The +10 lens gives a 2.5× magnification of anterior structures being examined.
3. Pupil dilation is essential for adequate visualization of the red reflex as well as the posterior portion of the eye, including the lens, vitreous, retina, and optic nerve. This can usually be accomplished by using a single drop of either tropicamide 1% or phenylephrine 2.5% or combination drops available commercially which contain these drugs. These drugs have proven safe in neonates; they are routinely used in the smallest premature babies in NICUs across the United States, Europe, and Asia.
4. Horizontal lines or striae within a cloudy cornea usually indicate that congenital glaucoma is present; vertical or near-vertical striae usually accompany trauma due to forceps during delivery.
5. When checking for strabismus, use of a light alone as a target is to be discouraged; babies usually do not fixate on lights as well as they do on a translucent toy (preferably with a face) into which a strong flashlight has been inserted. A fully awake very young infant should be able to follow such an object.
6. Test each eye individually, covering each eye in turn, comparing the reaction of each to the other. A difference in ability to fixate and follow usually indicates a very significant difference in visual acuity between the two eyes.
7. Culture of purulent matter from the eye rarely leads to a correct diagnosis. Rather, a scraping of the palpebral conjunctiva with a sterile micro-spatula or Calgiswab for culture studies is to be preferred strongly.
8. The normal "red reflex" can vary in color from a yellowish tan, usually in blond Caucasian babies, to an almost black color in darkly pigmented ones. The best way to look for an abnormal red reflex is to look at both pupils simultaneously through the direct ophthalmoscope. Whatever the color or

configuration, it should be the same on both sides.

9. In cases of suspected neonatal conjunctivitis, the character of the discharge can give immediate clues regarding the etiology of the infection. Frankly purulent yellow or white discharge is overwhelmingly likely to be due to bacterial conjunctivitis. Massive purulent discharge is most likely due to Neisseria conjunctivitis. The discharge in chlamydial conjunctivitis is white but scant and stringy that in viral conjunctivitis is usually watery or slightly cloudy. While purulent reflux with pressure on the nasolacrimal sac is seen in nasolacrimal duct obstruction, this is rarely true in the neonatal period. Thus, immediate antimicrobial therapy can be started on a presumptive basis with a high probability of success, long before culture or other laboratory results are available.

References

The references are not scholarly or technical articles for ophthalmologists but, rather, are summary articles, mostly available on the Internet and easily read by the practicing pediatrician

1. Russell HC, McDougall V, Dutton GN. Congenital cataract. BMJ. 2011 May 27;342:d3075.
2. Santana A, Waiswo M. The genetic and molecular basis of congenital cataract. Arq Bras Oftalmol. 2011) Mar-Apr;74(2):136–42.
3. Lloyd EC, Lamber SR. Congenital cataract, a concise guide to diagnosis and management: Springer International Publishing; 2017. p. 20–1.
4. Cassidy L, Taylor D. Congenital cataract and multisystem disorders. Eye. 1999;13:464–73.
5. Tuli SY, Giordano BP, Kelly M, Fillipps D, et al. Newborn with an absent red reflex. J Pediatr Health Care. 2013;27(1):51–5.
6. Katzman L, Reiser BJ. Pediatric Corneal Opacities: American Academy of Ophthalmology (2016). https://www.aao.org/pediatric-center-detail/pediatric-corneal-opacities.
7. Mallika PS, Asok T, Faisal HA, Aziz S, et al. Neonatal conjunctivitis – a review. Malaysian Family Physician. 2008;3(2):1985–2274.
8. Matejcek A, Goldman RD. Treatment and prevention of Ophthalmia Neonatorum. Can Fam Physician. 2013;59:1187–90.
9. American Academy of Pediatrics. Chlamydial Ophthalmia. Red Book (2015). Section 5.
10. Lueder G. Nasolacrimal duct obstruction. American Academy of Ophthalmology. 2015; https://www.aao.org/pediatric-center-detail/nasolacrimal-duct-obstruction-4.
11. Scheinfeld NS. Congenital clouding of the cornea. (2016). http://emedicine.medscpae.com/article/1197148-overview
12. Khaled K Abu-Amero, Edward DP. Primary congenital glaucoma. Gene Reviews, 2014. https://www.ncbi.nlm.nih.gov/books/NBK1135
13. Cibis GW. Primary congenital glaucoma clinical presentation. (2017). http://emedicine.medscape.com/article/1206081-clinical#b4.
14. Kozak A, Epley KD, Clark RA. Glaucoma, congenital or infantile. (2017). http://eyewiki.aao.org/glaucoma,_congenital or infantile.
15. Nixon RB, Helveston EM, Miller K, Archer SM et al. Incidence of Strabismus in Neonates. (1985) Amer J of Ophth;100(6):798–801.
16. AAP Schedule of Well-Child Care Visits. (Bright Futures) June 27, 2017. https://www.healthychildren.org/English/family-life/health-management/Pages/Well-Child-Care-A-Check-Up-for-Success.aspx.

Hearing Assessment in the Newborn Infant

21

Gilbert I. Martin, James S. Yeh, and Andrea C. Morris

Introduction

Universal newborn hearing screening (UNHS) is now legislated in most states (43 states) in the country, and in 2014, 98.4% of newborns were screened (CDC 2014 Early Hearing Detection; www.cdc.gov/ncbddd/hearingloss/2014-data/2014_ehdi_hsfs_summary_h.pdf) [1]. Legislative mandates were first passed in 1990, and since that time, with implementation of programs and public awareness, the need for newborn hearing screening has increased. The NIH Consensus Developmental Conference in 1993 recommended that all babies be screened for hearing loss before discharge. It has been estimated that treating hearing loss at birth will save more than $400,000/child in later education costs. If newborns are not identified with hearing loss and if appropriate management is not forthcoming, there is a potential impact on cognitive, intellectual, and social development of the child [2].

The incidence of sensorineural loss is estimated at 1–3 per 1000 live births in term neonates and increases to 2–4 per 100 in high-risk infants. The objective of UNHS is to identify children with all types of hearing impairment. It has been demonstrated that infants who are identified before the age of 6 months have better expressive and receptive language development [3–5].

Causes of hearing loss in the newborn include all of the following except:

1. Genetic disorders
2. Maternal drug use
3. Viral infections
4. Perinatal asphyxia
5. Exchange transfusion for hyperbilirubinemia

It is generally accepted that genetic and environmental factors are responsible for many cases of congenital hearing impairment. Among genetic defects, about 50 percent are due to a mutation in the connexin-encoding gene [5, 6]. There is a new technique using the gene-editing tool CRISPR-Cas9 which has shown promise in restoring hearing loss in mice. Nongenetic causes of hearing impairment include congenital infections (especially cytomegalovirus infection), asphyxia, hyperbilirubinemia, oto-

G. I. Martin, MD (✉)
Neonatal Intensive Care Unit, Citrus Valley Medical Center–Queen of the Valley Hospital, West Covina, CA, USA

Loma Linda University Medical Center, Loma Linda, CA, USA

J. S. Yeh, MD, FACS
Department of Surgery, Citrus Valley Medical Center–Queen of the Valley Hospital, West Covina, CA, USA

A. C. Morris, DNP, RNC-NIC, CCRN, CNS
Kaiser Permanente-Fontana, Fontana, CA, USA

G. I. Martin, W. Rosenfeld (eds.), *Common Problems in the Newborn Nursery*,
https://doi.org/10.1007/978-3-319-95672-5_21

toxic medications, and environmental factors (background noise). There has been no known association of maternal drug use and hearing loss.

Answer: 2

The technologies utilized for UNHS include evoked otoacoustic emission (OAE) and automated auditory brain stem response (AABR). Both of these screening technologies are noninvasive, easy to perform, relatively inexpensive, and portable.

Which of the following is not correct with regard to OAE?

1. OAE is faster than AABR.
2. The newborn does not need to be in a quiet awake or sleep state when the test is performed.
3. Has a higher fail rate (more false positives for hearing loss) than AABR.
4. Can detect auditory neuropathy.

Evoked otoacoustic emission (OAE) measures sound waves generated in the inner ear (cochlea) in response to clicks or tone bursts. OAE is affected by debris and/or fluid in the middle or external ear. When performing the OAE, a small probe is placed in the ear canal which delivers a sound stimulus. The sound is transmitted through the middle ear to the inner ear. The outer hair cells of the cochlea produce an active response (emission). These emissions are picked up by a microphone and analyzed. There is an automated "pass" or "refer" result. OAE testing is easier and faster to administer than AABR, and the baby does not have to be in a quiet state (asleep or quiet awake). Disadvantages include the problem that vernix or other debris in the canal or decreased mobility of the tympanic membrane may give a "fail" result. In addition, while OAE can pick up hearing loss due to conduction loss and cochlear or VIII nerve problems, it will not pick up auditory neuropathy (often associated with hyperbilirubinemia, asphyxia, viral infections, bacterial meningitis, and genetic disorders).

Answer: 4

Which of the following is not correct with regard to AABR?

1. Results are affected by debris in the ear canal.
2. Can detect defects in the VIII nerve.
3. Can detect defects in the cochlea.
4. Can detect defects in the brain stem.
5. Can detect auditory neuropathy.

AABR technology measures the electroencephalographic waves generated in response to clicks through earphones worn on both ears via electrodes pasted to the infant's scalp. The baby is required to be in a quiet state. AABR screening is not affected by middle or external ear debris. The AABR can detect impairment on the level of the cochlea, auditory nerve, and auditory pathway in the brain stem. The normal AABR takes the form of five successive neural waves labeled I–V. An infant's waveform is compared with standard template results, and a "pass" or "fail" result is determined (see Fig. 21.1).

Answer: 1

The provider in the nursery is often the first person informed regarding an abnormal hearing screening test and must be knowledgeable about

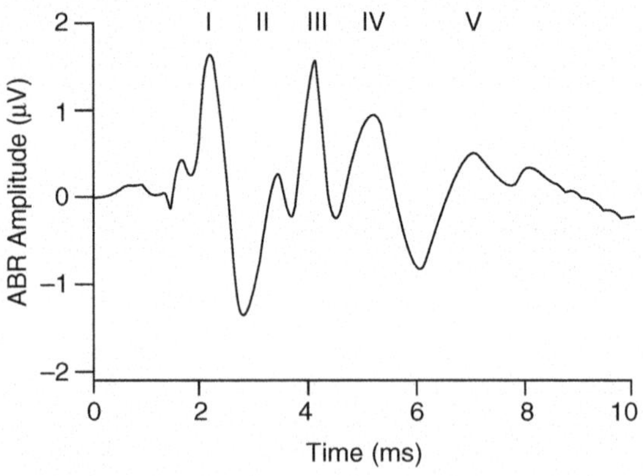

Fig. 21.1 Wave components of the auditory evoked response recorded with scalp electrodes and elicited by an acoustic click. The ABR waveform is usually described and integrated in terms of the latencies and amplitudes of these peaks

interpretation and appropriate follow-up. If the OAE is done in the nursery, the practitioner should understand that a false-positive result (failed hearing screening) can occur from a middle ear disorder (otitis media or effusion) or blockage in the ear canal (impacted debris) and an immature neurological system. Many nurseries have adopted a two-tiered screening procedure. Initial screening is done with OAE, and if it is a "refer," then an AABR is performed.

The failure rate for term newborns who have hearing screening is:

1. 1–2%
2. 2–4%
3. 4–6%
4. 6–8%

The failure rate for babies screened in the nursery is 1.6% (CDC 2014) [1].

Answer: 1

In addition, some children can pass screening who in fact suffer from a hearing deficit. The causes of this late-onset deafness are cytomegalovirus infection, genetic syndromes, neurodegenerative disorders, trauma, and neonatal meningitis. Rarely, AABR and OAE screening technology can miss some hearing loss in the mild or isolated frequency regions.

The hospital should provide training and monitoring of staff responsible for performing hearing screening, should establish a system which includes early detection and intervention, and monitors necessary follow-up. This regionalized approach will ensure access for all children with significant hearing loss to receive appropriate expert services.

Case Presentation

A 39 3/7-week 3100 g male is born by NSVD. Apgar scores were 9/9, and the baby has done well in the nursery. You have examined him on admission, and there were no abnormal findings. It is now day 3 of life, and you have just completed your discharge exam which is also normal. You check the results of the UNHS and find the baby has a "refer" on the OAE and a "fail" on the AABR.

Which of the following is a correct course of action:

1. Reassure the parents these tests have a high failure rate, and you will follow the patient in the office.
2. Tell the parents their baby has a hearing loss and needs to be referred for hearing aids.
3. Rescreen the patient in your office by 1 month.
4. Send the patient to audiologist who is qualified to perform more specific testing within 1 month.

While up to 2% of all neonates may not pass the initial screening, the true incidence of congenital hearing loss is 0.01–0.03%. This creates a dilemma for the practitioner in that they have a test with a high false-positive rate but a clinical situation which the American Academy of Pediatrics calls a "developmental emergency." There is wide consensus among the many organizations concerned about newborn screening that a well-defined program of follow-up for patients who fail screening be established. This program has been defined by the EDHI (Early Hearing Detection and Intervention) 1-3-6 guidelines formulated by the CDC. The guidelines call for screening within the first month of life (preferably in the birth hospital); newborns failing screening be rescreened by 1 month or sent directly to a qualified audiologist; newborns who again fail screening in the first month also need to be referred to an audiologist; diagnosis of hearing loss should be made by 3 months; and intervention services in place by 6 months. (www.pediatrics.org/cgi/doi/101542/peds.2007-2333) [7].

Answer: 3 or 4

Case Presentation

A 3300 g male infant born at 39-week gestation has increased vernix over his body. You are called by the nurse on day 2 of life when the baby fails the otoacoustic emission (OAE) test. Examination of the baby reveals dried vernix on the upper half of the body.

You should:

1. Order an automated auditory brain stem response (AABR).
2. Repeat the OAE immediately.
3. Ask the nurse to re-bathe the baby and redo the OAE.

Conductive hearing loss limits the amount of external sound that gains access to the inner ear.

Vernix caseosa is a waxy, cheese-like white substance which coats the skin of the newborn. It is primarily composed of sebum and shed lanugo hair. When vernix is present in the ear canal and dries, it can cause an abnormal hearing screen. Re-bathing the infant with special attention to the ear canal should remove the vernix. A repeat OAE should be normal. There is no need to consider doing an AABR.

Answer: 3

Case Presentation

A 2800 g female infant was born at 32 weeks by emergency C-section delivery due to fetal indications. At birth the infant was found to have microtia on the right side. The OAE was found to be abnormal. Normal results were found for the left ear. You are called to evaluate. Your examination of the ear canal was limited due to the small size of the ear canal.

You should:

1. Wait and repeat OAE in 2 weeks.
2. Examine the ear canal with appropriately sized speculum, and remove all debris before repeating OAE.
3. Perform AABR.

Microtia is part of congenital aural atresia, which is a developmental malformation of the external ear and may include the ear canal and middle and inner structures [8]. The degree of deformity can vary from mild to severe complete absence of the external ear. It can also have varying combinations of deformities, including stenosis or absence of the ear canal as well as the abnormalities of the tympanic membrane, the ossicles, and the inner ear structures. Usually the pinna is underdeveloped. If this underdevelopment is incomplete, the defect is named "anotia." Microtia can be unilateral or bilateral. The incidence is 1/8000–10,000 births [8]. Hence, it can cause conductive as well as sensorineural hearing loss in the affected ear. A good examination of the ear is essential in determining the type and the degree of deformity involved. The ear canal may be absent, poorly developed, or occluded by debris, all which can lead to an abnormal OAE, which should be differentiated from middle ear abnormalities. In this case, if the OAE is a non-pass and the AABR is a pass, then this is most likely a conductive hearing loss. If the OAE and AABR are both a non-pass, then it may be sensorineural or a combination of both. The patient should be referred subsequently to a pediatric otolaryngologist for further evaluation. One of the medications taken during pregnancy which can lead to microtia is Accutane (isotretinoin) [9].

Answer: 3

Case Presentation

You are called to see a 2500 g male born by Caesarian delivery due to fetal indications. The infant was found to have Down syndrome, which was detected by prenatal screen. The infant currently is on intravenous ampicillin, gentamicin, and Flagyl for sepsis. The OAE and AABR were abnormal bilaterally. Your examination revealed small and narrow ear canals.

You should:

1. Counsel the parents regarding the hearing loss and refer to an otolaryngologist.
2. Continue the antibiotic treatment and recheck AABR in 2–4 weeks.
3. Discontinue antibiotics and repeat the AABR in 2–4 weeks.

In Down syndrome or trisomy 21, the patients can have different ear abnormalities, involving external, middle, or inner ears. Surveys suggest that 38–78% of individuals diagnosed with Down syndrome will have hearing difficulty at some point in their life [10]. The American Academy of Pediatrics suggests completion of follow-up assessments for congenital hearing loss by 3 months of age. If the child passes the screening studies, repeat evaluations should be performed at 6 months of age. Since the tympanic membranes are often difficult to visualize, interval ear examinations by the otolaryngologist every 3–6 months until the tympanic membrane can be visualized. A behavioral audiogram should be attempted at 1 year of age [11]. Inner ear dysplasia can also occur secondary to hypoplasia of inner ear structures [12]. Furthermore, they have a predilection for developing chronic otitis media, especially in the setting of palatal abnormalities. A "glue ear," where mucoid secretions accumulate in the middle ear, prevents the ossicles from vibrating freely leading to decreased hearing. In addition, children with Down syndrome have narrower Eustachian tubes, and there is reduced drainage [10]. Hence, they may present with conductive or sensorineural hearing loss or both. In babies with sensorineural loss, cochlear implantation may be utilized to improve hearing and hence language development [13]. For further evaluation, pure tone audiometry can be used in follow-up as the child gets older. An audiologist usually performs this test where specific sound frequencies and intensities are recorded. Normal hearing is recorded at 0–15 decibels (dB), where hearing loss is then graded as minimal (16–25 dB) to profound hearing loss (>90 dB) [10].

Answer: 2

Case Presentation

A recently born infant male was referred to you because the parents are concerned about the hearing of the child. The child passed the OAE and AABR screening in the nursery. This was a full term, spontaneous vaginal delivery without any complication. You found the child to have unremarkable physical examination. However, the parents revealed to you that one of the two other older siblings have unexplained hearing loss. You should:

1. Assure the parents that the child is of normal hearing and no further intervention is needed.
2. Repeat OAE and AABR.
3. Close monitoring of the child's hearing and consider a referral for genetic counseling.

This case demonstrates the importance of family history in hearing loss. Both OAE and AABR are very important tools in the screening of hearing loss in newborn. However, in some cases of limited frequency hearing loss, particularly in the low frequencies and especially if they are mild, OAE and AABR may fail to detect the abnormalities. Furthermore, some genetic hearing losses do not show up until later in childhood. Hence, the close monitoring of the child's language and cognitive development is essential. It is not unusual for the abnormalities to be found much later in school screening or by parents. Genetic counseling and testing may possibly reveal the presence of genetic defect and help to intervene early in the child's development. Approximately 50% of hearing loss involves genetic factors. There are many genes which are associated with hearing loss, and there are two main categories: non-syndrome hearing loss (hearing loss with no other clinical symptoms) [14] and syndrome hearing loss, where there are no other clinical symptoms [15]. In addition, there are several mitochondrial disorders associated with congenital deafness [15].

Answer: 3

Case Presentation

A 3200 g female infant born at 39-week gestation was found to have abnormal OAE and AABR. You are asked to evaluate the child in the nursery. When you examine the child, you found increased intercanthal distance, somewhat prominent and broad nose, and heterochromia of eyes. You should:

1. Repeat OAE in 1 week after irrigating the ears.
2. Repeat AABR in 1 month to confirm the loss.
3. Refer the patient to an otolaryngologist for consultation.

In this case, the infant has features suggestive of Waardenburg syndrome. It is important to identify abnormal physical features. There are more than 70 different genetic syndromes associated with congenital sensorineural deafness. Waardenburg syndrome is one of the most common. Inheritance in Waardenburg syndrome is usually autosomal dominant. The stigmata most commonly observed are dystrophic canthi and an abnormal intercanthal distance as well as a broad nasal root. In older patients one may see the classic white forelock and anti-mongoloid slant of both eyes. There are four recognized types of Waardenburg syndrome which vary, depending upon physical characteristics and genetic causes [16]. In addition to hearing loss, there are physical findings of abnormal pigmentation. These abnormalities are frequently noticed in the eyes where color can be different in either or both eyes. In addition there is often a "white forelock" (a patch of white hair) noted. Mutations in several genes are responsible for Waardenburg syndrome [16]. The principal abnormality is the formation of several cell types, especially melanocytes, which make melanin. Melanin is responsible for hair, skin, and eye color but also has a role in hearing abnormalities. The syndrome can produce profound deafness, which may not be treatable with conventional hearing aid amplification [17]. Cochlear implantation at an early age, as early as at age of 2, has been shown to improve the outcomes in speech and language development as well as other learning and social parameters. An early referral to a pediatric otolaryngologist will facilitate the coordination with other providers such as audiologists and speech pathologist in planning and in early intervention.

Answer: 3

Clinical Pearls

1. The technologies utilized for universal newborn hearing screening include evoked otoacoustic emission (EOAE) and automated auditory brain stem response (AABR).
2. Causes of hearing loss in the newborn include genetic disorders, congenital viral infections, perinatal asphyxia, hyperbilirubinemia, ototoxic medications, and environmental factors.
3. EOAE is affected by debris and/or fluid in the middle or external ear.
4. ABR screening is not affected by middle or external ear debris.
5. Microtia is a developmental malformation of the ear and may include the ear canal and middle and inner structures.
6. Down syndrome has several different ear abnormalities which are complicated by the predilection for developing chronic otitis media.
7. Approximately 50% of hearing loss involves genetic factors, and there are also mitochondrial disorders associated with congenital deafness.
8. A common genetic syndrome associated with congenital sensorineural deafness is Waardenburg syndrome.
9. Referral to a pediatric otolaryngologist will facilitate coordination with other providers (audiologists and speech pathologists) in planning early intervention which can include conventional hearing aid amplification or even early-age cochlear implantation.

References

1. 2014 CDC EHDI Hearing Screening and Follow up Surveys (HSFS).
2. Early Identification of Hearing Impairment in Infants and Young Children. NIH Consens Statement 1993 Mar 1–3;11(1):1–24.
3. Katbamna B, Crumpton T, Patel DR. Hearing impairment in children. Pediatr Clin N Am. 2008; Oct;55(5):1175–88.

4. Kenna MA. Neonatal hearing screening. Pediatr Clin N Am. 2003, Apr.;50(2):301–13.
5. Wroblewska-Seniuk KE, Dabrowski P, Szyfter W, Mazela J. Universal newborn hearing screening: methods and results, obstacles, and benefits. Pediatr Res. 2017;81:415–22.
6. Mayberry RI, Lock E, Kazmi H. Linguistic ability and early language exposure. Nature. 2002;417:38.
7. Year 2007 Position Statement. Principles and guidelines for early hearing detection and intervention programs. Joint committee on infant hearing. Pediatrics. 2007;120(4):898–921.
8. Kountakis SE, Helidonis E, Jahrsdoerfer RA. Microtia grade as an indicator of middle ear development in aural atresia. Arch Otolaryngol Head Neck Surg. 1995 Aug;121(8):885–6.
9. Dolan AM Accutane and birth defects. Medscape OB/Gyn. 2004;9(2). Medscape.
10. Shott ST. Hearing loss in children with down syndrome. International Journal of Pediatric Otorhinolaryngology. 2001;61(6):199–205.
11. Bull MJ and the Committee on Genetics. Health supervision for children with down syndrome. Pediatrics. 2011;128(2):393–405.
12. Blaser S, Propst EJ, Martin D, et al. Inner ear dysplasia is common in children with down syndrome (trisomy21). Laryngoscope. 2006 Dec;116(12):2113–9.
13. Eyzawiah H, Suraya A, Sama A. Down's syndrome with abnormal inner ear: is it suitable for cochlear implantation? International medical review on Down's syndrome. Rev Med Int Sindr Down. 2013;17(2):25–8.
14. Schrijver I. Hereditary non-syndromic sensorineural hearing loss. J Mol Diagn. 2004;6:275–84.
15. Zhao, Hong-Bo. Congenital deafness. American Hearing Research Foundation. March 2007.
16. Waardenburg syndrome. NIH. U.S. Library of Medicine Genetics Home Reference.
17. Song J, Feng Y, Acke FR, et al. Hearing loss in Waardenburg syndrome: a systemic review. Clin Genet. 2016;89(4):415–25.

Index

G. I. Martin, W. Rosenfeld (eds.), *Common Problems in the Newborn Nursery*,
https://doi.org/10.1007/978-3-319-95672-5

C

D

The manufacturer's authorised representative in the EU is Springer Nature Customer Service Centre GmbH, Europaplatz 3, 69115 Heidelberg, Germany. If you have any concerns regarding our products, please contact ProductSafety@springernature.com

Printed and bound by CPI Group (UK) Ltd, Croydon, CR0 4YY
30/09/2026
02225232-0018